Introduction to Nursing
Concepts, Issues, & Opportunities

INTRODUCTION TO NURSING
CONCEPTS, ISSUES, & OPPORTUNITIES

Janice B. Lindberg, RN, MA, PhD
Associate Professor of Nursing
Associate Dean for Student Affairs
Interim Chairperson for Medical – Surgical Nursing
The University of Michigan School of Nursing
Ann Arbor, Michigan

Mary Love Hunter, RN, MS, CS
Assistant Professor of Nursing
The University of Michigan School of Nursing
Head Nurse
The University of Michigan Hospitals
Ann Arbor, Michigan

Ann Z. Kruszewski, RN, MSN
Assistant Professor of Nursing
Interim Coordinator
Registered Nurse Studies
The University of Michigan School of Nursing
Ann Arbor, Michigan

J. B. Lippincott Company
Philadelphia
Grand Rapids   London
New York   Sydney
St. Louis   Tokyo
San Francisco

Acquisitions Editor: Patricia L. Cleary
Editorial Assistant: Nancy Lyons
Project Editor: Grace R. Caputo
Coordinating Editor: Lori J. Bainbridge
Indexer: Ellen Murray
Design Coordinator: Ellen C. Dawson
Interior Design: Ellen C. Dawson
Cover Design: Terri Siegel
Production Manager: Carol A. Florence
Production Coordinator: Kevin P. Johnson
Compositor: Digitype
Printer/Binder: R. R. Donnelly & Sons Company

RT
41
.L728
1990

6   5   4   3   2   1

Library of Congress Cataloging-in-Publication Data

Lindberg, Janice B.
    Introduction to nursing / Janice B. Lindberg, Mary Love Hunter,
Ann Z. Kruszewski.
        p.   cm.
    Includes bibliographies and index.
    ISBN 0-397-54745-5
    1. Nursing.   I. Hunter, Mary Love.   II. Kruszewski, Ann Z.
III. Title.
    [DNLM: 1. Nursing.   WY 16 L742t]
RT41.L728   1990
610.73—dc20
DNLM/DLC
for Library of Congress   89-2713
                                                                          CIP

Any procedure or practice described in this book should be applied by the health-care practitioner under appropriate supervision in accordance with professional standards of care used with regard to the unique circumstances that apply in each practice situation. Care has been taken to confirm the accuracy of information presented and to describe generally accepted practices. However, the authors, editors, and publisher cannot accept any responsibility for errors or omissions or for any consequences from application of the information in this book and make no warranty, express or implied, with respect to the contents of the book.

Every effort has been made to ensure drug selections and dosages are in accordance with current recommendations and practice. Because of ongoing research, changes in government regulations and the constant flow of information on drug therapy, reactions and interactions, the reader is cautioned to check the package insert for each drug for indications, dosages, warnings and precautions, particularly if the drug is new or infrequently used.

REVIEWERS

Connie S. Austin, RN, MAEd, MSN
Assistant Professor of Nursing
Azusa Pacific University
Azusa, California

Maymie B. Proctor, MA, MS, RN
Assistant Professor
Hampton University School of Nursing
Hampton, Virginia

Joyce S. Willens, RN, MSN
Instructor
College of Nursing, Villanova University
Villanova, Pennsylvania

PREFACE

Introduction to Nursing is intended for anyone who anticipates being a professional nurse in the 21st century. Nurses differ in their backgrounds, education, and individual aspirations. Each, however, has the potential for professional growth through both formal education and lifelong learning. Nursing is both an art and a science. As an art, nursing is as old as civilization; as a science, it is relatively new. Professional nursing practice now is developed on a scientific and theoretical foundation. It involves sophisticated decision making and proficiency in certain skills. For both novices and practitioners, this book explores the development of futuristic nursing practice on a scientific foundation that enhances nursing art. Through concepts, issues, and opportunities, *Introduction to Nursing* details professional nursing practice involving decision making and skills beyond those traditionally associated with nursing.

The conceptual framework of the book is the conceptual framework underlying nursing as a science and a profession. The book introduces four concepts that are basic to nursing science: nursing, person, health, and environment. The book also presents additional concepts that shape nursing as an art and a profession: nursing process, the problem-solving process of nursing practice, communication, learning and teaching, and ethics and legal aspects. Other important ideas such as adaptation, culture, research, and spiritual aspects of persons are woven throughout the text. Although the four major concepts are those generally acknowledged to provide a theoretical base for nursing, the authors recognize that emphasis on concepts may vary from institution to institution.

Introduction to Nursing is divided into five parts. Part One is a single overview chapter that briefly represents the conceptual and practical chapters that follow.

Part Two sets forth the conceptual framework by introducing the four basic concepts that are the foundation for nursing science. Chapters 2 and 3 are devoted to *nursing*, the one concept unique to the profession. Chapter 2 presents an historical perspective of nursing as a prelude to the present. Chapter 3 details a current view of nursing as art, science, and profession. Part Two concludes with individual chapters dedicated to person, health, and environment, the other major concepts.

Part Three focuses on nursing practice in the real world of health-care delivery. Chapter 7 provides an overview of the health-care delivery system today. The remaining four chapters demonstrate how nurses communicate, solve problems and practice inquiry through nursing process, facilitate learning for their clients, and encounter ethical dilemmas and legal aspects of practice. In other words, this section demonstrates actual application of the basic concepts. In the spirit of person-centered care, clients in the clinical examples are referred to by name rather than by initials. Because ethical practice requires maintaining client confidentiality, the names are, of course, fictitious. In actual learning situations, students refer to their clients by initials when writing reports and case studies so that no name-linked information leaves the nursing unit, where care is given.

Part Four is a single concluding chapter detailing prospects for the future. Selected opportunities and challenges highlight the incentives to be a nurse in a promising health-care profession. These opportunities and challenges are intended to provide answers to questions prospective students might raise and also to offer food for further thought.

Nursing can be understood on a number of levels. Our presentation aims to make this possible for you. The reader may have had previous nursing experience but this is not assumed. As practitioners, educators, and administrators in nursing service and education, we share with you our experience of what makes nursing unique as a profession. You will learn how there is room for creativity in the practice of nursing as both art and science. You will discover what nursing, the health science of caring, offers to its practitioners.

JANICE B. LINDBERG, RN, MA, PhD
MARY L. HUNTER, RN, MS, CS
ANN Z. KRUSZEWSKI, RN, MSN

ACKNOWLEDGMENTS

An introductory nursing text reflects the motivation and commitment of many experienced nurse clinicians and educators. *Introduction to Nursing* grew out of such vision for and belief in nursing's contribution to health and society. Many ideas came from faculty colleagues and students through years of learning and growth. These ideas, shared through clinical practice, research, and teaching, form the nucleus of many chapters. Some of these colleagues shared their experiences as contributors to a previous text:

Bobbie Bloch, RN, MN, Sylvania, Ohio

Martha Keehner Engelke, BSN, MPH, CS (Medical-Surgical), Greenville, North Carolina

Sue V. Fink, RN, MS, Dearborn, Michigan

Marguerite Babaian Harms, RN, MS, Ann Arbor, Michigan

Sharon Hein Jette, RN, MSN, MPH, Andover, Massachusetts

Evelyn Malcolm Tomlin, RN, MS, CCRN, Big Rock, Illinois

Terry M. Vanden Bosch, RN, MS, Ann Arbor, Michigan

The authors gratefully express appreciation to certain individuals who offered objective critique and special expertise:

Kathy Grijalva provided that rare combination of editorial assistance and word-processing wizardry that brought the manuscript to fruition.

Diana Intenzo, Nursing Division, J. B. Lippincott Company, has been a consistent and enthusiastic ally.

Patti Cleary, Senior Editor, Nursing Division, J. B. Lippincott Company, recognized the window of opportunity open for nurses preparing for the future. More importantly, she provided the faith and encouragement to complete the project.

Sandra Garr, RN, MSN, Assistant Professor of Nursing, The University of Michigan, shared her perspective on nursing's past.

Lillian M. Simms, RN, PhD, Associate Professor of Nursing, The University of Michigan, contributed her ideas about nursing's future.

Many photographs were furnished by various offices at The University of Michigan.

Finally, we offer a special thank you to our families, whose patience and enduring support have assisted us immeasurably.

CONTENTS

PART ONE

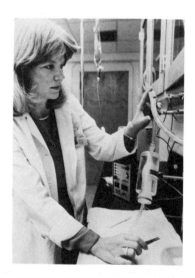

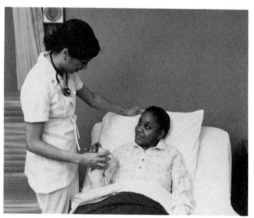

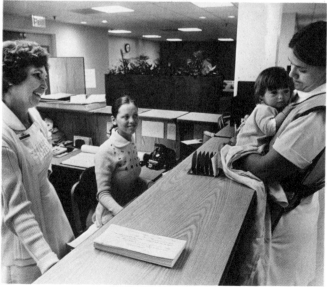

1 | THE PRACTICE AND PROFESSION OF NURSING

KEY WORDS	After completing this chapter, students will be able to:
Adaptation	Identify the expertise of the profession of nursing.
Caring	Identify common elements of several leaders' definitions of nursing.
Client	
Communication	Explain the concept of caring in relation to nursing practice.
Environment	
Health	Identify the elements of person-centered nursing care.
Illness	Describe the connotations of the terms *patient* and *client*.
Nursing	Identify concepts basic to nursing practice.
Nursing ethics	
Nursing process	
Patient	
Person	
Wellness	

Can you tell which occupation meets the criteria listed below?

- Is both new and old
- Claims elements of art, science, and profession
- Is in worldwide demand currently, foresees universal demand in the future, and yet provides job opportunities in virtually every hometown
- Has current and future personnel needs that exceed all projections of supply
- Offers life-long career opportunities without changing fields
- Serves society's health and well-being
- Offers participation in life's major events
- Offers interpersonal interaction in a high-technology world
- Develops self-understanding
- Provides immeasurable personal satisfaction
- Confronts issues of humanism, ethics, legalities, and economics that shape public policy
- Encourages entrepreneurs in the business of health
- Offers wide diversity in career possibilities

Nursing can certainly be an answer to the above question. Nurses are a scarce human resource in today's society. Although nurses are greatly admired by persons who have directly benefited from their services, nurses and their profession often are not understood by those who have not experienced nursing care directly.

This text is an introduction to the profession of nursing. There are many ideas about what nursing is. Common to many definitions of nursing is the idea of helping persons. Throughout history, the potential for helping was shaped by the influences of society, by forces within the health-care delivery system, and by visions within nursing. Today this helping takes many forms and is bounded primarily by the vision of nurses themselves. Indeed, nursing today is both like and unlike nursing of the past.

Nursing has always been the art of caring. Now nursing is becoming known as the health science of caring. Yesterday's nurses were found most often at the bedside of ill persons. Although grateful patients acknowledged nurses' skills in promoting, maintaining, and restoring health, nurses' unique expertise for health received little emphasis.

Today's nurses are still found at the bedside. The need for their expertise in caring for ill persons is at an all-time high. Traditionally and in many ways, nursing has emphasized its technical aspects. There is currently, however, much room and need for creativity within professional nursing practice. Such innovation occurs at the bedside and elsewhere. Today's nurses also enjoy practice opportunities as creative entrepreneurs, managers, administrators, teachers, and research scientists. Although practice at any level provides an important service to society, practice at different levels accommodates individual nurse's interests, different ability levels, and varying career investments.

In this chapter, we present an overview of what nursing is, both from our own perspective and from the writings of nursing leaders. This chapter also discusses concepts that are essential to nursing as a science: nursing, person, environment, and health. Additional concepts related to the practice of nursing within the health-care delivery system are also defined: nursing process, communication, learning and teaching, nursing ethics, and legal aspects of practice.

Before beginning a detailed discussion of the individual concepts, it is important that we have a clear understanding of how these concepts relate to nursing. To do this, we must first have a firm understanding of what *nursing* is. Beginning nursing students may now be saying to themselves, "But I know what nursing is. I learned that from my aunt who is a nurse (or from books, television, volunteer work in hospitals, guidance counselors . . .)." When asked to define nursing, most beginning students respond that it involves helping people. Our own concept of nursing is similar, for we believe that the essence of nursing is caring for *persons*. This is the approach to nursing that inspires this textbook. This chapter presents the concepts that we believe are essential to nursing practice. We hope to provide our readers with an appreciation of the philosophy that underlies this text.

| PERSON-CENTERED NURSING CARE

There are many professions in today's society. In this wide array, nursing is viewed as one of the health professions. Although the term *profession* has many common meanings, some writers have tried to ascribe a more strict definition to it. Schein and Kommers have identified certain criteria of a true profession, including a body of knowledge on which expert skills and services are based (1972, p 8). The other criteria related to professional status are discussed in detail in Chapter 2. In Table 1–1 we list some of the groups that are considered professions and identify their expertise.

TABLE 1–1
PROFESSIONALS AND THEIR FIELDS OF EXPERTISE

Professional	Expertise
Lawyer	Law
Pastor or minister	Spirituality
Physician or doctor	Illness, disease
Psychologist	Mind, behavior
Social worker	Societal support systems
Nurse	Caring for persons

The emergence of professional nursing is usually attributed to the influence of Florence Nightingale, who practiced in the last half of the 19th century. Thus, nursing as a profession is relatively young in comparison to the other professions we have listed. Nursing is an *emerging* profession trying to fulfill the criteria that define a profession. What is the expertise that nursing claims? We believe that it is *caring for persons*.

Caring as a Basis for Nursing

Nurses constantly use the term **caring**: "I'm caring for seven patients today," "Mr. Jones needs complete care," "Mrs. Smith doesn't require much care." When this text uses the term "caring," it does so with a specific meaning in mind. Caring should involve more than just carrying out nursing procedures such as bedmaking and treatments. True caring is based on an attitude of nurturing, of helping another to grow. Mayeroff, a philosopher who explored the nature of caring, stated, "To care for another person, in the most significant sense, is to help him grow and actualize himself" (1971, p 1). He continued, "In caring, I experience the other as having potentialities and the need to grow" (p 6).

Jean Watson is a nurse-theorist who described nursing as the science of caring. Watson contrasted care with cure. With cure activities, the end is treatment and elimination of disease. In caring, one assists the person to grow toward his or her potential. Watson stated:

> Human care . . . consists of transpersonal human to human attempts to protect, enhance, and preserve humanity by helping a person find meaning in illness, suffering, pain, and existence; to help another gain self-knowledge, control, and self-healing wherein a sense of inner harmony is restored regardless of the external circumstances. (1985, p 54).

Watson identified factors integral to the caring process, including the following:

- Cultivation of sensitivity to self and others
- Development of a helping-trusting relationship
- Promotion of acceptance of positive and negative feelings
- Provision for a supportive, protective and corrective mental, physical, sociocultural, and spiritual environment
- Assistance with human needs gratification
  (1985, pp 9–10)

Chapter 3 describes Watson's theory of caring in further detail.

Leininger, a nursing leader, believed that caring is essential to human development, growth, and survival. Leininger described the following caring behaviors:

Comfort	Nurturance
Compassion	Presence
Concern	Protective behaviors
Coping behavior	Restorative behaviors
Empathy	Sharing
Enabling	Stimulating behaviors
Facilitating	Stress alleviation
Health consultative acts	Succorance
Health instruction acts	Support
Health maintenance acts	Surveillance
Helping behavior	Tenderness
Interest	Touching
Involvement	Trust
Love	(1981, p 13)

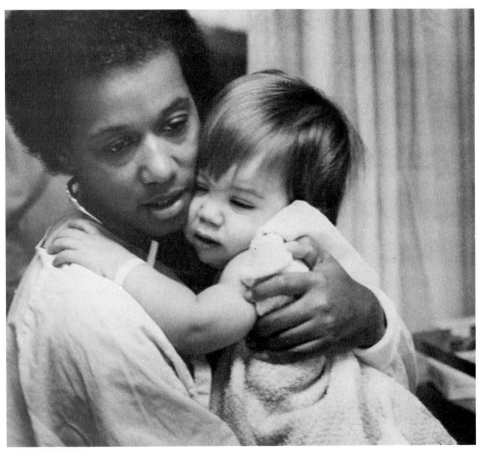

Nursing is the health science of caring.

The expression of caring varies across cultures. The priority of a caring behavior, its form of expression, and the needs that the behavior satisfies may differ from culture to culture.

Caring nurses recognize that persons have strengths as well as needs and that they possess worth and potential to grow. Rather than seeing persons as helpless because they need care, caring nurses respect them as autonomous in their own right. Caring nurses assist a person because of a desire to foster growth and independence. They want to enhance their clients' abilities to manage their own health needs as a result of the care received. As Mayeroff said, "To help another person grow . . . is to help that other person come to care for himself" (1971, p 10).

Definitions of Nursing

Thoughts on the caring nature of nursing are reflected in many of the definitions of nursing put forth by nursing leaders. Table 1 – 2 summarizes definitions of nursing from Nightingale, Henderson, Levine, King, Roy, Orem, and Martha Rogers. This summary shows that the theme of helping or caring is inherent in each of their definitions. Likewise, other common themes in these writings are the nature of persons, environment and health, the concepts on which this text is based.

Since nursing is a profession experiencing growth of its own, we think there is no single definition of nursing. You might develop a new definition of your own while reading this text. Whatever your definition, we hope that the element of caring for or nurturing persons is a motivation for your interest in nursing.

None of these thoughts on the definition of nursing is new. Nurses have always valued the idea of caring for persons; this is what attracts many nurses to the profession. Unfortunately, nurses sometimes lose sight of this goal in the reality of practice. For example, beginning students may find at times that they are so concerned about their own nursing skills that they forget that the person for whom they are caring may have anxieties. Even experienced nurses may become so overwhelmed by the complex technology involved in nursing care, or by institutional demands, that they lose sight of the person who is the object of their activities. Nursing texts frequently focus on concepts or techniques without considering how those techniques will relate to the persons who will benefit from them. For this reason, this text uses the term *person-centered nursing* as a reminder that caring for persons is the organizing focus for all aspects of nursing. Each of the concepts in the text is presented within this context. We have attempted to emphasize the person in each of our discussions, whether person means the nurse or the client.

Elements of Person-Centered Care

What is person-centered care? Carl Rogers provides us with many thoughts that can be applied to nursing. Rogers was a psychotherapist who challenged the manner in which traditional psychology is concerned with human behavior, particularly behavior that is considered abnormal. Rogers thought that rather than emphasizing what is wrong with a person, psychotherapists would do better to concentrate on strengths in order to facilitate personal growth toward one's highest potential. He believed that all persons are in the process of "becoming" — that is, moving toward their potential — rather than representing finished products. He also believed that persons move in a basically positive direction toward growth. Related to this belief is an appreciation of the value or worth of each person. Rogers stressed that facilitating optimal growth requires a strong interpersonal relationship between the therapist and the client. Through his experiences in psychotherapy, he came to believe

TABLE 1–2
DEFINITIONS OF NURSING

Definition	Thoughts on Caring	Related Nursing Concepts
Nightingale		
It is quite surprising . . . how many behave as if the scientific end were the only one in view or as if the sick body were but a reservoir for storing medicines into and the surgical disease only a curious case the sufferer has made for the attendant's special information (1859, p 70). What nursing has to do . . . is put the patient in the best condition for nature to act upon him (p 75). Nursing . . . ought to signify the proper use of fresh air, light, warmth, cleanliness, quiet, and the proper selection and administration of diet—all at the least expense of vital power to the patient (p 6).	The patient, rather than the disease process, should be the primary focus of health professionals.	Maintenance of a healthful environment is a primary concern for nursing. Health is achieved by enabling natural processes to work.
Henderson		
Nursing is primarily assisting the individual (sick or well) in the performance of those activities contributing to health or its recovery (or to a peaceful death) that he would perform unaided if he had the necessary strength, will, or knowledge. It is likewise the unique contribution of nursing to help the individual to be independent of such assistance as soon as possible (Harmer, 1955, p 4).	Caring is assisting persons in performance of activities they would accomplish independently given the necessary resources.	The person is a unique individual. Nursing as a profession makes a unique contribution to society.
Levine		
Patient-centered nursing means individualized nursing care . . . every man is a unique individual, and as such he requires a unique	Caring recognizes the uniqueness of individuals. Nursing is an interpersonal process.	Nursing care maintains or supports persons' adaptations through active participation in their environment.

(Table 1–2 continued)

Definition	Thoughts on Caring	Related Nursing Concepts
constellation of skills, techniques, and ideas designed specifically for him (1973, p 23). The nurse participates actively in every patient's environment, and much of what she does supports his adaptations as he struggles in the predicament of illness. Nursing intervention means that the nurse interposes her skill and knowledge into the course of events, which affects the patient (p 13).		

King

The focus of nursing is the care of human beings (1981, p 10). Nursing is defined as a process of action, reaction, and interaction whereby nurse and client share information about their perceptions in the nursing situation . . . leading to goal attainment (p 2). Nurses are concerned with human beings interacting with their environment in ways that lead to self-fulfillment and maintenance of health (p 3).	Caring for persons is the focus of nursing practice and is an interactive process.	Health is defined as dynamic life experiences of a human being which implies continuous adjustment to stressors in the internal and external environment through optimum use of one's resources to achieve maximum potential for daily living (p 5). Persons are open systems interacting with the environment (p 10).

Roy

Nursing focuses on persons and how they maintain well-being and high-level functioning whether sick or well (1984, p 5). Nursing aims to increase persons' adaptive responses and to decrease ineffective responses. An adaptive response is behavior that maintains the integrity of the individual (p 37).	The focus of nursing is persons and increasing their adaptive responses.	The person is an adaptive system (p 289). The environment is internal and external stimuli or all conditions, circumstances, and influences surrounding or affecting the development and behavior of persons and groups (p 28). Health is a state and a process of being and becoming an integrated and whole person (p 28).

(Table 1–2 continues)

(Table 1–2 continued)

Definition	Thoughts on Caring	Related Nursing Concepts
Orem		
Nursing is deliberate action; a function of the practical intelligence of nurses . . . is action to bring about humanely desirable conditions in persons and their environments. Nursing is distinguished from other human services and other forms of care by the way in which it focuses on human beings, i.e., by its proper human object (1984, p 15). Nursing has as its special concern the individual's need for self-care action and the provision and management of it on a continuous basis in order to sustain life and health, recover from disease or injury, and cope with their effects (p 54).	Nursing's concern is persons and their self-care actions.	Health is used to describe living things when they are structurally and functionally whole or sound (p 173). The physical, psychological, interpersonal, and social aspects of health are inseparable in the individual (p 174). Each human being is a substantial or real unity whose parts are formed and attain perfection through differentiation of the whole during processes of development . . . (who moves) toward maturation and achievement of (his or her) human potential (pp 179–180)
Rogers		
Professional practice in nursing seeks to promote symphonic interaction between man and environment, to strengthen the coherence and integrity of the human field and to direct and redirect patterning of the human and environmental fields for realization of maximum health potential (M. E. Rogers, p. 122). Nursing exists to serve people (1970, p 122).	Caring involves promoting optimum human–environment interactions. Nursing's focus is human beings and their worth.	Human beings are irreducible wholes that cannot be understood when reduced to their parts. Human beings and environment are energy fields that are integral with one another and are constantly evolving toward their higher potentials (M. E. Rogers, 1987, pp 141, 143).

"that it is the *client* who knows what hurts, what directions to go, what problems are crucial, what experiences have been deeply buried. It began to occur to me that . . . I would do better to rely upon the client for the direction of movement in the process" (1961, pp 11–12). Thus, his "client-centered" approach to psychotherapy began.

Some attributes of the therapist's use of a client-centered approach include the following:

- Trustworthiness
- Ability to communicate unambiguously (verbal behavior matches nonverbal behavior)
- A positive attitude toward the client built on a respect for his worth
- Ability to convey empathic understanding
- Acceptance of the client's feelings
- Ability to remain separate from the client (avoiding sympathy)
- Ability to allow the client to remain a separate person (avoiding taking over for the client)
- Acceptance of the client as a person in the process of becoming rather than as a fixed product or psychiatric diagnosis
  (C. Rogers, 1961, pp 11–55)

Abraham Maslow, a psychologist who shared this humanistic view of persons, defined categories of basic needs ranging from the most fundamental (food, oxygen, shelter) to the highest level (self-actualization or the desire for self-fulfillment). His approach is also person-centered because it focuses on assisting persons to meet basic needs, thereby freeing them to grow and achieve their potential (1970).

Attributes of the Person-Centered Nurse

Many of the beliefs about nursing presented in this text evolved from Carl Rodgers' and Abraham Maslow's philosophies. Because nursing is an interpersonal process, much of their work is applicable to our profession. We believe that nurses who give person-centered care will act as follows:

1 Appreciate that each person is a unique product of heredity, environment, and culture. This means that we must interact with our clients on an individual basis even though their health-care needs may appear to be similar.

2 Believe that persons strive for their highest potential. Nursing's function is to assist persons to achieve growth in relation to their health needs.

3 Respect the worth of each individual. We appreciate each person's potential no matter how impoverished or ill he or she appears to be. We recognize that even the sickest or poorest of persons have strengths that can be mobilized to meet their needs and achieve their potential.

4 Recognize one's own humanity. Nurses are persons, too, with unique strengths and needs. To care effectively for others, nurses must have self-awareness to recognize what they can offer another and what their own personal limitations are.

5 Be genuine. Rogers used the term *congruence* to describe a condition in which a person is "without 'front' or facade; that . . . feelings . . . are available to his awareness and he is able to communicate them if appropriate" (1961, p 61). A nurse cannot be truly genuine without the self-awareness just described. Rogers believes that congruence is essential to an effective helping relationship.

6 Allow control to remain with the client. Nurses who are truly genuine and who are aware of and comfortable with their own feelings will be able to let

clients be themselves. These nurses will not need to feel authority over their clients; rather, they will view clients as partners in the helping relationship. They will see the process of nursing as facilitating clients to meet their own needs. They will feel comfortable allowing the clients to express their needs freely and to set their own goals for nursing care.

7 Recognize that persons have basic needs and are motivated to fulfill these needs. For this reason, a person's behavior is the result of his or her needs. This is an important idea, for it implies that each person's behavior has meaning, no matter how different or "wrong" this behavior may appear.

8 Because all behavior has meaning, nurses should appreciate that a person's actions communicate messages about his or her feelings, beliefs, or physical functioning. The nurse should respect the meaning of a person's behavior and avoid such labels as "wrong," "bad," or "weird," even though the behavioral manifestations may be perplexing or difficult to deal with.

Person-centered care can be given to any age group from infancy through old age, from birth through death. This kind of caring is nursing's unique contribution to the health profession.

The best example of caring that we can present comes from a beginning nursing student. She described her relationship with a client whom she had been visiting for 12 weeks. This client was an elderly woman with severely impaired vision due to cataracts. The student had been working with this woman in her home.

"I began by developing a trusting relationship with Edith Butler. I worked to maintain an open atmosphere and encouraged her to discuss her visual impairment and the problems that had arisen due to her condition. This led to a significant exchange, by both parties, of personal feelings and opinions concerning Miss Butler's problems. A trusting and open relationship such as this helped her to express any uncomfortable feelings of confusion, dismay, and loneliness, or any good feelings of happiness, contentment, and relief to a person who could lend support and understanding.

In the course of our relationship, Miss Butler revealed many of her strengths to me. I picked out and reinforced these strengths to help her adapt and to make her aware of her many positive attributes. I let her know how I admired her ability to learn to do such things as cooking, crossing streets, and becoming involved in outside activities in a different way than she had before.

From the beginning, Miss Butler revealed a need for increased self-esteem. Self-esteem is extremely important to adaptation. Self-esteem provides motivation to change, makes a person feel worthwhile, and gives them a reason to be. Therefore, I found it extremely important to incorporate an intervention to satisfy Miss Butler's self-esteem need. I allowed her to give me advice and to use her "nurturing" qualities to help me in any way she could. In this way, she could feel that she was needed, accomplishing something worthwhile. Second, I let her know the "helping" relationship was mutual. Even though I was assigned to her as the student nurse, to spend time with her and help her in any way, I made it clear that I got just as much help out of the relationship by talking with her and learning from her. In addition, I periodically spoke highly of her. For example, I gave her a compliment or a pat on the back, and I encouraged a positive response from her. In this way, I could bring out Miss Butler's many good traits and reinforce them in an attempt to make her feel more important and valuable. Finally, I was a good listener and let her know that I was interested in her and in what she had to say. I did all of these things in an attempt to boost her morale and to make her feel better about herself as a whole.

Finally, I set goals with Miss Butler leading to change and optimal adaptation. I encouraged her to do new things, such as exercising with barbells, taking walks in front of her house, and listening to tapes specially made to entertain the visually impaired. I also determined the degree of independence at which Miss Butler would like to be functioning and encouraged her to attain it. At the present, Miss Butler is adapting and is working to become adapted. By setting goals, she has something to strive for, to work harder for, to live for. Such a healthy attitude can only promote adaptation to its fullest."

(O'Shea K: Adaptation to Visual Impairment. Unpublished manuscript, 1980)

THE PERSON AS A RECIPIENT OF CARE: PATIENT VERSUS CLIENT

You will note that throughout this book the word *person* is used when referring to anyone for whom nursing care is provided. On occasion, the word *client* may also be used and, even more rarely, *patient*. There are some important distinctions to be made among these words, as indicated by their definitions.

The Patient

A **patient** is "a person awaiting or under medical care and treatment; the recipient of any of various medical services." To be **patient** is to "endure pains calmly and without complaint; to hold steadfast despite difficult circumstances."

Looking at the above definitions of patient may help us realize that while a person receiving health care and treatment may not behave in the manner described, that description represents what we, as health-care providers, often expect. We wish for our patients to be cooperative, to behave themselves, to do as they are told, and generally to provide us with little trouble in this cumbersome business of getting them well. As you progress through the book, you may recognize that health-care providers become distressed when their patients do not behave patiently. It is with this idea in mind that we have attempted to underscore the notion that the person receiving care is more healthy than ill and more capable of strength than weakness. Persons who seek health care remain unique human beings who, although sharing some characteristics with other persons, nonetheless have their own individual thoughts, feelings, and ways of responding. That some persons may be patient during an illness is more a characteristic of their individual personalities than of their roles as ill persons.

P. D. James, in her novel *The Black Tower*, described this point quite clearly. The scene is a patient's hospital bedside. Present are the patient himself, a consultant physician, a nurse, and several medical students. The physician is speaking:

"We've had the most recent path. report and I think we can be certain now that we've got it right . . . It isn't acute leukemia, it isn't any type of leukemia. What you're recovering from—happily—is an atypical mononucleosis. I congratulate you, Commander. You had us worried."

"I had you interested; you had me worried. When can I leave here?"

The great man laughed and smiled at his retinue, inviting them to share his indulgence at yet one more example of the ingratitude of convalescence (1975, pp 9–10).

Although this attitude is expressed by a physician, it should be recognized that nurses are capable of similar responses to persons seeking their help. This example provides us with several interesting insights. We note that the patient is called *Commander*, indicating that he has some level of personal achievement. We can assume that he is intelligent, probably educated, and has been given a great deal of responsibility in some organization or other. Even if we did not have the name *Commander* to give us an idea of the character, we could see his individuality clearly in the response he gives. The last statement points out that the provider of services—in this case, the physician—does not think his patient is behaving very well.

The Client

At this point we should examine the word *client*. A **client** is "a person who engages the professional advice or services of another; a person served by or utilizing the services of an agency."

A client is a person who has contracted for services from another who is qualified to provide those services. There is an assumption that this kind of relationship is a negotiated partnership and that clients are capable of taking the information provided and using it in some fashion or other. Should they decide that it is not useful, they generally feel free to take their business elsewhere. Although some persons approach health care with the same sense of independence, most simply do what they are told, including going into the hospital when so directed. They may feel incapable of physically "taking their business and moving elsewhere." The fact that we, as health-care providers, are well aware of this passive type of response is reflected in the name we have so frequently given these persons—patients—and the way in which we have often assumed control over so many facets of their lives.

You may not be aware that this inequitable relationship often exists between a person and the provider of health services. We suggest that you accept a challenge to note this inequality as you explore the world of health-care delivery. You are challenged, moreover, to look first at yourselves to become aware of the degree to which you share these attitudes, many of which are rooted in our history as a people and in our cultural value systems. Indeed, the receiver of health-care services may be as likely to expect (and even want) control from the provider as the provider is likely to exert it.

It is our belief, however, that if nurses are to provide care that encourages each person to grow, we must view those who seek our services as unique beings. We must appreciate their worth, recognize their strengths, and offer a caring relationship in which they may truly be partners in this growth process.

CONCEPTS BASIC TO NURSING PRACTICE

As noted earlier, this text identifies four major concepts that are essential to nursing. They are nursing, person, environment, and health. The concepts have been identified by most theorists and can be found in the definitions of nursing that were presented in Table 1–2. In addition, several other basic concepts can be identified that are critical to the practice of professional nursing: health-care delivery, nursing process, communication, learning and teaching, and nursing ethics and legal aspects. Let us examine each concept briefly.

Nursing

The word *nursing* has its roots in the Latin term *nutricia*, which means to nurture or nourish. Nursing has been called the oldest of the arts and the youngest of the sciences. Art may be viewed as the systematic application of knowledge or skill. The art of nursing is the art of caring related to the health of persons, the "imaginative and creative use of knowledge in human service" (M. E. Rogers, 1987, p 140). Nursing as an art has its origin in the caretaking activities of ancient man. Donahue wrote, "From the dawn of civilization, evidence prevails to support the premise that nurturing has been essential to the preservation of life. Survival of the human race, therefore, is inextricably intertwined with the development of nursing" (1985, p 2).

Science, conversely, is an organized body of knowledge covering general truths or the operation of general laws obtained and tested through research. For many years, nursing "borrowed" its science from related disciplines such as medicine, psychology, and sociology. Chapter 2 presents an historical perspective of nursing as a prelude to the present.

During the last two decades, nursing research has come of age, assisting to identify a body of knowledge that is unique to the profession of nursing. Chapter 3 details a current view of nursing as art, science, and profession.

The nursing leaders listed in Table 1–2 included aspects of the art and science of caring for persons in their definitions of nursing. Although they may view caring differently, each author agrees that nursing is an art and a science that focuses on persons and their needs for care.

Nursing has been called a developing profession. This presents challenges to current and future nurses to facilitate the growth of the profession. To attain this end, we must commit ourselves to professional involvement and lifelong learning. Professional involvement is not only appropriate but also mandatory if nursing is to be acknowledged as a profession. Only nurses know how nursing ought to grow and develop; we cannot leave this decision to others. Students are asked from the start to assume responsibility for nurturing their profession as well as their clients. Nurses must also appreciate that learning does not end with a degree. As professional persons, we are maximizing not only our clients' potentials but also our own. You must care well for your profession: Who else will be concerned about nursing if nurses are not?

Person

Because **persons** are the focus of nursing care, professional nurses need to be "person experts." Theories from biology, psychology, sociology, and philosophy have attempted to explain aspects of persons. Because persons are greater than the sum of their parts (implying that we cannot learn about persons by viewing their components in isolation; the interactions of all of the parts are what makes persons unique), nurses need knowledge in all of these areas. They also need an awareness of how all the parts of an individual interact. Nursing theories attempt to explain these relationships.

This text provides commonly used nursing and non-nursing conceptual frameworks and theories, such as those related to growth and development, basic needs, and values. In this book you will discover how persons are alike and different in the ways that are uniquely significant for nursing. Through your studies in nursing and through your interpersonal interactions with the persons who are your clients, we hope that you will gain increasing appreciation of the dignity and unique potential of human beings.

The concept of person is sometimes referred to as the concept of the human being, that is, persons as a collective group. Such reference recognizes that the nurse's client is often a family, a group, or the community. In small group situations, persons in the group are treated as individuals. Even in larger groups when this is not possible, our knowledge of person as a concept will influence our notion of community. The detailed discussion of person in Chapter 4 helps us to understand how persons develop across the life span. Similarly the discussion of sociocultural environment in Chapter 5 broadens the idea of person beyond focus on the individual.

Environment

Just as we must view the parts of a person in relation to the whole being, we must consider persons in relation to their world. Major nursing theorists agree in their view of persons constantly interacting and changing within an ever-changing **environment**.

In the late 1800s, Florence Nightingale believed that the environment was a major determinant of the health of persons and that the most important nursing actions involved providing a healthful environment. Today we are beginning to realize the role of environmental factors such as stress and pollution on health.

The concept of environment means more than the physical surroundings. Social environment is now recognized as another variable that affects health. Nurses need knowledge of the physical, social, and human-made environments and how these aspects interact with persons to produce wellness or illness. Chapter 5 presents such an approach to the concept of environment.

Health

In nursing, we are concerned with persons' health. **Health** represents optimal biological, psychological, and social functioning. The concepts of health and adaptation are closely related. **Adaptation** is the process of changing in response to the environment; successful adaptation leads to health and growth. For instance, when we feel the sensation of thirst, we adapt by drinking. If we ignored this stimulus, we would soon die of dehydration. Because the environment is constantly changing, we are all in a continuous process of adaptation. By our constant adaptations, we move toward attaining our potential; that is, we continue to grow as individuals. The goal of nursing is to assist individuals to adapt to changes in their environments. Through our nursing care, we hope to promote optimal functioning and growth (biological and psychosocial for each person).

Health has sometimes been described as a continuum with **wellness** at one end and **illness** at the other. Because a person has many dimensions, he can be healthy (functioning at his optimum) even when elements of illness are present. Most beginning students think of health as the absence of disease. They also tend to think of physical well-being rather than mental health. Psychological well-being is important to mental health and, therefore, total health. Even the dying person who is functioning at his or her optimum may face death with a healthy sense of peace and well-being. Some would suggest that spirituality, a unique essence of person, contributes much to health when physical energy and resources are exhausted. Chapter 6 introduces a broad, multidimensional view of health.

Health-Care Delivery

Nurses do not practice their profession in a void, but rather we are members of complex health-care delivery systems. In the United States, our current systems for delivering health care are diverse and complicated, involving many settings and professionals. Frequently, the quality of health care delivered suffers from poor coordination between settings and providers. In many instances, the health-care system functions to meet its own needs at the expense of the consumer. Because nurses contribute an essential service to the health-care system, we need to be aware of its complexities and its current problems.

Nurses must recognize the needs of clients who are consumers of health care and act as their advocates. This may mean helping clients make informed choices about health care, assisting them through the maze of the health-care system itself, and ensuring that the clients' rights are respected.

Nurses face another problem within our current system. Much effort continues to be directed toward illness care (restoring wellness to ill persons) rather than wellness care (health promotion and maintenance). If the goal of nursing is the promotion of personal growth through optimal biopsychosocial adaptation, we are in potential conflict with the goals of most health-care systems. Today we need caring nurses who are concerned about wellness and who are willing to work on influencing health-care delivery so that it meets the *health* needs of consumers. Chapter 7 provides an introduction to today's health-care delivery system.

Nursing Process

Nursing process may be a mysterious term to beginning students, yet it is nothing more than the problem-solving process by which nurses meet a person's needs. It has its roots in the scientific method with which you are already familiar. You probably remember science projects in which you first used the scientific method. You began to study a problem by finding out all you could about its nature, proposing possible solutions, then testing the possibilities. The nursing process is quite similar, but the problems we deal with are persons' health-care needs. These problems are often referred to as the "nursing diagnoses." We work with our clients to identify all we can about their needs, we devise possible solutions with them, and then we assist them in testing approaches to meeting their needs. The nursing process is our professional method of assisting persons to achieve their highest level of functioning. The five component phases of nursing process—assessing, analyzing, planning, implementing, and evaluating—are explained and applied in Chapter 8.

The nursing process is a tool to help meet a client's needs. At the same time, however, it is important to identify a client's strengths. We draw upon strengths to assist each person to regain health. The nursing process, by focusing on the person who needs care, enables that person to express his or her perceptions of personal needs and to determine individual goals for health care to the level of his or her ability.

Because nurses care for persons (rather than working with scientific problems), we must work *with* our clients rather than *on* them. Caring nurses are less concerned with what clients should or ought to do than with supporting them to attain their goals. By providing the framework for respecting our clients' health and strength and their worth and individuality, the nursing process becomes not only our professional method but also a caring process as well.

Communication

Communication is the complex process in which messages are exchanged between or among persons. Because interaction between persons is the heart of nursing, nurses need a sound knowledge of the principles of communication. Communication assists nurses to build trusting relationships between themselves and their clients. Listening to our clients is often a way of showing we care. Communication is also used to assist persons to adapt to stressors, whether these affect physical, psychological, or social functioning. This kind of communication is called therapeutic — meaning communication that promotes healing or health. Nurses who deliver person-centered care value the rights of others to control their own health. Therapeutic communication is one way to achieve this end. For instance, a nurse might use this skill to help a client reduce anxiety about a heart problem and concentrate on learning about diet as one facet of self-care. Nurses who believe that persons have inherent ability to achieve optimal health will value communication as a skill that assists their clients to attain this goal. Chapter 9 introduces the nature and application of interpersonal communication in nursing.

Learning and Teaching

Teaching is a specific type of communication that focuses on facilitating learning for clients. *Learning* is a change in behavior in response to a stimulus. Nurses are concerned with the concept of learning because many clients need new skills or knowledge to adapt to their health needs. Nurses use their teaching skills to assist persons who have learning needs related to their health.

Teaching is significant only insofar as it promotes learning for clients. This principle is important because persons learn only what they perceive as having meaning for themselves, no matter how earnestly the nurse teaches them. Teaching is valued as a nursing activity because it assists persons to achieve control over their health and enables them to take better care of themselves. Because nurses recognize that each client is unique, they vary their teaching approaches to meet individual learners' needs. With emphasis on learning, Chapter 10 presents learning and teaching as a special kind of communication within the framework of the nursing process.

Nursing Ethics and Legal Aspects

Legal issues that deal with actions permitted or authorized by law affect the practice of nurses in many ways. The practice of nursing is legally regulated by individual states that are responsible for granting licenses to practice nursing, establishing criteria for licensure, and defining the scope of nursing practice. The malpractice crisis in health care has received much attention in the media. Although most of the publicity has centered around the high cost of malpractice insurance for physicians, nurses and hospitals are also being affected. Nurses need an awareness of the legal issues that affect their practice, not only for their own concerns but also to enable them to function as client advocates.

Ethical issues are those issues that relate to moral duties or obligations. Our society is changing its attitudes about major ethical issues. Nurses confront a variety of ethical issues in their practice and may find themselves in situations in which conflicts between value systems exist. Those conflicts may be among the nurse's own values, those of the client, those of the health-care institution, those of other health professionals, and those of the nursing profession. How does a nurse make decisions in these instances? Chapter 11 provides information on legal and ethical principles and examines the decision-making process for nurses' professional actions.

The prospects for the future of nurses and nursing have never been brighter. Chapter 12 explores some of the specific opportunities and challenges that await nurses preparing for the professional practice of nursing today and into the 21st century.

I CONCLUSION

This overview chapter provides an introduction for the rest of the text. The chapter has examined definitions of nursing, both from the perspectives of major nursing theorists and those of the authors. The notion of caring as a basis for nursing was explored as well as a set of beliefs about persons as the recipients of nursing care. The major organizing concepts of this textbook — nursing, person, environment, and health — were defined and other basic concepts of health-care delivery, nursing process, communication, learning and teaching, and nursing ethics and legal aspects of practice were discussed. As you continue reading, we, the authors, encourage you to examine your own thoughts about nursing and persons and consider how the ideas presented here might affect you as you begin your nursing practice.

I STUDY QUESTIONS

1   What is your definition of nursing? What common elements exist between your definition and those in Table 1 – 2?
2   How do you define "caring for persons"? Think of a nurse you know who exemplifies this definition. What attributes does he or she have?
3   Consider any of your family members who have received health care. In what ways were they treated as "clients"? As "patients"? As "persons"?

I REFERENCES

Donahue MP: Nursing: The Finest Art, an Illustrated History. St Louis, CV Mosby, 1985
Harmer B (revised by Henderson V): Textbook of Principles and Practice of Nursing, 5th ed. New York, Macmillan, 1955
James PD: The Black Tower. New York, Scribner, 1975
King IM: A Theory for Nursing: Systems, Concepts, Process. New York, John Wiley & Sons, 1981
Leininger MM: The phenomenon of caring: Importance, research questions, and theoretical consid-

erations. In Caring: An Essential Human Need (Proceedings of the three national caring conferences). Thorofare, NJ, Charles B Slack, 1981

Levine M: Introduction to Clinical Nursing, 2nd ed. Philadelphia, FA Davis, 1973

Maslow A: Motivation and Personality, 2nd ed. New York, Harper & Row, 1970

Mayeroff M: On Caring. New York, Harper & Row, 1971

Nightingale F: Notes on Nursing: What It Is and What It Is Not. London, Harrison, 1859. Facsimile edition: Philadelphia, JB Lippincott, 1966

Orem DE: Nursing: Concepts of Practice, 3rd ed. New York, McGraw-Hill, 1984

Rogers C: On Becoming a Person. Boston, Houghton Mifflin, 1961

Rogers ME: An Introduction to the Theoretical Basis of Nursing. Philadelphia, FA Davis, 1970

Rogers ME: Rogers' science of unitary human beings. In Parse RR (ed): Nursing Science: Major Paradigms, Theories, and Critiques. Philadelphia, WB Saunders, 1987

Roy C: Introduction to Nursing: An Adaptation Model, 2nd ed. Englewood Cliffs, NJ, Prentice-Hall, 1984

Schein EH, Kommers DW: Professional Education. New York, McGraw-Hill, 1972

Watson J: Nursing: Human Science and Human Care. Norwalk, CT, Appleton-Century-Crofts, 1985

Watson J: Nursing: The Philosophy and Science of Caring. Boston, Little, Brown, 1979

PART TWO

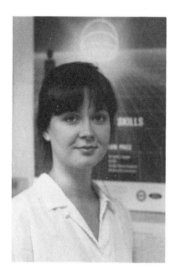

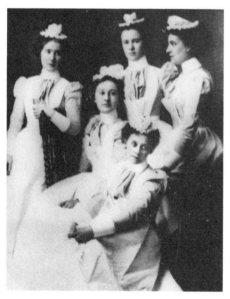

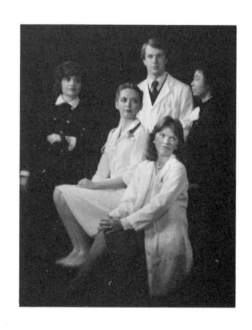

2 | NURSING THROUGH HISTORY: A PRELUDE TO THE PRESENT

KEY WORDS	After completing this chapter, students will be able to:
Accountability Art Career Certification Professional Professionalism Profession Science Standard	Describe how social and philosophical systems have affected nursing through history. Describe the highlights of nursing history. Describe nursing's historical progress as art, science, and profession. Describe nursing's status in relation to each of the characteristics of professions.

History reveals deep-rooted philosophical traditions and social forces that have shaped nursing. The term *nurse* has been applied to persons with a wide range of skills and educational backgrounds. Additionally, history informs us that the caring tradition of nursing encompasses both art and science (see Chapter 1).

To *nurse* is to nourish or look after carefully to promote growth, development, or other favorable condition. To *doctor*, by contrast, is to diagnose, treat, and cure disease. Florence Nightingale (1859) used this common definition of nursing when she declared nursing to be both an art and a science, and differentiated nursing from medicine.

Throughout history, medicine and nursing have been closely associated. "The nurse usually was the one who personally cared for the sick and helpless patient, attended to basic needs and afforded rest and comfort" (Simms and Lindberg, 1978, p 148). Not surprisingly, the nurse assumed the feminine care-giving role as the word "nurse" suggests.

| A PHILOSOPHICAL PERSPECTIVE

Hygeia of Greek mythology was the ancient goddess of health; nurses are described in Greek literature, though their gender is open to debate. However, as Donahue wrote, "The history of nursing first becomes continuous with the beginning of Christianity" (Donahue, 1985, p. 93).

Early values and beliefs created a philosophical base for the art and science that was to become nursing, the profession. Bevis described four philosophical periods of nursing

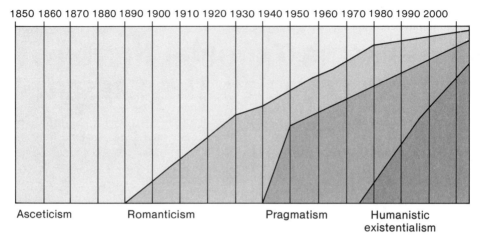

1850 1860 1870 1880 1890 1900 1910 1920 1930 1940 1950 1960 1970 1980 1990 2000

Asceticism   Romanticism   Pragmatism   Humanistic
                                                             existentialism

Figure 2-1 Chronology of four philosophical systems that affect nursing. (Bevis EO: Curriculum Building in Nursing: A Process, 3rd ed, p 36. St. Louis, CV Mosby, 1982)

history that have shaped the development of the profession and continue to influence nursing today (Fig. 2-1). Labels for these elements of nursing's value system are asceticism, romanticism, pragmatism, and humanistic existentialism (Bevis, 1982, p 36). These labels, which reflect several philosophical influences on nursing's collective consciousness, provide a strategy for understanding nursing today.

Asceticism originated in the days of Plato. It arose from the idealism that projected an ultimate spiritual reality beyond physical reality. Asceticism was associated with a life of self-denial and devotion to duty and spiritual calling. Perhaps the related salvation was as much the nurse's as the client's. Emphasis was on a service learned while doing. Learning was "training" rather than formal education. No wonder nursing originated as hard work with employer exploitation and few monetary rewards. There was a prolonged era when nurses themselves thought it was inappropriate to expect economic advantage from their calling. This period, despite Nightingale's introduction of rudimentary nursing science and formal education, dominated nursing until well into the 20th century. The influences of this period remain evident today. Nurses are often expected to make charitable contributions to society and health care.

Romanticism developed from the emphasis on materialistic realism that arose with the industrial revolution. Romanticism was the kind of escape from realism that created a fantasy experience. Romanticism is reflected in the 19th-century music of Tchaikovsky and Schumann and the romantic paintings of the Victorian painters and the impressionists.

Nurses were romanticized in dress, paintings, and literature. Severe and plain religious garb gave way to elaborate uniforms and fussy caps reflecting hospital school loyalty. Nightingale, rather than gaining wide recognition for her scientific and political acumen, was portrayed as "The Lady with the Lamp." If the Civil War dramatized the need for nurses, the later 19th and early 20th centuries romanticized their role. The romantic adventures of nurses in literature influenced young girls and women well into the mid-20th century. During this era of romanticism, nursing became medicine's loyal auxiliary. The lady-of-the-house role was assumed in hospitals where students provided much of the domestic care. Even though graduate nurses were nursing supervisors, they reported to physicians and hospital administrative authorities. Bevis argued that the romantic era greatly influenced nursing education programs until past the mid-20th century. Nursing content was parallel to medical content. It focused more on diseases than on the persons who were the recipients of care.

Throughout history, wars have reaffirmed the need for nurses. Not all wars, however, have had the same influence. World War I was a romantic war. World War II dramatically introduced a new era of realism that Bevis labeled *pragmatism*.

Pragmatism equated practical consequences with worth and truth. Bevis' philosophic interpretation of this era is particularly useful. Wartime casualties created an acute care shortage. It was during this era that a group of health-care workers, auxiliary to nurses, came to prominence. Aides, technicians, and "practical" nurses gave much of the actual nursing care. The better-prepared nurses were needed to supervise and to instruct. Medical specialties dictated the most efficient care of hospital patients. Both health-care delivery and nursing curricula were organized by disease. "The focus was on the problem, the disability, the disease, and the diagnosis, not on the person, his family, his needs, his wholeness, or his humanity" (Bevis, 1982, p 39). But eventually, toward the end of this era, practical realities dominated. The need for intensive care, rehabilitation, and ambulatory care units enabled nurses to return their focus for care to client or human need. This transitional period signaled a forthcoming era of humanistic existentialism.

Humanism is a mode of thought in which human interests predominate. Existentialism is a modern philosophic view that accepts that reality exists in the mind of the person. Reality is unique to each person who is a holistic being. The sum of a person is greater than the scientific study of his individual parts can reveal. Underlying this philosophy are choices for personal destiny and also accountability. This value system elevates care about others to a high priority for basic human reasons. The humanistic movement was popular in psychology as the "third wave" in the "me" era of the 1960s. Current humanistic values in nursing shape the view of persons for whom nursing care is provided. These values also influence nurse–client interactions, nurse accountability, and professional autonomy. This dominant philosophic notion ushers in an exciting new era for the nursing profession. Humanistic nursing care can balance and complement the high technology of health care and provide cost-effective options in an era of rapid cost escalation. As Naisbitt declared in *Megatrends*, "We must learn to balance the material wonders of technology with the spiritual demands of our human nature" (1984, p 36). This challenge awaits aspiring nurses.

With the background of this philosophic overview, we can highlight other historical influences on nursing's development.

| OTHER HISTORICAL HIGHLIGHTS

As Donahue wrote, "The roots of a movement toward the creation of religious orders of men and women with the primary motivation of nursing the sick began to occur in the late [1000–1500] Middle Ages" (1985, p 140). During the crusades to the Holy Land, knights served as nurses. These male military orders were called Hospitalers. During this time, charitable secular orders of women also nursed.

The Reformation ushered in a 300-year (1550–1850) dark period of nursing when nursing conditions changed markedly. Male nurses nearly disappeared. Although religious orders of women (e.g., the Deaconesses, Sisters of Charity, and Sisters of Mercy) came to prominence, women prisoners and prostitutes were also pressed into nursing service. Such were the times that preceded the era of Florence Nightingale.

Florence Nightingale's era (1820–1910) marks the advent of modern nursing. Nightingale, a well-educated English woman, was born of wealthy and influential parents. She entered nursing at age 25. "Called the founder of modern nursing, Nightingale was a strong-willed woman of quick intelligence who used her considerable knowledge of statistics, sanitation, logistics, administration, nutrition and public health not only to develop a new system of nursing education and health care but also to improve the social welfare systems of the time" (Kelly, 1985, p 26).

Florence Nightingale is credited with working miracles in the Crimean War and decreasing mortality in the Barrack Hospital to 1%. Her greatest miracle, however, was the reform of nursing education. To some, Florence Nightingale was a saint; to others, a strong-willed eccentric. Regardless of varying views, she was a most remarkable woman.

The nursing reform, which began in mid-19th century England, saw the establishment of three Nightingale Schools in the United States soon after the Civil War. The Civil War, like other wars, moved women from the home into the work force. As indicated earlier, "modern nursing," which originated during this Victorian era, prescribed women's roles as secondary to those of men and nurses' roles as secondary to physicians'. And, despite their prominence in nursing during the Middle Ages, men were discriminated against during the post-Nightingale era. Blacks and other ethnic minorities also suffered both discrimination and lack of recognition for their contributions. One recent documentation of black nurses' contributions was skillfully compiled by Mary Elizabeth Carnegie (1986), an outstanding black nurse-scholar. Ethnic minority groups within nursing contribute essential knowledge and sensitivity regarding cultural differences. A book by Orque and colleagues (1982), entitled *Ethnic Nursing Care: A Multicultural Approach*, presents just such knowledge.

Despite Nightingale's influence, early "training" for American nurses emphasized standard procedures, housekeeping tasks, and an ethic that supported medicine. Although nursing has a wonderful heritage, it also carries historical baggage that influenced its art and deterred its scientific development from occurring earlier.

Nursing's more recent history in the 20th century has also influenced its development. The divergence between medicine and nursing, which has occurred since Florence Nightingale's death, provides such an example. This divergence also contributes to an understanding about nursing's development as art, science, and profession.

Development of Medicine and Nursing: A Comparison

At the turn of the 19th century, there were many similarities between medical and nursing practice (e.g., similar knowledge and practitioners such as the country doctor and the private duty nurse). Early in the 20th century, medicine made a purposeful assessment of its social situation. This assessment resulted in a candid report (Flexner, 1910) on the condition of medical education in the United States. Criticism abounded and targeted the students, faculty, clinical facilities, and libraries of the current medical establishment. Medicine and society took corrective action, and medicine skyrocketed to a position of professional prominence not held previously.

As a result of the Flexner report, medicine began to standardize its education programs in colleges and research universities. The Flexner report had specifically identified that society would be deprived of appropriate health care unless it was scientifically based and delivered. Medicine began to give considerable attention to accreditation and licensing issues. The Flexner report also emphasized that society would need to pay for the necessary improved and sophisticated education of physicians. Thus, an econometric model of reimbursement was created for medicine. Long formal education and clinical experience was rewarded by generous fees for service.

Nursing, conversely, remained charitable about the services it provided and unassertive about its economic welfare. In 1923, the Goldmark Report identified the needs of nursing education and public-health nursing. This report was the first of many studies by, about, and for nursing and its advancement. Despite repeated studies, a variety of programs proliferated in nursing that did not clearly or uniformly identify the kind of practitioners that were being prepared. Finally, in the 1970s, two reports about the scope of nursing practice created a great deal of reaction within and outside nursing. These reports were "Extending the Scope of Nursing Practice," from the Health, Education, and Welfare Secretary's Committee (1971), and "An Abstract for Action," from the National Commission for the Study of Nursing and Nursing Education, chaired by Jerome Lysaught (1970). The reports validated the divergence of medicine and nursing and emphasized that nurses and nursing were not realizing their full potential. In 1980, Lysaught, describing the transformation of American medicine between 1900 and 1980 as a miracle, credited this fantastic change more to research than to technology itself. A nursing research effort aimed at improving nursing practice has just emerged since the 1970s and will be detailed below.

Table 2–1 depicts a summary of the divergence between medical and nursing practice in the 20th century. Clearly, the cornerstone of medical advance was education and research. This medical initiative was coupled with other scientific advances (e.g., the

TABLE 2–1
DIVERGENCE BETWEEN MEDICAL AND NURSING PRACTICE

1900 — Medical and Nursing Practice Similarities

- Based on similar knowledge
- Characteristic of the individual
- Benevolent

1990 — Medicine	1990 — Nursing
Members educated largely in postgraduate university programs	Most members without baccalaureate education
Established scientific base	Developing scientific base
Established research effort	Developing research effort
Career commitment of members	Chronic instability of workforce
Recognized professional autonomy and control of health care	Seeking professional autonomy and control of nursing
Strong professional organization	Struggling professional organization and some unionization of members
Prospective payment collected privately and through third-party payors	Cost of services often not identified or reimbursed through third-party payors
Dominated by men ?????	Dominated by women ?????

discovery of penicillin and technology for safer surgery). Medicine assumed a position of power to diagnose and to cure illness. Also, medicine built a cure system that was gratefully accepted by the public for decades. As the cure role grew for physicians, care and cure became further dichotomized between physicians and nurses. Dock and Stewart had defined nursing as "not only the care of the sick, the aged, the helpless and the handicapped but the promotion of health vigor in those who are well especially the young growing creatures on whom the future of the race depends" (1938, pp 4–5). The concern for the care of the healthy was overshadowed, however, by rapid advances in the care of the ill. This situation further reinforced nursing's role as care of the sick. Nursing of the sick necessarily involves many physical care activities. Therefore, nursing was often seen as primarily concerned with physical tasks (*doing*) or as artful caring, rather than mental activity or science.

| NURSING AS AN ART

Traditional nursing as **art** predominated in the first half of this century when nursing was largely the care of the ill in the hospital and the care of mothers and children in the community. Nursing was primarily the art of caring, based on intuition and skill training rather than on science. Influenza, wars, and depression produced their share of ill and dependent persons who needed care. Thus, although the seeds of nursing science had been sown by Florence Nightingale nearly a half century earlier, social forces supported the growth of nursing as art and constrained its development as science.

Caring, as one nurse colleague wrote, "depends upon the potential for expression of self" (Gold, 1978, p 107). Expression of self is, in turn, an element of art. The artistic or creative expression of self suggests the importance of developing unique aspects of personal ability. The intuitive nature of nursing has been identified and supported as the art of nursing. Purposely developing the creative aspect of nursing has often been minimized.

Donahue wrote, "Nursing is not merely a technique but a process that incorporates the elements of soul, mind, and imagination. Its very essence lies in the creative imagination, the sensitive spirit, and the intelligent understanding that provide the very foundation for effective nursing care" (1985, p 10). The art of nursing was exemplified beautifully in Donahue's classic volume *Nursing, the Finest Art — An Illustrated History*. The illustrations capture the beauty, appeal, and significance of interpersonal care, aid, and comfort across the ages. The book shows how individuals recognized as leading practitioners of the art of nursing have expressed themselves throughout history in the ministrations that gave them a prominent place in the annals of nursing.

Such creative nurses, too numerous to mention individually, include some names you may recognize:

- Florence Nightingale, the versatile genius who created modern nursing
- Lillian Wald who pioneered public health or community nursing
- Mary Breckenridge, who founded the frontier nursing service
- Virginia Henderson, who created a modern worldwide definition of nursing
- Martha Rogers, a contemporary catalyst for theory development

Other true artists of nursing toil with less recognition. However, they strive to use their unique personal attributes as they interact with clients of all ages in a variety of settings. In many ways, art is timeless as represented by human creativity throughout the ages.

After the mid-20th century, a renewed interest in art and creativity paralleled a growing interest in nursing as science and nurses as scholars. Scholarliness, as Meleis reminded us, ". . . by definition requires creativity . . . a leap of imagination" (1985, p 304). Certainly our nursing history has a heritage of creativity. Now, social and professional circumstances challenge us to rekindle that creativity to secure nursing's future and society's health. The future of nursing as art couples technological and scientific advances with artistic creativity. Together, these will enhance the precious vitality of the interpersonal interaction that has been the essence of nursing.

From a slightly different perspective, art is also the reflection of feelings and perceptions. Because the core and essence of nursing is interpersonal interaction, the art of nursing finds expression in many ways. These include, for example, both a nurse's sensitivity to and perception of the client or patient's thoughts and feelings. Also included are the nurse's expression of thoughts and feelings to the client. An example of the former could be a nurse's artistic sensitivity to a patient's nonverbal behavior indicating anxiety or pain. An example of the latter could be a nurse's unique expression of unconditional positive regard for a person based on his or her worth as an individual. Although these behaviors can be learned scientifically, they can also be learned through experience and practiced intuitively as art. Nursing practice as both art and science offers the best of both worlds to society and the widest range of practice expressions to nurses.

| NURSING AS A SCIENCE

Florence Nightingale (1859) is often recognized as nursing's first scientist/theorist for her writings, *Notes on Nursing: What It Is and What It Is Not*. She identified nursing as a scientific discipline separate from medicine. Perhaps her strongest action supporting this view was creating independent schools of nursing where nurses (rather than doctors) assumed responsibility for nursing education. Later, Nightingale claimed that, with nursing, both a new art and a new science had been created. The early science of nursing was not a separate and recognized discipline like chemistry or psychology. Instead, it was a loosely defined body of scientific facts and principles underlying physician prescribed nursing activities. For example, physicians taught nurses the knowledge of asepsis needed to perform the sterile technique of changing dressings and to assist with surgical procedures. In the early days, nurses were most often taught the scientific applications necessary to perform the delegated duties safely but taught to do so without question.

A major breakthrough for the discipline of nursing came when nursing schools moved into university settings and nurses began to study the basic sciences and humanities on which nursing was thought to be based. This preparation served two major purposes. First, it gave nurses the educational foundation necessary to make the scientific applications themselves rather than to take them on faith. Second, it gave nurses basic college credit in scientific disciplines related to nursing, which in turn prepared nurses to earn advanced degrees in a variety of biopsychosocial sciences. For example, nurses became psychologists, sociologists, anthropologists, and physiologists. Because there were a minimal number of programs within nursing to prepare scientists, theorists, and researchers, preparation in other fields was a necessity. This preparation taught nurses the processes of science and also the theories of other scientific disciplines. Additionally, this advanced preparation enabled nurses to teach other nurses. Nurses also learned that within other scientific disciplines, especially biological and physical sciences, there are specific laws and principles that give direction for making predictions within the discipline.

When nursing did not have doctorally prepared scientists within its own discipline, it also did not have the person power to develop and offer advanced nursing degrees. Only in recent years have nursing schools been able to recruit sufficient numbers of doctorally prepared nurses to offer the nursing Ph.D. in a large number of schools. Within the last decade, the number of nursing schools offering the doctorate in nursing has jumped from a mere handful to 50. Doctorally prepared nurses have the advanced research skills necessary to conduct independent scientific investigations and to contribute to nursing theory.

Considering nursing's short scientific history and the 20th-century divergence between medical and nursing practice, the last 40 years provide a startling contrast to earlier times. Selected highlights are summarized in Table 2–2.

TABLE 2–2
HIGHLIGHTS OF NURSING'S SCIENTIFIC HISTORY

1950s	1960s	1970s	1980s
▪ Code of Ethics adopted by the American Nurses' Association (1950).	▪ Postbaccalaureate programs in nursing specialty areas increase.	▪ Nurse-practitioners in expanded practice roles gain national visibility.	▪ Master's and doctoral programs in nursing proliferate.
▪ Nurses seek postbaccalaureate preparation in nursing; first graduate programs established for clinical nurse specialists.	▪ Nurses establish National Clinical Specialty nursing groups.	▪ Nurses' Coalition for Action in Politics (N-CAP) formed.	▪ Professional nursing journals increase remarkably (over 80 by 1985).
▪ The professional journal *Nursing Research* is first published (1952).	▪ Nursing researchers pioneer clinical investigations	▪ American Nurses' Association creates American Academy of Nursing to honor outstanding contributors to nursing.	▪ By 1984, more than 20,000 nurses nationally "certified" in 17 specialty areas of practice.
	▪ International Nursing Index categorizes worldwide nursing articles.	▪ Nursing theorists come into national spotlight.	▪ National Institutes of Health house a National Center for Nursing Research.
			▪ Sigma Theta Tau, international honor society for outstanding baccalaureate-prepared nurses, numbers 75,000 members at middecade.
			▪ Sigma Theta Tau launches 10-year plan, Focus on Scholarship, to increase the science of nursing and increase public awareness of research required.

Nursing as a Profession

Most of us use the terms **profession** and **professional** rather casually. In some instances, we intend to convey the impression that a person is an expert; in other instances, we use the term "professional" politely as a title of distinction. Accordingly, we describe someone as a professional athlete, musician, or engineer. We may ask someone, "What is your profession?" when we mean, "What work do you do?"

Professionalism is defined as professional character, spirit, or methods. Professionalism also encompasses teaching and activities found in various occupational groups whose members aspire to be professional.

Professionalization is a process of acquiring or changing characteristics in the direction of a profession.

The debate about whether nursing is a profession has stirred and divided nursing throughout its history. With attention focusing on educational preparation for entry into professional nursing practice, professionalism in nursing remains a current and pressing issue. Because the issues related to professionalism present implications and challenges for every nurse and recipient of nursing care, the topic is important to practicing and aspiring nurses as well as the public.

History informs us that the occupations traditionally accepted as professions are medicine, law, and the ministry. Many other occupational groups now seek the status that has been assigned to these professions over time. Whether society views these aspiring occupations as professions is another matter.

You may or may not consider nursing to be a profession. At the very least, you are probably being confronted with a view of nursing that is somewhat different from what you expected. Often, beginning students regard nursing primarily as the mastery of many technical procedures. Indeed, such technical mastery is important, but it is only a part of the larger scheme of professional nursing practice. To clarify the notion of professional practice in nursing, it is helpful to reflect on the general criteria for all professions.

General Criteria for Professions

In general, all professions have the following characteristics:

- A body of knowledge on which skills and services are based
- An ability to deliver a unique service to other humans
- Education that is standardized and based in colleges and universities
- Control of standards for practice
- Responsibility and accountability of members for their own actions
- Career commitment by members
- Independent function
  (Schein and Kommers, 1972, pp 7–14)

Let us consider each of these criteria for professions individually.

Body of Knowledge on Which Skills and Services Are Based

At one time in history, nursing skills and practice were based largely on intuitive knowledge. Today, as a practice discipline, nursing is called an applied **science**. If the person is the recipient of nursing and each person is a biopsychosocial being interacting with his or her environment, then nursing applies concepts from many different basic sciences. Some nursing leaders argue that nursing need not have a unique knowledge base. They believe nursing can be unique in its application of knowledge common to many disciplines. Other experts believe that nursing eventually will develop its own body of knowledge and its own theories.

Those who are particularly interested in nursing as science will be enriched by exploring further the work of nurse-philosophers, theorists, and researchers. The nature of knowledge development in many fields is changing—from a deductive, reductionist, mechanistic, and quantitative view to an inductive, holistic, qualitative, and social view. This change may signal an era of science that is more supportive of the scientific agendas that are important to nursing. As Meleis said, "It is a view that has shifted the focus from a causation to a more interpretive view" (1985, p 51). Meleis' book, *Theoretical Nursing: Development and Progress*, is an excellent resource for both a sophisticated scientific nursing perspective and extensive theoretical abstracts and bibliography.

Ability To Deliver a Unique Service to Other Humans

According to Henderson (1966) and as indicated earlier, the unique function of the nurse is to assist the person in performing activities contributing to health and recovery, or a serene death, which the person would do for himself or herself if he or she were able. Furthermore, the nurse does this in a way that encourages independence. The current emphasis on nurses' promoting self-care is consistent with Henderson's definition. In addition to a person-centered practice, the unique focus of nursing is often identified as health, not illness, which is the focus for medicine. Society validates its need for nursing by continuing to educate nurses. At present, however, it is foolish to argue that all persons termed *nurses* provide the same unique service.

Standardized Education Based in Colleges and Universities

As long ago as 1859, Florence Nightingale advocated training schools that would be educational institutions supported by public funds. Although she thought the schools should be closely associated with hospitals, she also believed that they should be administered separately.

In 1909, a Minnesota physician, Dr. Richard Beard, proposed and strongly defended university education for nurses. The first university school of nursing opened in Minnesota that year. A significant development regarding collegiate education for nurses occurred in the 1950s: Montag (1951) introduced associate degree (A.D.) programs to prepare nurse-technicians. The success of these programs, coupled with the general increase in numbers of community and junior colleges, resulted in a proliferation of such A.D. programs. In 1974, the New York State Nurses' Association proposed that by 1985 the baccalaureate degree become the minimal educational preparation for entry into professional nursing practice. This proposal generated controversy among nurses, other health professionals, and hospital administrators even though the suggestion of collegiate education was far from new.

In the last decade, there has been a decrease in diploma nursing programs and an increase in all other nursing education programs. Statistics from the National League for

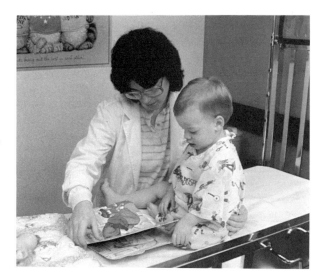

Nurses build trust and autonomy.

Nursing (1987), the organization that accredits educational programs in nursing, document this increase. In 1974–1975, there were 21,562 graduations from diploma programs, 32,183 from A.D. programs, and 20,170 from baccalaureate programs. In 1984–1985, there were 11,892 graduations from diploma programs, 45,208 from A.D. programs, and 24,975 from baccalaureate programs.

The questions of how nurses should be prepared and titled have been ones of long-standing debate. During the registered nurse shortages of the late 1980s, many questions arose about how and whom to prepare to do many of the basic tasks of nursing that had once been done by aides and licensed practical nurses. Whenever there are nurse shortages, the creation of other lesser educated nonprofessional health-care workers to fill in for nurses becomes an issue.

Control of Standards for Practice

A **standard** is an authoritative statement or criterion by which the quality of practice can be judged. In the late 1950s, the American Nurses' Association (ANA), nursing's professional organization, expressed formal concern for control of practice at a level above the legal minimum required for registered nurse (RN) licensure. The ANA first published *Standards for Organized Nursing Services* in 1965. These standards emphasized both systematic nursing plans providing for client participation and nursing actions to maximize health capabilities. The nursing practice standards assume individual nurse responsibility and accountability for meeting the standards.

The ANA recognizes excellence in practice through a process called **certification**. According to the Association's *Social Policy Statement*, "Certification of specialists in nursing practice is a judgment made by the profession, upon review of an array of evidence examined by a selected panel of nurses who are themselves specialists and who represent the area of specialization" (1980, p 24). Certification identifies persons who have obtained specialized knowledge and affirms professional achievement. Certification also carries with it the endorsement of professional colleagues.

Responsibility and Accountability of Members for Their Own Actions

Accountability is responsibility for the services one provides or makes available. The concept of accountability is not new to nursing. In fact, nurses are probably more concerned about accountability than many other professionals. Accountability has several dimensions, including legal, peer group, employer, and consumer accountability. Licensing boards can revoke licenses to practice for incompetence or certain violations of the law. Nurses are accountable to health-care colleagues with whom they are professionally associated, as reflected in the increasing use of peer review within the clinical setting. Such review may include evaluating the client's health record to compare actual practice to the ANA nursing practice standards. Because nurses are not generally independent practitioners, they are often also accountable to hospitals or other employing agencies. Increasingly, nurses describe themselves as directly accountable to their clients or patients. The concept of accountability implies both that one is responsible for the consequences of actions chosen and also that one accepts the consequences of choosing not to act in particular situations.

Primary care is a mechanism whereby health-care providers, including nurses, are accountable for the services rendered to specific clients. One usually thinks of accountability in this more narrow sense of specific care situations. In the broader sense, one is accountable for moving the profession toward professional goals. The individual is also accountable to oneself for achieving maximum potential.

Code for Nurses.   Another way professionals monitor conduct within their ranks is by formulating and enforcing a code of ethics. The Code for Professional Nurses was first outlined in the 1920s. It was finally adopted in 1950 and has been changed many times since (ANA, 1976). This code not only guides members but serves as a proclamation to the public served by nursing (Table 2–3).

Career Commitment by Members

A **career** is what you do as your major life work. It is sometimes described as the progress of a person through life. A career may be distinguished from a job, which is an individual piece of work done in the routine of one's trade or occupation. In earlier days, when women's life work was done primarily in the home, they had little opportunity for professional careers in the world of work outside the home. Today, most married women work outside the home.

This fact reflects both economic necessity and a change in society's attitudes toward women's work. As women today consider employment, the choice between job and career is no longer made based solely on the length of time one expects to remain in the work force. Most nurses who work probably do so for more than a quarter of a century, or a third of their lifetime.

The characteristics of jobs and careers listed in Table 2–4 may help distinguish between the two. The intent is not to imply that a career is inherently better than a job, nor is the contrast suggested as more than a guide.

Although there are more nurses than ever before (more than 2 million), the impact of this number is deceptive. Some nurses do not maintain a current license to practice. The yearly turnover rate of nurses in acute care settings continues to be high. Many of these

TABLE 2-3
AMERICAN NURSES' ASSOCIATION CODE FOR NURSES

1 The nurse provides services with respect for human dignity and the uniqueness of the client, unrestricted by considerations of social or economic status, personal attributes, or the nature of health problems.

2 The nurse safeguards the client's right to privacy by judiciously protecting information of a confidential nature.

3 The nurse acts to safeguard the client and the public when health care and safety are affected by the incompetent, unethical, or illegal practice of any person.

4 The nurse assumes responsibility and accountability for individual nursing judgments and actions.

5 The nurse maintains competence in nursing.

6 The nurse exercises informed judgment and uses individual competence and qualifications as criteria in seeking consultation, accepting responsibilities, and delegating nursing activities to others.

7 The nurse participates in activities that contribute to the ongoing development of the profession's body of knowledge.

8 The nurse participates in the profession's efforts to implement and improve standards of nursing.

9 The nurse participates in the profession's efforts to establish and maintain conditions of employment conducive to high quality nursing care.

10 The nurse participates in the profession's effort to protect the public from misinformation and misrepresentation and to maintain the integrity of nursing.

11 The nurse collaborates with members of the health professions and other citizens in promoting community and national efforts to meet the health needs of the public.

(American Nurses' Association: Code for Nurses with Interpretive Statements. Kansas City, MO, American Nurses' Association, 1985)

nurses (almost one third) are employed part-time. Increasingly, more nurses are employed in nontraditional community settings.

Independent Function

During the first half of the 20th century, a view of nurses as handmaidens or assistants to physicians pervaded American thinking. The reason for this perception probably related more to deeply ingrained social values than to any inherent characteristics of nursing practice. State nursing practice laws generally do not prohibit nurses from behaving more

TABLE 2-4
CHARACTERISTICS OF A JOB VERSUS A CAREER

Job	Career
A piece of work; may or may not be long-term employment	Life work; long-term commitment, long-term planning important, possibly involving a mentor
Variable initial training	Long training or education
Part-time or full-time	Usually full-time
Intermittent retraining possible	Lifelong learning necessary
Job selects person	Person selects career
Administrator evaluation primarily	Peer evaluation primarily

independently in ways consistent with their knowledge and skills. At the same time, nurses are clearly restricted in diagnosing illness and in prescribing independently for its treatment. These two functions are currently the prerogative of medical practice.

As currently practiced, nursing has acknowledged independent and interdependent functions. Occasionally, nurses set up private practices outside a formal health-care institution and practice independently. Society also receives great benefit from nursing's independent practice in the form of voluntary service or charity. In fact, society often expects nurses to provide free advice and service in their neighborhoods and communities. It does not ask the same of law or medicine, in which most of the practitioners are men.

Additional Criteria

Two additional criteria of American professions identified by Lysaught (1980) are an active and cohesive professional organization, and acknowledged social worth and contribution. In 1984, the ANA — the official professional organization — consisted of only 180,716 nurses, that is, less than 1 of 7 in practice. Probably a comparable number belonged to other organizations such as specialty groups or honor societies. The membership of these combined organizations accounted for about one quarter of all registered nurses.

Professionalization is a dynamic process. Some people describe nursing as a semiprofession or an emerging profession. Others call it an aspiring profession. Just as the human being is viewed as being in the process of becoming, so might nursing be viewed. Thus, the terms *developing profession* or *aspiring profession* are useful because they convey a possibility of striving to achieve a potential. As the human being moves from basic needs to growth needs, so nursing must move from occupational to professional criteria before achieving full professional status. If the parallel drawn here holds true, nursing has perhaps reached early adulthood, not full maturity, as a profession.

| LESSONS OF THE PAST

The following are three lessons of the past worth learning:

1   Issues and problems facing nursing today are neither as new as we sometimes like to think nor as immobilizing as some might suggest.
2   Just as yesterday's issues are today's history, today's issues will be tomorrow's history.
3   In the past, as now, individual persons make things happen as they work alone and together for common causes. Ideas and actions begin with one person. Although society shapes the nursing profession, persons within nursing have and will determine much of what happens to nursing.

Historically, nurses were not always fully aware of their special contributions to health care. That is, they did not identify and articulate the essence of nursing. Sometimes nurses minimized their abilities to develop trust between themselves and those they nursed, to identify the health aspects of the person they were caring for, and to help individuals mobilize their own health qualities to achieve their personal potential. Nurses recognized that although people might have severe or even life-threatening physical problems, they were still unique individuals capable of growth. However, because nurses did not identify and articulate nursing's unique contribution completely, much of it was set aside as nursing entered an age of increased technology.

As technology flourished, much of nursing became "doing activities." Nurses and others measured their value by their skill in taking care of equipment. A unique nursing contribution was present in much of what nurses did, but it often seemed less important. It was not unusual for a patient to describe this appreciation of nursing care, and for the nurse to think or say, "But I didn't do anything!" Perhaps the nurse listened with trust and therapeutic purpose and helped the patient to rediscover control of his or her life, to regain a sense of self-esteem, and to view the future with hope or a sense of well-being.

In the 1970s and 1980s, nursing made enormous leaps in practice, education, and research. The decisions to be made in the 1990s are understood better from an historical perspective. For the same reason that cultures find their roots important, nursing is experiencing a surge of interest in the profession's roots. Today, a primary and specific purpose for considering history is to relate it both to the present and to the future. Some of the many works that do this well include Aiken (1982), Ashley (1976), Chaska (1983), Kalisch and Kalisch (1978), and Kelley (1985).

| CONCLUSION

Nursing began as an art, became a science, and is developing as a profession. A historical perspective was presented to illuminate this evolution. Nursing as a profession was considered in relation to the generally accepted criteria for professions. Contemporary nurses and aspiring nurses can learn much from nursing's history that will help them understand nursing today and for the future: deep-rooted philosophical traditions and social forces shaped nursing throughout history and influence nursing's continued development as art, science, and profession.

| STUDY QUESTIONS

1 How do you think nursing might have developed differently if

   a Most practitioners were men?

   b Most nurses were baccalaureate prepared?

   c All nurses accepted nursing as a career rather than as a job?

2 Using the criteria given, how do you rate nursing in comparison to other professions?

3 How has your awareness of professionalism changed?

| REFERENCES

Aiken LH: Nursing in the 1980s: Crises, Opportunities, Challenges. Philadelphia, JB Lippincott, 1982

American Nurses' Association: A Social Policy Statement. Kansas City, MO, American Nurses' Association Pub. Code NP-63 35M, 1980

American Nurses' Association: Code for Nurses with Interpretive Statements. Kansas City, MO, American Nurses' Association, 1985

American Nurses' Association: Standards for Organized Nursing Services. New York, American Nurses' Association, 1965

Ashley JA: Hospitals, Paternalism, and the Role of the Nurse. New York, Teachers College Press, 1976

Bevis EO: Curriculum Building in Nursing: A Process, 3rd ed. St Louis, CV Mosby, 1982

Carnegie ME: The Path We Tread: Blacks in Nursing 1854–1984. Philadelphia, JB Lippincott, 1986

Chaska N: The Nursing Profession: A Time to Speak. New York, McGraw-Hill, 1983

Dock LL, Stewart IS: A Short History of Nursing. New York, GP Putnam's Sons, 1938

Donahue MP: Nursing: The Finest Art, An Illustrated History. St. Louis, CV Mosby, 1985

Flexner A: Medical Education in the United States and Canada. New York, Carnegie Foundation for Advancement of Teaching, 1910

Gold H: Caretaking, giving care, caring for, caring. In Simms LM, Lindberg JB (eds): The Nurse Person, pp 105–111. New York, Harper & Row, 1978

Goldmark J: Nursing and Nursing Education in the United States. New York, Macmillan, 1923

Health, Education, and Welfare Secretary's Committee to Study Extended Roles for Nurses: Extending the scope of nursing practice. Am J Nurs 71:2346–2351, 1971

Henderson V: The Nature of Nursing. New York, Macmillan, 1966

Kalisch PA, Kalisch BJ: The Advance of American Nursing. Boston, Little, Brown, 1978

Kelly LY: Dimensions of Professional Nursing, 5th ed. New York, Macmillan, 1985

Lysaught J: Action on affirmation toward an unambiguous profession of nursing. Paper presented at American Nurses' Association Biennial Convention, Houston, TX, June 1980

Meleis AI: Theoretical Nursing: Development and Progress. Philadelphia, JB Lippincott, 1985

Montag M: The Education of Nursing Technicians. New York, GP Putnam's Sons, 1951

Naisbitt J: Megatrends. New York, Warner Books, 1984

National Commission for the Study of Nursing and Nursing Education: An Abstract for Action. New York, McGraw-Hill, 1970

National League for Nursing: Nursing Student Census. New York, National League for Nursing. Pub. No. 19-2175, 1987

Nightingale F: Notes on Nursing: What It Is and What It Is Not. London, Harrison, 1859. Facsimile edition: Philadelphia, JB Lippincott, 1966

Orque MS, Bloch B, Monroy LA: Ethnic Nursing Care: A Multicultural Approach. St. Louis, CV Mosby, 1982

Schein EH, Kommers DW: Professional Education. New York, McGraw-Hill, 1972

Simms LM, Lindberg JB: The Nurse Person: Developing Perspectives for Contemporary Nursing. New York, Harper & Row, 1978

3 | NURSING TODAY: THE HEALTH SCIENCE OF CARING

KEY WORDS	After completing this chapter, students will be able to:
Authority Career option Caring Conceptual frame- work or model Function Health Nursing Nursing research Nursing theory Politics Power Science Scientific method Theory	Recognize the concepts of nursing, human or person, environment, and health as the subject matter common to all theories of nursing. Recognize several nurse-theorists who have contributed to developing conceptual frameworks for nursing. Recognize the contributions of nursing theory and nursing research to the development of nursing as a profession. Describe contemporary nursing issues. Describe individual and group strategies for increasing nurse self-actualization and influence.

To understand fully the career opportunities available in nursing today, it is necessary to look at nursing from several perspectives. This chapter provides an introduction to the concept *nursing* that shapes nursing as art, science, and profession. The chapter provides a basic foundation for understanding the many intellectual and interpersonal skills that nurses use. It also provides a context for understanding the many technological aspects of nursing that are necessarily a part of nursing education as well as professional nursing practice. *Professions* are applied sciences whose theoretical knowledge must be used to achieve practical ends because one important characteristic of professions is their service to humankind.

The discussion of nursing as a theoretical science includes information that will be beyond the perceived need for some readers and insufficient for others. Likewise, some readers will not initially identify with the importance given to nursing research in an introductory text. However, the material included suggests a full range of nursing's potential scope.

The final portion of the chapter, Leadership and Literature, suggests strategies for increasing both nurse self-actualization and nursing influence. These individual and group strategies enumerate ways that aspiring nurses can influence their own professional development and that of nursing.

As indicated in Chapter 2, people have always needed nursing care. As society evolved, attempts to meet nursing care requirements evolved. These changed from familial and informal caregiving to caregiving based on formal education, state licensing, and national credentialing. Now, society has declared that the need for nursing is expanding. In addition, nationally unmet nursing need has reached crisis proportions. In fact, the U.S. Department of Health and Human Services has projected a deficiency of 600,000 nurses prepared at baccalaureate and higher levels by the year 2000 (Rosenfeld, 1987). This projected deficiency raised cries of both crisis and doom in the late 1980s. Some who looked to the future, however, foresaw an era of golden opportunity previously unequaled for the profession of nursing.

History demonstrates that when society recognizes a pressing unmet social need, it may mobilize social forces to correct the situation. Thus, social need can create a window of opportunity to benefit both society and the professional group addressing the social need. In the present nursing care crisis, society has made a case for an overall shortage of nurses *and* also for a deficit of "advanced" practitioners. The current demand is simultaneously for greater numbers and higher levels of specialized practice. Not only does society need expert technical nurses, but it also values appropriately prepared professional nurses who practice nursing as *the health science of caring.*

| THE NURSING CONCEPT EXPLORED

Nursing is gaining professional and public recognition as the health science of caring. Caring is perhaps the one word or phenomenon most clearly associated with nursing over time. **Caring** means to have thought or regard for as a person. It also means to give watchful oversight or to advocate for or assist when the individual is unable to tend to his or her own personal needs. Caring is practiced: parent to child, lover to lover, well to ill, fortunate to less fortunate, or professional to client. Caring is the most intimate, tender, protective, and growth producing of interpersonal interactions. The difference between caring and caring as science, however, is a real difference.

To call nursing the health science of caring is to value health and its promotion, to emphasize the science of nursing as well as the art; and to acknowledge that caring is a prime interpersonal interaction open to study. Caring is also an interpersonal interaction that transcends time, gender, and technology. In that spirit, nursing, the health science of caring, is a service basic to society. This service was born in the days of earliest humankind and has the potential to serve human needs as long as people inhabit the earth and the universe beyond.

A century after Nightingale, Virginia Henderson wrote:

> The unique function of the nurse is to assist the individual, sick or well, in the performance of those activities contributing to HEALTH or its recovery (or to peaceful death) that he would perform unaided if he had the necessary strength, will, or knowledge. And to do this in such a way as to help him gain independence as rapidly as possible. This aspect of *her* work, this part of *her* function, *she* initiates and controls; of this *she* is master. In addition *she* helps the patient to carry out the therapeutic plan as initiated by the physician. (1966, p 432; emphasis added)

Henderson's emphasis on the nurse as "she" reflected an accepted reality but one that overlooked a valuable human resource for society and nursing. In the 1980s, men's caring abilities finally received recognition and social approval. This recognition and approval may encourage men to choose nursing in greater numbers.

Another more current, definition of nursing comes from the Model Practice Act published in 1982 by the National Council of State Boards of Nursing. It states:

> the "Practice of Nursing" means assisting individuals or groups to maintain or attain optimal HEALTH throughout the life process by assessing their HEALTH status, establishing a diagnosis, planning and implementing a strategy of care to accomplish defined goals, and evaluating responses to care and treatment. (p 2)

Also in the early 1980s, the ANA (1980) issued a social policy statement with an emphasis on the importance of health. In fact, a few brief words from this statement took on the status of a national definition for nursing, namely, that nursing is "the diagnosis and treatment of human responses to actual or potential health problems" (p 9).

Notice that these last two definitions make no gender reference for nurse. All of these definitions suggest the need to clarify several terms to understand nursing as the health science of caring.

Health is such an important concept for nursing that we have devoted an entire chapter to its elaboration. At this point, however, a few brief comments will be enough to introduce the subject. Clearly, the definition of health is changing over time. **Health** is now considered to be a condition of the life cycle that is dynamic, adaptive, responsive to both internal and external stimuli, and influenced by the behaviors of the "person." Health has, as subconcepts, wellness and illness components. Health and illness often coexist in the same person. This latter thought illuminates an important point: all people have health needs. These are needs to promote, retain, or regain health according to individual and varying potentials.

These health needs exist across the life span in both well and ill persons. Anywhere nurses encounter persons with health needs is a setting where nursing care can and should be delivered. For generations, the health-care system in the United States has been primarily an illness-care system that treated illness while downplaying wellness promotion, health maintenance, and illness prevention. Interestingly, the nurse shortage is finally coming to be described as a health hazard as well as a deficit in illness care.

That nursing is now designated a health science will be expanded on later. At this point, we can begin by saying that **science** is, as everyone knows, knowledge gained by systematic study. Science is also a particular branch of knowledge. An alternate and once-popular definition of science — that is, knowledge as skill resulting from training — is no longer adequate. This adaptation is easily illustrated in nursing: What was once referred to as *nurses' training* is now called *nursing education* and takes place along with other higher education in colleges and universities. Nursing theory and the scientific knowledge gained by research help nursing gain recognition as the health science of caring.

| NURSING THEORY

What Is Nursing Theory?

Nursing theory is the systematic abstraction or formation of mental ideas about nursing practice reality. Its purpose is to describe, explain, predict, and control nursing action (caring) to achieve certain nursing practice outcomes. Theories interrelate concepts to provide new ways of looking at nursing care and improving nursing practice. Theories assist in increasing the general body of knowledge within the discipline through the research implemented to validate (confirm) them (Torres, 1980).

Theories can be characterized according to their scope of focus. For example, a *grand theory* of nursing would be very broad and encompass supposedly everything a nurse needed to know. A *middle-range theory*, on the other hand, would be concerned with a limited aspect of nursing, for example, a nursing theory of pain management. Theories may have even more limited scope, but then they risk having trivial impact. Many other ways to describe theories are beyond the scope of these introductory remarks.

Importance of Nursing Theory

Sciences develop and mature as the knowledge in the discipline increases and becomes unique, organized, and more complex. Nursing must create a theoretical science that is distinct and unique. The science must describe, explain, predict, and control the outcomes of nursing practice. Only then will nursing be fully recognized as a separate scientific discipline and a true profession.

Apart from the intellectual reasons for developing nursing theory, one might ask the logical question, "How does theory relate to nursing practice?" The basic answer is that practicing nursing from a theoretical perspective gives a scientific credibility to practice. Theory provides a framework or paradigm to direct the action of practice. As Erickson and colleagues indicated:

> Basic needs can often be met in a very few actual minutes of care, assuming that a clear and purposive theory and paradigm [framework] are employed. If a substantial block of time IS taken, it may in the long run preserve the nursing staff from even greater investments of time and energy extended over numerous future times. More strenuous efforts become necessary when complications occur that might otherwise have been avoided. (1983, p 242).

A brief example contrasts two ways of looking at clinical situations, that is, with and without a theoretical perspective:

Angry, anxious, frightened patients constantly call the nurse. The nurse can respond *without theory* and be exasperated, angry, disgusted, tired, bored, avoiding, and feel helpless. This approach may lead to the nurse's complaining, scolding, or avoiding such patients. Or, the nurse can respond *with theory* and recognize patients' inability to maintain an image of the nurse when they cannot see him or her caring about them, be aware of the patients' feelings of insecurity in hospital settings, understand the grief process, and consciously plan theoretically based nursing care for patients.

Both nursing theory and nursing research have as their purpose to suggest answers to puzzling questions from nursing practice. These puzzling questions are concerned with

1   *Description* — clarifying ideas, phenomena, experiences or circumstances that are not well understood, for example, describing what pain really means to patients. This is accomplished by presenting new information.

2   *Exploration* — exploring how ideas of interest are related, for example, what is the relationship between pain and patients' physical and psychological conditions?

3   *Explanation* — explaining, often within the context of an existing theory, the whys of events or occurrences, for example, why does pain occur more

frequently and severely in persons whose physical and psychological resources are impoverished or reduced?

4   *Prediction and control* — knowing and foretelling correctly what will happen and also how to make it happen on command and with some regularity, for example, in what specific ways can the nurse control the severity of pain for patients?

If nursing is the science of caring, caring is a critical phenomenon of both theoretical and practical interest. Therefore, as nursing science develops, nurses will be better able to predict and control this caring phenomenon. Such control will benefit individual patients and clients and society in a unique way. Belief in nursing's extraordinary contribution to society has been the driving force that leads nurses to create nursing science and theories that are indeed singular to nursing. Scientific theories are built on concepts or general abstractions. Below are defined some of the words we have already used and will be using in our discussion of theories:

- **Concept** — a mental image or classification of things and events in terms of similarities. In nursing, person, health, environment, and nursing itself are concepts of primary interest to theory and practice. Scientific concepts are the building blocks of theory and refer to the abstracts notions that are related within a theory.
- **A conceptual framework or model** — a structure composed of concepts associated in such a way as to form a whole, for example, a developmental model with concepts of infant, child, adult.
- **Theory** — a group of concepts, definitions, and statements that present an organized view of phenomena (e.g., caring) by specifying interrelationships among concepts with the intent of describing, explaining, predicting, or controlling these phenomena. A now well-recognized theory that has moved from the realm of science to that of everyday life is Einstein's theory of relativity: $E = mc^2$.

Additional definitions related to theoretical ideas include the following: *laws*, for example, laws of physics, chemistry, or nature; and *principles*, for example, principles of sterile technique or thermodynamics. Perhaps nursing will have its own laws someday and its principles will be based less on traditions and more on research and theory. (See Levine's principles in the section Selected Contributors to Nursing's Theoretical Knowledge, below.)

Many theories within the same and different scientific disciplines share similar notions or general concepts. Different sciences use the same or similar concepts in different ways. The concept of *human* is used differently by those in the discipline of anatomy than by those in psychology, for example. Anatomy is concerned with the human being's body and the physical structure of its parts; in contrast, psychology is the science of human behavior and also is concerned with mental states and processes. Likewise, scientific nursing is built on common concepts, the most frequent of which are nursing, person, health, and environment. Except for nursing, all of these concepts are also pertinent to some other disciplines. Theory within a science shows how the science uses concepts uniquely. Theory differentiates one science from others that are built on some of the same or similar concepts.

Theory is important to nursing both to increase and to organize nursing's knowledge. Theory also helps establish nursing's credibility as a legitimate scientific branch of knowledge.

Considerable debate exists within nursing about the proper use of the terms *conceptual model* and *theory*. Fawcett correctly made the point that "a conceptual model is not a theory, nor is a theory a conceptual model" (1984, p 25). As she noted, the primary distinction between the two is the level of abstraction. A conceptual model is more abstract or less concrete than a theory. In reality and to date, nursing science has created mostly conceptual models, which are being used to guide and organize nursing knowledge in educational programs, research, and practice. Recognizing this point is especially important for all nurses, including new professionals who often experience frustration in dealing with abstract ideas. Because conceptual models are so abstract, they can be mentally taxing. They may seem to have nothing to do with the real world of nursing care. True, they do not directly answer questions for practice and research. The fact remains, however, that vague conceptual models and beginning efforts at nursing theories are the state of nursing science at the present time. Also, conceptual models and theories are more scientific than mere intuition. Theories and models provide many challenges. They also define the tasks yet to be accomplished by current and future nurse-scholars if nursing is to become a true science and full profession.

Learning about theory is sometimes avoided or theory is dismissed as unimportant. Aspiring nurses should recognize the herculean efforts of a few especially valued nurse-scientists. These nurses take risks and blaze trails in nursing theory development. Some scholars have pioneered the way in nursing theory because of their dedication, conviction, and commitment. They value nursing as an important and distinct scientific discipline. They also value nursing as a practice profession that society needs. These nurse-scientists have boldly shared their conceptual models, what Fawcett (1984) called formal presentations of their private images of nursing. Although it is not necessary that we all be theorists, it is necessary that we work together to push nursing forward and help it develop as both a mature science and profession.

Theoretical Foundations From Related Sciences

Nursing has borrowed or used theories from other related sciences as the foundation for nursing. A major reason for this borrowing is the lack of well-developed nursing theories. Many problems arise when borrowing bits and pieces of theoretical foundations from related sciences. In this age of knowledge specialization, nurses cannot maintain the expertise across a wide range of disciplines that scientists within those fields have. This lack can lead to incomplete, inaccurate, or obsolete knowledge. It also leads to problems synthesizing or putting together information appropriately. Additionally, theoretical notions are meant to be used within the context of the specific theory and discipline for which they were designed. They may or may not be appropriate or compatible with other notions outside the theory. A theory that holds in non-nursing reality may not represent reality with the same accuracy in a nursing situation. The trick, of course, is to understand enough to make both reasonable judgments and appropriate synthesis, which is one reason nurses need a liberal education.

Examples of many kinds of theories from other disciplines have been applied to nursing with varying success, including, but not limited to, theories of stress, development, and learning. Such borrowing will continue until nursing has its own unique and well-developed theories that are sufficient not only for describing outcomes and actually controlling results of our area of interest, nursing practice. Even then, some suggest, we will continue to adapt theories from other discrete disciplines but will make unique linkages within a nursing context.

It is not surprising that "nursing," the one concept unique to our discipline, is also the one concept that is least well developed in relation to the others we use. Nursing's interest in and application of any of the concepts it shares with other disciplines are different from those of the other disciplines, including medicine. For example, a nurse's interest in anatomy, physiology, and pathophysiology is not to gather data for making medical diagnoses. Rather, nurses assess the functional disabilities and remaining strengths of persons to understand and to predict responses to altered health states. In turn, this understanding enables nurses to plan nursing care to enhance health.

Where disciplines overlap—for example, nursing and medicine or nursing and psychology—the overlap is significant because of common shared knowledge. What is often understood in other disciplines but misunderstood in nursing is that the area of no overlap between sciences is what becomes the content unique to a discipline. It is this area of no ovelap—that is, what is unique to nursing—that will prove most fruitful in the development of nursing theory and science.

One Theory or Many?

In its present state, the developing science of nursing needs to approach theory building on many fronts. For some time to come, theories will continue to be borrowed from other disciplines. There are many reasons why multiple theories or conceptual frameworks will be pursued: the conceptual frameworks now prominent require considerable development as theories to be truly useful in research and practice with any regular consistency; the scope of nursing is such that mid-level theories will be more realistic to construct and use; and the diversity of practice within clinical areas (which is also one of nursing's most attractive features) supports theoretical diversity.

Common Theoretical Themes

Stevens's contrast of the themes of the recent past with emergent themes (Table 3–1) can be useful in understanding both the direction of theory development in nursing and the career opportunities this new science offers.

The subject matter common to all theories of nursing includes the concepts of nursing, human or person, health, and environment. Any combination of these concepts and others may be approached or developed in a variety of ways to create models that are primarily concerned with systems, human development, or interpersonal interaction.

Selected Contributors to Nursing's Theoretical Knowledge

This section presents in table form a brief overview of selected contributors to nursing's theoretical knowledge. The authors assume responsibility for inclusion of some but not all of nursing's acknowledged theorists. At the end of the section, the reader is directed both to the detailed works of these and other theorists and to some of the works of nursing leaders who have thoughtfully critiqued nursing's experience with theory development.

TABLE 3–1
CHANGING THEMES IN NURSING

Themes of the Recent Past	Emergent Themes
Subservience to the discipline of medicine	Growth of nursing as an independent practice
Quasiprofessional status	Movement toward full professional status
Practitioner rewards occurring through effective one-to-one relations with clients	Rewards occurring through advancement of nursing knowledge
Hands-on care and psychomotor tasks as the major domain of nursing	Planning and cognitive tasks as the major domain of nursing
Acceptance of ideal nursing care for each patient as an appropriate goal	Care goals constrained by limited resources and contextual factors

(Stevens BJ: Nursing Theory: Analysis, Application, Evaluation. Boston, Little, Brown and Co, 1984, p 102)

Florence Nightingale (1820–1910)

Nightingale's writings about nursing predated nursing's concern with either theories or concepts identified as such. However, Nightingale's writings show her interest in the concept of environment with attention to the subconcepts of ventilation, warmth, effluvia (smells), noise, and light. Nightingale's ideas relate closely to current scientific theories of adaptation, needs, and stress (Torres, 1980). Nightingale wrote of treating persons rather than disease through providing a better environment. She clearly thought, as history has demonstrated, that hospitals of her time did not generally promote health.

Virginia Henderson (1897–   )

Virginia Henderson's classic book, *The Nature of Nursing* (1966), provided us with a definition of nursing that was translated into many languages. It was also the definition of nursing accepted earlier by the International Council of Nurses (1961). This definition, along with a list of functional abilities she outlined for clients, provided a view of the scope of practice she thought nurses could initiate and control.

> The unique function of the nurse is to assist the individual, sick or well, in the performance of those activities contributing to health or its recovery (or peaceful death) that he could perform unaided if he had the necessary strength, will or knowledge. And to do this in such a way as to help him gain independence as rapidly as possible. (1966, p 15).

The activities, not unlike those performed by many nurses today, include the following:

1   Breathe normally.
2   Eat and drink adequately.
3   Eliminate body wastes.
4   Move and maintain desirable postures.
5   Sleep and rest.
6   Select suitable clothing — dress and undress.
7   Maintain body temperature within normal range by adjusting clothing and modifying the environment.
8   Keep the body clean and well groomed and protect the integument.
9   Avoid dangers in the environment and avoid injuring others.
10   Communicate with others in expressing emotions, needs, fears, or opinions.
11   Worship according to one's faith.
12   Work in such a way that there is a sense of accomplishment.
13   Play or participate in various forms of recreation.

14 Learn, discover, or satisfy the curiosity that leads to normal development and health and the use of the available health facilities.
(Henderson, 1966, pp 16–17)

Henderson was concerned with nurses assisting clients in meeting their personal needs, and her ideas relate closely to Maslow's hierarchy of basic needs. She claimed to have been influenced by Claude Bernard, a physiologist, and Jean Broadhurst, a microbiologist. Within nursing, she cited as influential persons Ida Orlando and Ernestine Weidenbach. Generations of nurses began their basic study of nursing using the classic text *Principles and Practice of Nursing*, written by Bertha Harmer and Virginia Henderson (1955).

Myra E. Levine (1920–   )

Person was a central concept of Levine's model which focused on the holistic individual. Her theory drew from many theories and concepts in various sciences and humanities. As the author of *Introduction to Clinical Nursing* (1973), she was much concerned with the scientific concepts that provided the rationale for nurses' actions with dependent ill persons in acute care settings. She saw adaptation as the process by which the individual changed to meet the internal and external environmental demands. Although the person was dependent in her model, his or her uniqueness and input were as important as the underlying scientific knowledge. Levine (1967) advocated nurse and client participating together, creating a view of nursing as interactions. Her theory is unique for its conservation principles and the use of the word *trophicognosis*.

The four conservation principles are as follows:

1 Nursing intervention is based on the conservation of the individual patient's energy.
2 Nursing intervention is based on the conservation of the individual patient's structural integrity.
3 Nursing intervention is based on the conservation of the individual patient's personal integrity.
4 Nursing intervention is based on the conservation of the individual patient's social integrity. 1967, pp 45–59)

The word *trophicognosis* is of particular interest given the recent emphasis in nursing on *nursing diagnosis*, a term Levine rejected. Trophicognosis was suggested as a new term and an alternative to nursing diagnosis. Trophicognosis described the method used to establish an objective and scientific basis for nursing care and also to implement that care in a specific setting according to established standards. It is appropriate to note that while she rejected the term *nursing diagnosis*, perhaps for semantic and legal reasons, Levine supported the scientific process applied to nursing.

Levine also wrote, "Patient-centered nursing care means individualized nursing care. It is predicated on the reality of common experience: every man is a unique individual, and as such he requires a unique constellation of skills, techniques, and ideas designed specifically for him" (1973, p 23).

Hildegard Peplau (1909–   )

Peplau's major theoretical work was *Interpersonal Relations in Nursing* (1952). Her focus was the therapeutic interpersonal relationship between nurse and patient. The four sequential phases of interpersonal relationship as identified by Peplau were orientation, identification, exploitation, and resolution. They were essentially problem-solving processes paralleling the steps of the nursing process (see Chapter 8) although they preceded delineation of nursing process per se. Prominent psychosocial theories of the time, Harry Stack Sullivan's interpersonal theory and Sigmund Freud's work, undoubtedly influenced her work, which is also consistent with Maslow's emphasis on a hierarchy of needs over a lifetime. Peplau's emphasis on interpersonal process and psychosocial aspects continues to influence nursing today.

Imogene M. King (1923–   )

Her first book, *Toward a Theory for Nursing: General Concepts of Human Behavior* (1971), proposed what the author called a conceptual framework for nursing. Her more recent book is titled *A Theory of Nursing: Systems, Concepts, Process* (1981) and is a derivative of a systems approach. Her writings indicate how theoretical ideas develop over time. She offered an example of how inductive and deductive reasoning shape theory. Using person as a major concept, King included three dynamic interacting systems: individuals, groups, and society. King's description of individual growth and development included thoughts of both Jean Piaget and Erik Erikson. She believed, as do nurses today, that mutual goal setting by nurse and client is a condition of achievement of goals within the nursing process. King's underlying general assumption is, "The focus of nursing is human beings interacting with their environment leading to a state of health for individuals which is an ability to function in social roles" (1981, p 143).

Betty Neuman (19   –   )

Neuman's systems model was first put forth in 1972. Her more recent book is entitled *The Neuman's Systems Model* (1982). One assumption regarding the concept of person is of particular interest: "Though each individual is viewed as unique, he is also a composite of common 'knowns' or characteristics within a normal, given range of response" (1974, p 101). Selye's conceptualization of stress influenced Neuman's model, as did clinical observations in mental health (inductive thinking) and synthesis of scientific knowledge from other disciplines (deductive approach). Neuman's 1982 model speaks specifically to both nursing diagnosis and the client's perception of stressors. Additionally, the model emphasizes variations from wellness. Interestingly, Neuman considered her model applicable to other health-care disciplines.

Martha Rogers (1914–   )

Rogers' conceptual model of nursing was presented first in her 1970 book *An Introduction to the Theoretical Basis of Nursing* and later as "Nursing: A Science of Unitary Man" in J. P. Riehl and C. Roy's *Conceptual Models for Nursing Practice* (1980). In the spirit of Nightingale, she emphasized the knowledge base for nursing and also, in a more universal way, was concerned with the relationship of the man and the environment. Rogers was one of the first nurse theorists to specify man or person as the major focus of nursing concern.

Rogers defined her unitary man as an energy field of four dimensions, showing the influence of Einstein in incorporating the space-time dimension into her model. As Rogers herself stated in her first book:

> Descriptive, explanatory and predictive principles give substance to nursing's conceptual system and make possible knowledgeable nursing practice. Principles derive from the imaginative synthesis of available data. General patterns and regularities characterizing the phenomena under study are identified and provide a means for systematically anticipating future events. (p 95)

In this spirit she put forth her provisional principles of reciprocy, synchrony, helicy, and resonancy, also in her 1970 work.

The first principle, *reciprocy*, assumes "the inseparability of man and environment and predicts that sequential changes in the life process are continuous, probabilistic revisions occurring out of the interactions between man and environment" (p 97). The principle of *synchrony* asserts that "change in the human field depends upon the state of the human field and the simultaneous state of the environmental field at any given point in space-time" (p 98). Often compared to a coiled children's toy, *helicy* is "a function of continuous innovative change growing out of the mutual interaction of man and environment along a spiralling longitudinal axis bound in space-time" (p 101). Finally, Rogers' principle of *resonancy* holds that "change in pattern and organization of the human field and the environmental field is propagated by [energy] waves" (p 101).

Although many students and practitioners are turned off by the unusual terminology and mind-stretching ideas voiced by Rogers, her influence as a prototype of nurse scholar remains strong and other nurses including Newman (1979) and Parse (1981) have developed theories based on her conceptual model. With increasing interest in space travel, parapsychology, and predicting the future, Rogers' ideas seem less foreign today than when they were first expressed.

Dorothea Orem (19 –   )

Orem (1959) is credited with the first explicit use of the term *self-care* in nursing. Interestingly, the impetus for such a model was the education of practical nurses. Nursing intervention was recognized as needed when persons had self-care limitations. Orem believed that self-care was a human requirement for both life maintenance and optimal functioning. The persons who needed the nurse's assistance with self-care were adults with health-related limitations, the young, the aged, the ill, and the disabled. Furthermore, Orem thought that self-care needs could be classified as universal (i.e., like Maslow's basic needs), developmental (i.e., a range of life events and developmental processes), and health deviation needs. Some terms associated with Orem's theory include *therapeutic self-care demand*, the self-care actions necessary to meet requirements for self-care; *self-care agency*, referring to who performs the activity, which may be either nurse or client (ability to nurse is nursing agency); and *self-care deficit*, the discrepancy between the patient's need requirements and patient ability, a discrepancy that must be met by nurse or other care-giver if the client is unable.

A self-care theoretical approach is clearly person centered, consistent with the international definition of nursing, and places increased emphasis on the consumer of health-care services. Orem's approach to nursing process delineates three steps: diagnosing and prescribing or determining agency deficit as listed above, designing and planning what she calls a system of nursing assistance, and producing and managing the systems. A more recent book is *Nursing: Concepts of Practice* (1985).

Sister Callista Roy (1939 –   )

Roy's adaptation model has undergone refinement and revision by the author since its first publication in 1970. She identifies the influence of other nurse theorists including Martha Rogers and Dorothea Orem. Her later text is *Introduction to Nursing: An Adaptation Model* (1984).

The focus of nursing in Roy's model is on the individual as an adaptive system (see Chapter 4). The model can also be applied to family or community and used in a variety of settings. The adaptive behavior involves the whole person, who is seen as having great potential for self-actualization. The person is conceptualized as having two internal subsystem mechanisms for coping with internal and external stimuli. One of these — the "regulator" — works primarily through the autonomic nervous system, while the other — the "cognator" — acts by conscious and unconscious psychosocial means. The environmental stimuli are designated as focal (immediate), contextual (background), and residual (extraneous, unvalidated). The activity of the two subsystem mechanisms is demonstrated by coping behavior in four specific "adaptive modes," that is, physiological needs, self-concepts, role function, and interdependence. The nurse intervenes through nursing process to promote adaptation in these four modes by modifying stimuli as needed.

Jean Watson (1940 –   )

Jean Watson's theoretical work, *Nursing: The Philosophy and Science of Caring* (1979), presents a philosophical orientation that seeks to balance science and humanism. Watson identified the 10 primary carative factors that form a structure for studying and understanding nursing as the science of caring:

1   The formation of a humanistic-altruistic system of values.
2   The instillation of faith-hope.
3   The cultivation of sensitivity to one's self and to others.
4   The development of a helping-trusting relationship.

5   The promotion and acceptance of the expression of positive and negative feelings.
6   The systematic use of the scientific problem-solving method for decision making.
7   The promotion of interpersonal teaching-learning.
8   The provision for a supportive, protective, and/or corrective mental, physical, sociocultural, and spiritual environment.
9   Assistance with the gratification of human needs.
10 The allowance for existential-phenomenological-spiritual forces (1979, p 10).

Regarding what she called a phenomenological orientation to nursing, Watson went on to say the following:

1   It concerns itself with the unique subjective and objective experiences of the individual (or family or group).
2   It adopts a holistic, gestalt attitude toward the understanding of one's self and others.
3   It holds the individuality of the person as its most important concern.
4   It values people because they are inherently good and capable of development.
5   It values the total person context or gestalt as a more important determinant of health-illness care than the patient's bacteria, organic pathogens, or disorders alone. (1979, pp 208–209)

Not surprisingly, Watson considered caring as the moral ideal of nursing. A later book by Watson is *Nursing: Human Science and Human Care: A Theory of Nursing* (1985).

M. M. Leininger (19   –   )

The definitive theoretical works of Leininger include a book, *Transcultural Nursing: Concepts, Theories, and Practices* (1978), and two shorter works, "Caring: A Central Focus of Nursing and Health-care Services" (1980) and "The Phenomenon of Caring: Importance, Research Questions and Theoretical Considerations" (1981). Leininger stated, "One of the reasons I have been pursuing cross-cultural studies on caring behaviors and processes is that scientific knowledge of care is limited; and yet, I hold it is the central concept and essence of nursing" (Watson, 1979, p xii). Caring behaviors as identified by Leininger encompass, but are not limited to, comfort, facilitating, health instruction, protective and restorative behaviors, and support.

Helen Cook Erickson (1936–   )
Evelyn Malcolm Tomlin (1929–   )
Mary Ann Price Swain (1941–   )

The definitive work of these theorists is *Modeling and Role-Modeling—A Theory and Paradigm for Nursing* (1983). They acknowledged synthesizing the work of theorists from other fields: Erik Erikson, Abraham Maslow, Hans Selye, George Engel, and Jean Piaget.

Modeling is the process or means by which the nurse develops an image or understanding of the client's world from his or her frame of reference. Modeling is both art and science and involves the intake and analysis of information about the client and his world. *Role-modeling* is the planning and implementation of nursing interventions uniquely for the client based on his model of the world.

Erickson, Tomlin, and Swain believed that the role of the nurse "is to nurture biophysical, psychosocial, spiritual beings" (1983, p 2).

The final nurse-theorists (Watson, Leininger, and Erickson and colleagues) have perhaps received less attention than those detailed earlier. They typify nurse-scholars' willingness to struggle with humanistic theoretical ideas that may have great potential for nursing as it moves toward the 21st century.

RELATIONSHIP OF THEORY, RESEARCH, AND PRACTICE

Both nursing science and nursing practice need theory and research. To *theorize* is to conjecture or construct the framework of a discipline or science. And theory systematically shows specific interrelationships for the purpose of describing, explaining, predicting, or controlling nursing practice.

Similarly, to *research* is to search into or to investigate thoroughly. Nursing practice and nursing research advance the discipline or science of nursing by shaping the theory. Conversely, the theory, knowledge, and research advance the quality of care and its delivery. As Chinn and Jacobs wrote, "There are two major approaches to interrelationships between practice and theory: how nursing practice contributes to the process of theory development and how theory contributes to nursing practice" (1987, p 169).

Nursing research links **nursing theory** to practice in various ways. Sometimes theories give rise to hypotheses (hunches) that can be tested through research (experiments) in practice. Depending on whether the hunches are supported in the real world of practice, the theory is strengthened or weakened. A theory describes or explains a phenomenon, and research aims to test the description or explanation in either a simulated or natural setting. Or, a theory predicts an outcome and research attempts to demonstrate that prediction as true.

Sometimes notions generated from practice and tested through research become the concepts that in turn can build theories. As may be obvious, the process of theory development requires many well-coordinated research studies over time.

Many realities cloud the theory-practice relationship. It is partly because nursing is a developing science and profession that the questions about these relationships are so persistent. Theory, because it does not bring immediate answers to practice problems, is often considered impractical if not useless. Also, the reflective thinking of theory is often at odds with the "doing" activities of nursing practice.

But many nurses, if they reflect thoughtfully on their practice activities, will recognize the kind of observations that are important to theory — that is, how do their patients respond similarly and differently to both health situations and nursing interventions. Concepts that come from practice are the mental images that become the building blocks of theory. This working inductively — that is, from specifics to generalities provides a way to generate theory from practice (see the aggregation discussion in Chapter 8). Unfortunately, although trained to be careful observers, nurses often do not take the reflection and thinking time necessary to organize and synthesize their observations beyond individual care situations.

The term *grounded theory* has been used to identify one such type of theory created inductively from systematic observation, analysis, and synthesis. In a famous study using this approach, Barney Glaser and Anselm Strauss (1966) studied dying patients and related personnel to understand their shared reactions. The importance of their study was the light it shed on death as a reality that health-care workers must accept.

Rather than create theory themselves, most nurses are concerned with how others' theories assist their practice. Because nurses desire to improve practice and recognize that theory contributes to this end, they are tempted to make immediate application and expect immediate results. Reality demands considerable caution. Again, research is a necessary intervening step to test possible applications to practice before implementing them full scale.

Theories suggest general guidelines and possible outcomes. Research demonstrates how more-specific guidelines actually fare in particular test situations. A particular conceptual framework or nursing theory used for research will guide the nature of the problems and how they are studied. For example, using Orem's conceptual model, Denyes (1982) created a tool to measure adolescents' ability to care for self (Orem's self-care agency). The Roy Adaptation Model has also proven useful in guiding nursing research: Fawcett (1981) used the adaptive modes of the Roy Adaptation Model to classify survey data measuring fathers' responses to cesarean birth of their children.

In addition, several of the theoretical notions discussed earlier have been applied to a wide variety of practice situations. A few brief examples follow: Backsheider (1974) used Orem's model in a diabetic management clinic, Galligan (1979) described use of Roy's concept of adaptation to care for young children, and Utz (1980) wrote of applying the Neuman model to nursing practice with persons with elevated blood pressure.

As indicated earlier, nursing has borrowed many of its theories and its research methods from other disciplines. Furthermore, theory development and nursing research are often associated more closely with academic nursing than practice. Too often, the networking that could link theory, research, and practice does not exist. Perhaps in the future, nursing's conceptual frameworks will become well-developed theories unique to nursing. Ideally, increasing sophistication in research will yield better methods to measure results of holistic nursing interventions: nursing needs to demonstrate how these interventions, derived from theories, make a difference in the health of persons and have economic value. In 1988, a new refereed journal, *Applied Nursing Research (ANR)*, billed itself as "devoted to uniting the efforts of all professional nurses to advance nursing as a research-based profession." When the theory-research and theory-practice relationships become clearer to all nurses, then theory will move from the realm of textbook discussion and academia into the center of professional nursing activity.

Nursing Research for Scientists and Practitioners

Nursing research is scientific study or investigation about nursing practice. Nursing research provides a purposeful way of seeking answers to questions about the specifics of nursing practice. Individual research studies do not prove or disprove scientific hunches. Multiple studies over time may provide strong evidence to support or refute educated scientific guesses about practice. Nursing research aims to answer both exploratory and complex questions. Exploratory questions concern the nature of nursing concepts (health, person, environment) or events (activities of daily living like sleeping). More-complex questions ask about what will happen if specific nursing actions are practiced.

In this section, readers will find that research in nursing is based on the scientific method common to other scientific fields of study. A brief introduction to the various kinds of nursing research is provided. Also, readers will learn that although research is a relatively new activity for nurses, it is of rapidly increasing importance for nursing education, science development, and practice.

A decade ago, nursing research conferences were unusual. Today, they are commonplace in both schools of nursing and practice settings. The ANA and Sigma Theta Tau International, the nursing honor society, have become moving forces behind both nursing scholarship and research. But nursing research concerns not just nursing scholars. Increasingly, nurses of all educational backgrounds and clinical specialties must see the political necessity of elevating nursing research to a priority of the profession. An important mandate regarding nursing research is clear: without an adequate research foundation, the unique knowledge of nursing science cannot be identified and developed. Because nursing is also a developing profession, it needs scientific research to further its growth as a profession. Without research, nursing will not maximize its scientific, professional, or social potential.

Development and enhancement of the profession of nursing is realized through knowledge acquisition. As Polit and Hungler (1985) wrote,

> The scientific approach is the most advanced method of acquiring knowledge that humans have developed. The scientific method incorporates several procedures and characteristics to create a system of obtaining knowledge that, though not infallible, is generally more reliable than alternative problem-solving approaches. (p 5)

Scientific Method

The format of the **scientific method** is much the same whether used in physics, psychology, medicine, or nursing. The scientific method is the most advanced approach to acquiring knowledge, but it has limitations. It cannot answer ethical or value questions. Neither can the scientific method overcome current inabilities to measure some of the concepts of interest to nurses. Furthermore, applying the scientific method in the real world of health care is much more difficult than in the confines of the laboratory.

The scientific method can also be purposefully used in both everyday and research situations to find an answer to a problem or perplexing question. The steps of the scientific method, which will be considered individually, include

- Define the problem.
- Collect data from observation and experimentation.
- Devise and execute a solution.
- Evaluate the solution.

Define the Problem

A basic but sometimes forgotten principle is that if you intend to solve or investigate a problem, you must know what the problem is. As described by de Bono (1970), a *problem* is the difference between the existing situation and a more ideal situation. Most problems are complex or multidimensional. Therefore, a general problem area may contain several related questions. Problems are often phrased in the form of *what* and *how* questions, but other words like *who, when, where,* and *why* may also be appropriate. Questions asked this way, rather than in a way that anticipates a yes or no answer, lend themselves to exploring alternative solutions, an important element of the scientific method.

Because beneath their individual differences people are alike in many ways, it is also possible to identify problems that apply to people collectively. This generalizability is the rationale for applying the scientific method to research, that is, being able to identify so-called researchable problems or problems that are of potential interest to large groups of people. For example, a general problem area of interest to both nurses and physicians may be that of how the risk of heart attack can be minimized for apparently healthy persons. Depending on the scientific and professional background and also the hunches of the investigator, a variety of more specific problems (e.g., related to medication, diet, or exercise) might be identified.

Collect Data from Observation and Experimentation

Experts in any scientific field are distinguished by their ability to use decision-making processes based on scientific principles. There is a large body of scientific knowledge about normal human functioning in all areas previously mentioned (i.e., biological or physiological, psychological or intrapersonal and interpersonal). In health care, identifying problems of deviant function involves comparison with what a healthy or "normal" person should be able to do. The health-care professional compares the information (data) received from the person to known standards or norms. Because persons are so complex, this task requires comparison with many normalcy standards. The definition of normal itself changes over time as scientific knowledge is added to a discipline: for example, information about what changes to expect in physiological function with age. A full health history, physical examination, and laboratory tests, as well as an in-depth interview about how the person sees his or her current life situation, may yield valuable information to clarify the problem further. Such "experiments" as controlled tests of heart function may furnish additional information for comparison with normal expected values for persons of similar age, sex, and so on.

For a particular situation, information (data), problems, and solutions may seem confusingly interwoven. Indeed, a certain amount of data collection precedes being able even to identify a general problem. Also, although we often diagram the scientific method in stepwise fashion, the process is less straightforward and more circular than usually imagined.

Devise and Execute a Solution

The solution or potential solution of a problem will depend on the specific problem identified. Executing a solution is a process of selecting from among the alternatives those that seem likely to lead to a desired goal. Consider the problem and goal as two points and imagine a large number of paths linking them. Alternative courses of action provide paths or bridges between problems and goals. Considering alternative solutions forces choices among options. Problem statements that are too broad or too narrow can interfere with the discovery of alternative solutions. It is rare that a problem has only one solution. Some solutions, of course, will be more likely, less costly, and easier to execute than others. In research terms, alternative solutions are sometimes called scientific hunches or, more technically, hypotheses to be tested.

Evaluate the Solution

The scientific method does not guarantee the results of a problem-solving solution. Evaluation, although appearing to be a final step in the scientific method, is really a point in a circular process. Evaluation requires judging outcomes against specific criteria to determine the effectiveness of actions. Essentially, outcomes result from executing a problem solution. To be successful, an outcome must be a resolution, an alleviation, or a prevention of the original problem. This reality is both a reason for stating problems precisely and also evidence of the circularity of the process. Evaluation challenges the problem solver to move on to new problems or to readdress old ones.

Where Do Research Problems Come From?

A common question about nursing research is where do the problems investigated in research originate? A previous discussion indicated that nursing practice and nursing theory generate problems for scientific investigation. As one head nurse in a busy acute care hospital put it, "Reality, i.e., practice, must drive both research and theory." To use these sources most effectively requires readiness to reflect on practice. Curious professionals also scour the nursing periodical literature to learn what others are thinking and doing. Perhaps the most important source of problems is less obvious: problems come also from the mind or imagination of the nurse-researcher. The tendency is to minimize this source when we think of problems as coming from practice or theory. Problems do not materialize out of thin air. Whether they originate from theory or from practice, they are shaped in the mind of the practitioner-researcher.

Problems are the difference between the ideal and the real, and someone must identify them as such. Dumas (1963) made such an identification in a pioneering nursing study about the effect of nursing on postoperative vomiting. She envisioned the ideal as no postoperative vomiting for her patients, but observed the reality to be frequent postoperative vomiting. In a controlled experiment, she intervened with some patients and found that her intervention decreased the incidence of postoperative vomiting. This study, based on Orlando's theory of interaction, illustrates that a research problem can be based on an abstract theory, made concrete for study, and yield results that can be generalized to a broad population for some practical application.

Since Dumas' early clinical study, research has repeatedly demonstrated that nursing can make significant differences in both mortality and quality of life. In September 1981, before a national health policy audience (the American Academy of Nursing meeting in Washington, DC), Fagin eloquently summarized many research examples of nursing effectiveness when she presented a paper entitled "Nursing's Pivotal Role in Achieving Competition in Health Care." Unfortunately, such information often escapes widespread professional or public awareness. Lack of broad communication about significant nursing research results is a weak link in nursing's research chain.

Increasingly and fortunately, individual nursing studies are finding their way into national journals. A landmark study demonstrating nursing's economic value was published in the *New England Journal of Medicine* by Brooten and colleagues in 1986. The study also made news in *The Wall Street Journal* and *The New York Times*. Nursing assessment and care by nurse-specialists enabled premature infants to be discharged safely to home care, saving a single hospital hundreds of thousands of dollars yearly. Similar early discharge programs are being tried in other health-care centers and with other populations, for example, elderly patients.

The particular problems chosen for nursing investigation will determine how the problems are best studied and also will suggest the appropriate research methods to be used. Just as there is no one "best" theory of nursing, there is no one correct way to research all nursing problems. An important and ultimate aim of research in nursing is to enable clinical practitioners to improve care by being able to predict the patient outcomes of intervention (what will happen if _____?) and thereby develop prescriptions to achieve goals (how can I make _____ happen?).

The variety of research approaches used in nursing parallels those used in other sciences. Four research approaches are mentioned briefly as a point of departure for further exploration. For detailed discussion of research methods, the reader is referred to such texts as Polit and Hungler's *Essentials of Nursing Research: Methods and Applications*.

Research Approaches

Nonexperimental Research

Nonexperimental research is often labeled ex post facto (after the fact) or descriptive. Descriptive theory and research in nursing also contribute important and necessary foundations for advanced research and theory development.

Experimental Research

Experimental nursing research, that is, true experiments with random selection of subjects to differing care, is often difficult to carry out in real-life situations and in hospital settings. Nurses and health-care administrators must weigh economic and ethical considerations in doing such experiments. Additionally, nurses must be able to control the experimental conditions. Because of these real difficulties, many nursing studies have been studies about nurses rather than about nursing, or they were nonexperimental. In recent years, the nursing profession has given the highest priority to studies that are central to clinical practice, be they experimental or nonexperimental. Such studies clarify the effectiveness of specific nursing interventions, show the impact of nursing care on certain health problems and illnesses, or indicate the appropriate environment for effective nursing practice methods. Well-educated nurses are confident about how to study the phenomena that interest them.

Qualitative Research

A basic principle of research is that the nature of the problem will dictate the nature of the investigation needed to answer the research question. Much scientific research uses quantitative analysis, that is, processing of numerical data for the purpose of describing phenomena and inferring relationships among them. With recent interest in humanistic nursing by such theorists as Watson and Leininger, it seems likely that qualitative research will increase in nursing. A qualitative approach organizes narrative or words to discover themes and also relationships among concepts in a nonnumerical way. Examples of such qualitative research strategies may have names like human sciences research or phenomenological approach.

An example of a qualitative study using a human science approach is Boodley's 1986 dissertation, "A Nursing Study of the Experience of Having a Health Examination." She sought to discover the meaning a person attaches to the health examination experience. Her rationale for this interest was quite simple:

> The health examination is probably the most frequent reason for a layperson's contact with the health-care system. Many basic expectations about how the health-care system functions and the person's role within it come from the experience of having a health examination. If nurses hope to understand more about the context for nursing practice they must begin with an understanding of the meanings clients find in this common health-care experience. (1986, p 5)

Interestingly, such a research focus is consistent with "person" as a major theoretical concept. Swanson and Chenitz (1982) reminded us that the monumental scientific works of such scientists as Darwin and Einstein came not from counting but from observing.

Certainly, this fact gives us reason to be open to a variety of research approaches for nursing.

Historical Research

Another very different research method is worthy of consideration before we begin the section on nursing as a profession. It is historical research, which also may be called the literary or critical approach. This approach is a past-oriented research method seeking to illuminate a current question by an intensive study of material which already exists. In the historical approach, the researcher uses original or primary data whenever possible. Most data are gathered from actual historical documents. You may be familiar with the Kalisches' research on the image of nurses in the media. The Kalisches used a clipping service to gather articles from newspapers to ascertain nurse image at particular times. Their writings include such titles as "When Nurses Were National Heroines: Images of Nursing in American Film, 1942–1945" (1981), and "How the Public Sees Nurse-midwives: 1978 News Coverage of Nurse-Midwifery in the Nation's Press' (1980).

In many ways, the image of the nurse has changed immensely since Nightingale's time. A place now exists in nursing for professionals who want to be researchers and scientists studying health and people's adaptation to changes in their health. True, nurses have long been data collectors for physicians doing medical research. The emphasis in this section, however, has been on nurses doing nursing research. Nurses also work with physicians and other health-care professionals to do collaborative research. Increasingly, government and private funding agencies are looking for evidence that health-care professionals are working together to solve priority health-care problems.

Nursing Research Comes of Age

Nursing is just coming into its own in developing both its scientific base and research visibility. You may have heard of the National Institutes of Health (NIH), which is largely concerned with disease. It was not until 1986 that nursing found a home in the established research halls of NIH. This development occurred when the National Center for Nursing Research was created by a congressional override of a presidential veto. To have key legislators speak to the value of nursing research was a major victory for nursing. It seems only logical that nurses should have such a visible national center; they are, after all, the nation's largest group of health-care professionals.

Ensuring funding for nursing research is an important beginning and supports the work of nurse scientists. The next step is to bring nursing research and nursing practice closer together so that nursing research becomes a reality for practitioners. Pioneering work in this area was done by Horsley and colleagues in the 1970s and reported as *Using Research to Improve Nursing Practice: A Guide* (1983). Horsley emphasized the importance of working from a conceptual base and identifying particular clinical problems from which would come specific innovations that could be clinically evaluated. This model clearly followed the steps of the scientific method. Progress, however, comes slowly. In the mid-1980s, Butler (1987) investigated how innovations actually get used or ignored in nursing service organizations.

While research may still seem mysterious, it is learnable and exciting to those who participate. Research progress in nursing has been slower than many nurses would like, but advances in the last decade have been quite dramatic. Nurses who enter the profession

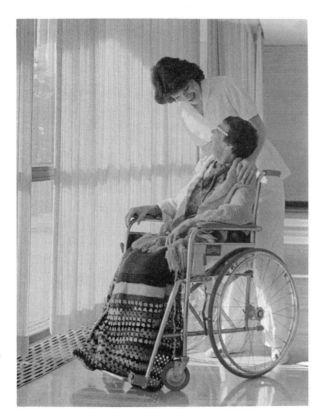

Nursing is caring across the life span.

today should anticipate that they will encounter many research opportunities to enrich their careers. When nursing research becomes a usual and ordinary professional activity, rather than an extraordinary event, nursing will have come of age as a science.

| NURSING AS A PROFESSION

The criteria for professions and the brief historical perspective of nursing's development presented earlier can help us understand modern nursing and its relation to other professions and society at large. We might conclude the following about nursing as a profession:

1   Nursing has a briefer professional history than the traditional professions of law, medicine, and theology.
2   Nursing has been and continues to be primarily a woman's occupation.
3   Nursing's ranking on the criteria commonly used for professions is the subject of considerable debate.

This final point argues for the individual growth and activities of nurses as crucial to the continuing professionalization of nursing. Current and aspiring nurses who are the present and future nurse leaders will need to be the ones who provide, preserve, and develop today's nursing for tomorrow.

Problems Common to Nursing and Other Professions

If nurses are to control the service they provide to society, some current problems and issues will need to be addressed vigorously by nurses. In general, the problems faced by nurses and other professionals originate from the characteristics of professional occupations (as discussed previously). These qualities include autonomy and independent decision making, career commitment, collegial relationships, and professional worth or rewards. Issues, in contrast to problems, are larger questions for which no consensus exists about a right answer. Issues, therefore, are questions not easily answered with a simple yes or no.

Contemporary Nursing Issues

Control of Nursing Practice

One of the largest issues facing nursing is that of who shall control nursing practice. Control is a primary issue determining whether nursing will continue its professionalization toward independence and autonomy. Forces both within and outside nursing challenge the obvious answer that nursing should control its own practice. For example, medicine and health services administration would gain much from controlling nursing, and some nurses are unwilling to assume this responsibility. If nurses do not assume control of nursing, all issues related to future practice will be decided by whatever group does control it.

Control of nursing practice has led to controversy about the so-called extended and expanded roles for nurses. A *role* is a pattern of behavior associated with a distinctive social position. An *extended role* is a role lengthened in a unilateral manner. For example, the role of the physician is extended through the use of another health worker. In this case, the authority base for extension is from the physician. *Role expansion* is a multidirectional spreading out. For example, an expanded role for the nurse may involve some extension into the physician's role, but this is a lesser part of the expansion. The authority base of expansion is primarily nursing knowledge and clinical expertise.

The boundaries among medicine, nursing, and other health professions will be altered as sciences develop and practices change. Boundaries will also be affected by a surplus of some health-care professionals (MDs) and a scarcity of others (RNs). Roles in particular practice areas may be especially affected, for example, anesthesiologists (MDs) and nurse anesthetists (RNs), or obstetricians (MDs) and nurse-midwives (RNs). The issues may be ones not only of professional control but also of consumer preference for certain health-care choices. It may be to nursing's advantage that its professional care better fits both client pocketbooks and consumer priorities.

Relationship of "Control" to Other Issues. Other important issues will continue to affect nursing as a developing profession. They are the following:

1 What services should nurses provide?
2 How should nurses be educated?
3 How should nurses receive payment for their services?
4 What should be the influence of organized nursing on American health-care policy?

If nursing demands its autonomy and retains control, then nurses, with their clients and society, will decide these issues together. Answers to the above questions, in turn, will influence organized nursing's impact on even larger national and international health policy issues. Many issues are more intertwined than they may appear to be on first inspection.

What Services Should Nurses Provide?

Those who contend that nursing is moving toward professionalization would argue the following principle: the profession, with help from the society it serves, should decide what services to offer. Other considerations are listed below.

First, we must recognize that the health-care needs of society are changing because of changes in the nature of the population, technological advances, disease patterns, and life-styles. This reality affects or should affect the way health-care services are organized and delivered and also the scope of practice of various health-care professions, including nursing (ANA, 1979, p 8).

Second, health is an umbrella concept covering services of many professional and technical health-care providers. Health care is not solely medical care. Many health-care problems, especially chronic conditions, require other than medical management. The number of persons who require supportive nursing services to adapt to the lengthening life span will continue to increase greatly.

Third, nurses need to make known the nature of the service they are able to deliver. Both the recipients of nursing care and other health-care professionals need this information. The authority for professional nursing practice legitimately comes from the skill and knowledge of the nurse provider.

How Should Nurses Be Educated?

Differences in education now undermine unity and development of the profession. Although the baccalaureate degree is advocated as the preferred professional preparation, associate degree programs prepare approximately half the graduating RNs.

Two interesting points have been made about the preparation for the inevitable increase in health-care technology. One is that as technology in health care increases, more — not less — humanistic nursing is needed. The other point is that technological development may mandate that bioengineering technicians, rather than nurses, monitor equipment. Currently, some people believe that baccalaureate programs do not place enough emphasis on technical skills. Others believe that BSN programs continue to place too much emphasis on technical skills. Although many employers do not differentiate among RNs in the workplace, baccalaureate graduates should seek employment that will use their skills fully and compensate them for their additional preparation. Of course, nurses who have undergone a more expensive education should offer something obviously different and important.

Although there is a shift in education to the graduate level for other health-care disciplines, only a small percentage of RNs are prepared with either master's degrees or doctorates. A need exists for master's-prepared nurses as clinicians, administrators, educators, and researchers. Doctorally prepared nurses are needed as leaders in all nursing areas. If one assumes that each facility in which nursing care is provided would benefit from having doctorally prepared nurses to stimulate research and practice, the shortage becomes apparent. Imagine a hospital or health-care agency with only one medical doctor! It will be increasingly difficult for nurses to be peers with other health professionals who are educated beyond them.

These issues present both challenges and opportunities. Therefore, it is important to consider the educational opportunities and requirements for future nurses (see Changing Images, below).

How Should Nurses Receive Payment for Their Services?

The whole health-care payment scheme has changed in recent years. Retrospective reimbursement or governmental payment of actual cost after the fact is now becoming prospective prepayment. Such prepayment for hospitals and physicians is limited to "reasonable" cost based on averages because health-care cost containment has become a critical national economic issue. Most nurses are hospital employees and will continue to be so. Increasingly, nurses employed by hospitals are entering into negotiated contracts with their hospital employers. The state professional organization, a branch of the ANA, may serve as a local bargaining agent.

Salaries for entering nurses are competitive with those in other service occupations. Because nursing provides around-the-clock service, shift differential wages usually prevail. And few other health or social service fields offer comparable earning power while pursuing advanced career preparation. Although differences in basic education may not affect initial earning power, advancement to better-paying positions favors those persons with advanced degrees. These persons will assume leadership positions of increased responsibility in specialized practice, management and administration, teaching, and research. Although salary increases over time are somewhat compressed in nursing, there are other economic compensations: expanding job markets, especially in advanced positions; favorable conditions of supply and demand at all levels; and long-range job security. Some nurse-administrators in large organizations make salaries in the six-digit range.

Opportunities for nurses as health-care entrepreneurs are increasing daily. A detailed discussion of creative practice options in unlimited settings as well as opportunities for being a health-care entrepreneur is found in Chapter 12.

Clearly, some of the rewards for service are not monetary. As one colleague wrote, "Aren't we truly blessed in being able to contribute to others and our profession through our knowledge and experience?"

What Will Be the Influence of Nursing on Health-Care Policy?

Despite the many issues facing the profession and the occasional lack of organized nurse power, nursing is beginning to value equally the caring and scientific components of the profession. Nurses are recapturing the autonomy and independence that many of our nursing ancestors had. We are learning to put forth a nursing model of health care so that we will be viewed as colleagues of other health professionals rather than as extensions of them. We could learn much about influence from some of our nurse predecessors: Florence Nightingale, Margaret Sanger, and Lillian Wald did not sidestep the issues of their day as they intervened to halt the miseries of the battlefield, unwanted pregnancies, and urban poverty. They neither always agree with nursing or medical colleagues nor found support from them. They persevered because they believed they were right about the essence, nature, and value of nursing service to society.

We need to remember that nursing is not the only profession with problems of confusion about unique services, educational preparation, and payment for services. Medicine is oversupplied in certain specialties; increasingly, physicians are being salaried rather than receiving unrestricted fees for professional services. Dentists, once in great demand, are finding society has greatly diminished needs for traditional dental services. Nurses should also remember that issues and crises can be growth producing. Nursing is growing as a profession and its practitioners can grow as professional persons. From this perspective, many professional issues can be understood better as having maturational and situational aspects, as do other crises. Optimistically, nurses are taking the best of nursing art and melding it with scientific nursing to create a better health-care future.

| CHANGING IMAGES

National Need

Need for professional nurses exceeds supply in all geographic and specialty areas. The need is particularly great in acute care settings. Nurses are the largest health-care personnel category partly because they provide around-the-clock coverage. Because of the sharp enrollment declines in nursing schools in the mid-1980s, a national shortage will continue for years to come. Additionally, the demand for intensive care nurses at all stages of the life cycle is growing. For example, premature neonates, who only a few years ago would not have survived, need one-to-one around-the-clock intensive care. Frail elderly, who might not previously have survived a medical crisis, may now be candidates for major surgical intervention and postsurgical nursing care in the hospital or home.

Because most nurses are white and female, there is a great need for minority persons and men, in nursing. Job availability, security, and mobility—which have attracted men and minorities in the past—continue to be attractions.

Basic educational programs in nursing prepare nurses for generalist, entry-level staff nurse positions. After graduation from state-approved schools, nurses take a state licensing examination before receiving recognition as RNs. All RNs are expected to have certain basic skill competencies. Increasingly, hospitals recognize the gap between the best of educational preparations and the demands of nursing in the real world. It is in the best interest of hospitals to bridge this gap, which they do with extensive orientation programs. Many nursing schools and service settings provide internships or opportunities to work as nursing assistants while completing basic programs. In addition to increasing competency, these opportunities provide wages while learning. Until recently, experience as a general staff nurse usually preceded assignment to a specialty area. Indeed, the changing image of nursing is well reflected in the growing number of areas for specialty practice and nontraditional career options.

Specialty Areas of Practice

The specialty areas of practice for nursing are of two basic kinds: clinical specialty and functional specialty. The former parallels the increasing specialization that has occurred in medicine and other components of the health-care delivery system. There are nurse specialists for the following specialties:

1 Age groups—that is, pediatric, adult, and geriatric
2 Illnesses—for example, coronary disease, diabetes, cancer
3 Abilities or disabilities—for example, midwives, sexuality, burns, rehabilitation
4 Locales—for example, ambulatory care units, operating room, emergency room or trauma center, home-care coordinator, and community health

Some specialists in clinical areas are certified. Certification may be public within state licensure or private, that is, voluntary, such as through professional organizations.

Functional specialty refers to the following activities: clinical practice, as described above; management or administration; research; and teaching. All clinical specialty areas offer opportunities for nurses to combine a clinical specialty with a functional one. In fact, in recent years the trend has been to consolidate positions so that to practice solely as a clinical nurse-specialist without taking on functional responsibility (e.g., as a coordinator for staff or patient education) is unusual.

Traditional and Nontraditional Career Options

Traditional **career options** exist in acute care settings and community health and parallel the traditional medical specialty areas: medical and surgical nursing, obstetrical and pediatric nursing, psychiatric mental health nursing, operating room, and others as indicated earlier.

Several trends related to practice options are listed below:

- More practice options are available and possible than ever before.
- The trend is toward more advanced preparation [i.e., Bachelor of Science in Nursing (BSN) or Master of Science in Nursing (MSN)].
- External barriers (traditions and legalities) to practice options are presently decreasing but have the potential to go either way.
- Increasing attempts are being made at collaborative practice among health professionals.
- The increasing movement toward community and home health care provides tremendous potential for autonomous practice.
- There is increasing emphasis on wellness programs in schools, residential living communities, and industry.

Several commonly confused labels relate to practice options. The following are definitions that may be useful in understanding some common practice options.

Nurse-practitioner is defined in some states as any nurse who renders service to a recipient. This term is also used to refer to an ambulatory care nurse with advanced skills in assessment of the physical and psychosocial health and illness statuses of persons in a variety of settings, through health and development interviews and physical examination. In addition, the term may be used to describe a nurse functioning in an expanded role, such as a pediatric nurse practitioner. Nurse practitioner will probably be a general title describing the nurse of tomorrow, for whom the now-special practitioner skills will become commonplace.

A *clinical nurse specialist* is an expert in a particular practice, such as psychiatric mental health or medical-surgical nursing. This person gives direct and expert nursing care, models expert behavior for other nurses, and serves as a consultant or coordinator for persons needing nursing care in the area of specialty. This nurse usually has a master's degree and may have clinical nursing research skills, which are used directly or offered in consultation with other practicing nurses.

A *physician's assistant* (PA) is a dependent health worker who is selected by a physician and administratively reports to the physician. This position is an example of what was earlier described as role extension. The authority for this role comes from the physician, which is why the PA is a dependent worker. Under direction of an MD, this person is capable of performing routine functions now usually performed by physicians, for example, physical and diagnostic examinations and treatment of common diseases. Many of the first

PAs were military corpsmen. It is not uncommon for physicians employing PAs to increase their practice size and income with relatively little cost to the physician.

The *Nurse clinician* was first described by Reiter in 1966. This specialist was denoted primarily as a bedside or direct-care expert with an area of specialty and, possibly, advanced preparation. Today, nurses designated as clinicians are usually baccalaureate prepared. In many large health-care centers, a clinical ladder of advancement provides a meaningful reward to expert nurses remaining in direct patient care. A nurse wishing to be identified as a clinician may present a specific proposal or petition to be so designated and recognized. The request is acted on by a peer review board.

Nurse-midwife, although recently more publicized as a practice role, has been in existence for much longer than other practitioner roles: the first midwifery school opened in 1931. The American nurse-midwife, although professionally licensed, functions within a physician-directed health service and is not considered an independent practitioner.

The *nurse anesthetist* usually functions under direct or indirect supervision of an anesthesiologist (medical specialist) whenever anesthesia is given. Preparation includes about 2 years in a school of anesthesia, which may or may not give credit toward an advanced degree.

A new practice option called *case manager* or *clinical manager* is coming to prominence. In many health-care settings, this role is seen as the domain of nurses. "Nursing Case Management" (ANA Pub. No. NS-32) describes a health-care delivery process whose goals are to provide quality health care, decrease fragmentation, enhance the clients' quality of life and contain costs ("Nursing Case Management," 1988, p 5). Some might argue that nursing case management has long been a general function of nurses. But new emphasis on cost containment compels even greater care efficiency. Nurses may hesitate to choose these roles out of concern that management efficiency will erode clinical nursing care. If nurses do not assume case management, however, others will do it in the name of efficiency. Nurses should view this reality as an opportunity to exert control over nursing practice, influence health-care policy, and demonstrate both efficiency and effectiveness of nursing care. Master's-prepared nurses with advanced clinical and management skills may be ideally suited to this role.

Future of Practice Options

Nurses themselves must take the leadership role in deciding what part of health care is nursing and then follow through to control that nursing care as illustrated earlier. Given the size of the health-care industry, this leadership must come not just from nurses prepared in graduate programs, with master's and doctoral degrees, but from baccalaureate graduates as well. Never before have more practice options existed for beginning nurses, especially those prepared at the baccalaureate level.

Although some employers do not differentiate among associate degree, diploma, and baccalaureate graduates, nurses need to find or generate job opportunities that allow them to practice as prepared and to grow to their full potential. Many students begin to explore practice options through part-time employment as a nurse assistant during their formal education. The realities of the workplace look different from the student and the employee perspectives. The opportunity to observe how a variety of nurses practice in different ways can be most instructive.

Nursing's Independent, Interdependent, and Dependent Functions

Nursing has independent, interdependent, and dependent functions. Remember that health care is medical and nursing care. Medicine and nursing are separate but not always distinctly so. Traditionally, nursing has assumed a subordinate position in health care and has performed functions auxiliary to medicine. The current image of the professional nurse, as advanced by nurse leaders, is that of a baccalaureate graduate who is an independent career colleague of the physician.

Function is the kind of action or activity proper to a person. To describe someone's function, we would note the person's behavior. Let us look at what characterizes independent, interdependent, and dependent behavior in nursing.

Independent nursing behavior is initiated as a result of the nurse's own knowledge and skills, rather than as a result of delegated authority from the physician. Although some nurses may practice independently, it is not the norm for practice options. Even if most nurses do not believe that independent practice is currently feasible or something they want to do, they may be interested in independent behavior.

Mundinger preferred the term *autonomous* nursing practice to *independent* nursing practice. She believed that although nursing may encompass some physician-directed activities, both nursing theory components and unique nursing practice will be involved. Mundinger differentiated autonomous function from dependent function in the following way.

> Knowing why, when, and how to position clients and doing so skillfully makes the function an autonomous therapy. But, if physicians order it, how can it be autonomous? If physicians order an action nurses would not do in the absence of those orders, if they do not know why or when to do so, it is probably a dependent rather than autonomous function. But if the nurse has the knowledge and the skill to initiate and carry out the actions and answer for the results, then it is autonomous. (1980, p 4).

If nursing is a profession, most of the practice should consist of independent functions!

Interdependent nursing behavior designates overlapping functions shared between nursing and medicine, and speaks to the desirability of collegial relationships in which each profession contributes according to its knowledge, skills, and focus. Overlapping gray areas may occur, especially in critical care units and primary care centers. Often, activities seem more independent only because they are more like physician behavior, such as monitoring complex equipment or ordering diagnostic tests. However, strict regulations or prior agreements about steps to be taken in special circumstances may leave little room for autonomous decision making.

Dependent nursing behavior is performed under delegated medical authority or supervision or according to a priori routines. Routine administration of prescription medications might be an example of a dependent nursing behavior. Much of traditional nursing activity has been giving care or doing treatments according to the dictates of physicians' or doctors' order book.

Nursing as a profession has only recently begun to assert its autonomy. This fact means nursing must find ways to expand practice options to accommodate independent behavior of students now being prepared. Ways to function within the hospital setting without loss of professional identity and the desire for independent behavior should be researched more vigorously by the profession. At any time, some 75% of nurses are hospital employed. Nurses generally do practice in acute care settings on graduation, because of job availability and also to obtain valuable experience.

Educational Opportunities and Requirements

Just as aspiring nurses should know about practice options, they should also know about the educational opportunities and requirements in nursing. Nursing is one of the few fields where such a range of formal programs educate practitioners who have the same legal registration, that is, RN. In the past, the opportunity to enter licensed practice in nursing has been available to persons with little if any formal education beyond high school. Such programs preparing licensed practical or vocational nurses, however, are being phased out or increased to 2-year programs.

Currently, the minimal educational preparation for RN licensure is 2 years of college study culminating in an associate degree. Such programs are widely available in community or junior colleges. Associate degree programs in nursing may also be available in colleges and universities offering the baccalaureate degree. A widespread move is underway to require the baccalaureate degree for eligibility to receive professional licensure in the future. With this move has come a clear intent to "grandfather in" persons who do not have this educational preparation but who were already practicing as RNs prior to the change, which would mean that whenever such legislation might go into effect, all those persons previously prepared for this level of licensure with lesser education will be accepted as "professional" by grandfathering. A similar grandfathering provision has been made for persons who practiced a clinical specialty before the introduction of specialty certification requirements.

Diploma or hospital schools once offered the most common programs to prepare nurses for RN licensure. Today, most nurses are being prepared with associate degrees in institutions of higher education offering regular college credit. For those persons who are academically qualified and economically able, initial enrollment in a college or university program leading to the baccalaureate degree with a nursing major (B.S.N.) is highly recommended. Other so-called generic baccalaureate programs may offer the Bachelor of Science (B.S.) or Bachelor of Arts (B.A.). Undergraduate programs also exist that enable persons who are already RNs to complete the baccalaureate in nursing through curricula with such names as RN studies or RN completion programs. Because nursing as a profession values mature practitioners, increasing numbers of universities are offering the first professional degree at the graduate level. These programs enroll persons who are not RNs but who already hold an undergraduate degree in another field.

A variety of educational opportunities are available beyond baccalaureate preparation in nursing. They usually require 1 or 2 additional years of full-time study (or equivalent) for completion of a master's degree.

Nurses who intend to advance significantly in clinical nursing are expected to receive advanced educational preparation in clinical nursing as opposed to some other functional specialty, for example, business administration. The purpose of master's degree education in nursing is to prepare nursing leaders for advanced clinical practice, teaching, and administrative positions. Nurses obtain degrees that are basically of two kinds: professional and academic. The professional degree, often the Master of Nursing (M.N.), may require fewer credits and tends not to have a research emphasis. Academic degrees are commonly the Master of Science (M.S.) or Master of Arts (M.A.). These graduate degrees usually take 1 to 2 years of full-time study (or equivalent) and have a research emphasis, possibly requiring a formal project or thesis. Although full-time study may be educationally preferable, most nurses have multiple responsibilities and find part-time study necessary.

Nurses who expect to do independent research or teach in colleges offering graduate degrees should expect to be doctorally prepared. The Doctor of Philosophy (Ph.D.) is the most common academic doctoral degree in nursing. Doctoral education emphasizes theory development and research skill. Doctoral programs in nursing have recently added postdoc-toral fellowship programs that are comparable to those available in other sciences. An additional variety of educational opportunities are available at the doctoral level. Some common graduate professional degrees earned by nurses include the Doctor of Nursing Science (D.N.S.), Doctor of Nursing (D.N.), or in other fields such degrees as the Juris Doctor (J.D.), Doctor of Education (Ed.D.), or Doctor of Public Health (D.P.H.).

Perhaps most exciting and significant, regarding educational opportunities in nursing, is that today all major educational opportunities essential to professional nursing practice are available within nursing education.

Leadership and the Literature

Leadership by nurses is needed for both nursing and health care. As Kelly said, leadership in many ways defies definition but, "in its simplest context, it is the ability to influence others, to lead, guide, and direct" (1985, p 362). Nursing needs leaders to advance the art, science, and profession. Society needs nurses to exercise leadership in shaping health care to meet society's need in a humanistic way. A number of strategies can be used for increasing nurse self-actualization and influence.

Strategies for Increasing
Nurse Self-Actualization and Influence

Interrelatedness of Self-Image, Public Image, and Nursing Influence.   A strat-egy is both a plan and action; it is the means to an end or goal. We are interested in the individual goal of self-actualization because we believe nurses themselves have inherent self-actualization tendencies just as their patients do. We are interested in the professional goal of influencing health-care policy because we believe nurses will move policy in the direction of helping other persons — namely, clients of health-care delivery — to realize their inherent potential. According to Lysaught (1980), 75% to 90% of the social worth of a profession is based on the profession's view of itself. The profession's view of itself arises from the self-image of individual practitioners. Each nurse needs to consider self-concept and its relationship to personal growth, the profession's image, and nursing's influence on health-care policy.

In the lay view, all nurses tend to be the same. In the past this view has sometimes considered nursing as a part of medicine. Public media have also tended to portray the nurse more often as a sweet young woman than as a mature practitioner.

For nursing to influence health-care policy is a big order. You may have heard nursing scorned by feminists as traditional women's work done by unassertive workers. Sometimes, perhaps, this has been so. It is true that nurses have not always banded together to use their personal power as have feminists. Neither have they regularly demonstrated the use of coalition strategies that politicians find so successful. These circumstances suggest that both individual and group strategies can and should be used by nurses of both sexes to achieve personal self-actualization and to influence health-care policy.

Individual Strategies

Use of Information.   Most professionals are generally well informed about society and the world. They appreciate and understand society's development, its potentials, and its perils. They may have both a strong national consciousness and a humane view of world problems. Individual practitioners understand how their unique professional service to society relates to a larger scheme. Professionals recognize that knowledge is power, whether in science, economics, or politics. Some nurses have seen little need to be informed beyond their small sphere of practice. Yet nurses need to be informed about nursing specifically, health care generally, and the world beyond.

One of the ways the community of professionals maintains and advances its subculture is through an information network. The formal communication network consists of books, journals, organization newspapers, and so on. These outlets provide for the scholarly expression of group goals and ideas. Much professional literature is available through both service and educational institutions. Increasingly, the scientific journals of nursing are *referred journals*, meaning that the articles within them are reviewed by peers in the nursing science community before publication. Remember, the scholarly writing of today lays the groundwork for the nursing practice and research of tomorrow. Using a variety of abstract periodicals available in reference libraries will give nurses access to both the original basic science research and other health science literature.

Planning Ahead.   Being well-informed is necessary for the strategy of effective planning. All the strategies suggested here are intended to be points of departure for later professional growth and development. If you are tempted to explore such strategies more fully now, many books like those of the Kalisches, including *Politics of Nursing* (1982), will be of interest. Well-informed nurses need to learn much about leadership, change theories, economics, and politics to achieve individual and professional goals.

At this point in your studies, it is probably difficult to imagine planning many years ahead. It is probably also true that few people in any field reach either their personal or professional goals unless they identify goals and plan appropriately. As Henning and Jardin (1978) suggest, taking a long-range look and deciding what you want can be the difference between surviving and winning.

Know yourself. Unless you know what you want personally, it is unlikely you will get it. To control both your personal and professional lives, you must be active rather than reactive. Already you can ask yourself many questions. Do you anticipate working for most of your life? Most nurses who do work can expect a career of more than 30 years! Economists suggest that most women will continue to work for economic reasons alone. You might ask yourself what work you imagine yourself doing a decade from now. What must you do to reach that goal?

One reason for setting goals is to be able to identify obstacles in reaching them. With planning, it is possible to maintain a career focus even if you work part-time or anticipate time away from a career because of family or child-care responsibilities. Planning assists you to exercise freedom of choice and in that way take control. An analogy may be made between the control we advocate for your career life and the control nurses urge clients to assume for their health and self-actualization. Similarly, just as nurses plan short- and long-term goals for clients, it is appropriate to do the same for yourself.

Not all persons who make long-term career commitments anticipate the potential personal conflicts that career decisions may provoke. A profession such as nursing, with expanding science and practice horizons, needs persons who are not reluctant to seize the available opportunities.

When external barriers to independent behavior are removed, such as when laws and policies are changed, internal barriers like lack of confidence and low self-esteem assume increased importance. Such unrecognized psychological barriers make some persons reluctant to plan and accept responsibility for their decisions. After all, hapless victims of circumstances are seldom held accountable for events beyond their control. Do you share your planning and aspirations with your significant others to gain their understanding, support, and encouragement?

Participation.   Being informed and planning ahead are dead-end strategies unless they are accompanied by active participation. Sometimes the personal focus of nursing tempts nurses to judge participation by satisfaction in relationships rather than by achieved outcomes. Several questions to ask yourself about participation follow:

- Are you using your abilities and assets? To the fullest? To what end?
- Do you give positive feedback and unsolicited support to peers for accomplishment?
- Do you recognize the urgency of research participation by all nurses?

Contrary to what you might have expected, Mauksch (1980) suggests that the research roles in nursing involve supporting research, being a participant or collecting data, initiating research, or being a consumer implementer. Any nurse, whether student or practitioner, can perform three of the four research functions. As indicated earlier, broad research participation is needed to aid nursing's development and scientific credibility and, hence, its influence.

Experienced practitioners of nursing are always finding ways to participate as nurses beyond nursing. Increasingly, nurses are becoming appropriately visible in the media. One nurse-gerontologist we know persisted until the local newspaper ran her column, "Ask Your Gerontologist." Other nurses are taking the story of nursing's contribution to health care to radio, television, and popular magazines.

Participation involves risk-taking behavior. It implies conviction about goals and willingness to be identified with them. Sometimes participation leads to activities that fail to achieve their potential. Under these circumstances, the participant accepts failure as a characteristic of the activity not of the individual person involved. Participants come in many varieties. "Gray-shadow joiners" may be participants in name only, whereas "movers and shakers" seldom lack stimulation and a piece of whatever action happens. By definition and tradition, professionals are self-starters, initiators, and generally assertive persons. As Hein (1966) queried, "Living is the thing you do now or never . . . which do you?"

Demonstration of Competence.   Competence is both an individual strategy and a goal. One definition of *competence* is proper qualification or adequacy. Although the competence asked of learners is different than that expected of the licensed practitioner, the underlying concept is the same. Given your professional intent, are your skills sufficient for the purpose? For example, how are your writing and speaking abilities? As an informed and interested person, you can help others understand what nursing is trying to accomplish for health care. Nurses need to demonstrate competence in very public ways in order to change the media image of nurses and nursing. Such change is critical to making nursing a potent force in shaping health-care policy. A major public relations campaign is being waged to advertise nursing's unique contribution to health care and also its independent functions.

Sometimes we use the term *competent* to mean taking responsibility for your own actions and making appropriate decisions. You need to feel a certain fundamental personal competence to be personally powerful and to control your own life. In this sense, personal competence is basic to any professional competence. An extension of this competence is an ability to adapt to personal and professional stresses. Nurses need management skills to maintain the equilibrium necessary for their own adaptive living. Ideally, they also ought to be able to model the adaptive coping strategies they are advocating for their clients.

Recognition of nurses' competence may provoke a variety of responses. Nurse competence may challenge physician control explicitly and, when nurses are female, challenge masculinity implicitly with male physicians. Yet, it is in their everyday settings that individual nurses who have expertise and competence can anticipate making their initial and informal impact. Competent practitioners, managers, and leaders will be more effective change agents for improved health-care delivery. Selected individual strategies for increasing self-actualization and nursing influence are summarized in Table 3–2.

Group Strategies

Informal Peer Groups. Informal peer groups are built from personal relationships. Because *peer* means equal, you will probably initially define your peer group to be your classmates—perhaps friends in the same class studying for the same examination. As professional identity matures, nurses come to identify other nurses and other health professionals as peers. Tomorrow, your informal peer group may be an interdisciplinary team with common research interests. Perhaps such informal peer groups of practicing nurses and physicians can counteract some of the misunderstanding that occurs between health professionals under more formal circumstances.

TABLE 3–2
SELECTED INDIVIDUAL STRATEGIES FOR INCREASING SELF-ACTUALIZATION AND NURSING INFLUENCE

Use Information	Plan Ahead	Participate	Be Competent
Use person resources	Know yourself	Learn independently	Write and speak well
Gain access to professional literature through indexes and abstracts	Set goals Share aspirations	Interact with other health professionals	Project a professional image
		Join health organizations	Assume accountability
		Mobilize support	Document practice
Read widely *American Journal of Nursing* *Nursing Outlook* *Nursing '90* *Nursing Research* *Imprint*		Provide curriculum input	Commit yourself to lifelong learning
		Support research	Strive for excellence
		Find a mentor	
		Fight sex discrimination	

Another type of informal peer group combines neophytes and experienced mentors. In corporations, politics, and academia, such support groups are called, quite aptly, old-boy networks. They aid in climbing the corporate ladder or in moving from junior to senior ranks. Some of the stressors that students and practitioners alike experience as "burnout" could be managed through peer support systems. Persons who understand the structure and function of informal peer groups and networks know that they are the glue that holds formal bureaucracies together. They are essential to successful functioning in hospitals and other large health-care organizations.

Formal Organizations.   Formal organizations serve many important functions for professions, including providing social and moral support for individuals, setting standards, advancing and disseminating knowledge, and speaking for the profession (Merton, 1958).

Professional nursing organizations can form a significant power base. Until recently, the word *power* was foreign to nurses. Now nurses are working to assert power within the health-care delivery system. Unfortunately, nursing's primary professional organization, the ANA, has been fighting an uphill battle to build membership. Significantly more physicians belong to their professional group than is true in nursing. At least two reasons for the drop in ANA membership may not be readily apparent. First, beginning in 1968, nurses began to trade ANA membership for membership in specialty-nursing organizations that were more closely associated with their clinical interest. Although these smaller groups may have met the needs of individual nurses for clinical interest, they did not meet the need of the profession for a strong central organizational voice for nursing. Second, many nurses find a conflict between the ANA being both a collective bargaining agent and a professional organization.

Two professional organizations of special significance for students are Sigma Theta Tau International — the nursing honor society — and the autonomous National Student Nurses' Association. Another national organization that is concerned specifically with nursing is the National League for Nursing. Membership in this organization is not limited to nurses, although the organization aims to influence nursing education and practice. An encouraging development in recent years is that nursing organizations have formed coalitions to advance the profession of nursing and nursing's role in meeting the health-care needs of society.

Political Participation.   Most of us grew up believing in political action or decision making by majority vote. However, as children we also learned about decision making by authority. Even in the adult world, majority alone does not ensure **power**, the ability to secure a particular outcome. Power among adults also comes from authority. **Authority** is recognized as an assumed right to control, whereas **influence** is the power of producing effects by less visible means.

In its narrowest sense, political action means power in government. Increasingly, other kinds of political action or **politics** are advocated. For instance, in *Carl Rogers On Personal Power*, Carl Rogers described politics as power and control and the extent to which persons "desire, attempt to obtain, possess, share, or surrender power and control over others and/or for themselves" (1977, p 4). According to the Kalisches, "Politics concerns the promotion of one's interest group and the use of whatever resources are available to protect and advance that interest" (1976, p 30).

As a group, nurses have only recently become interested in political action. Nurses'

Coalition for Action in Politics is a nonprofit, nonpartisan program to improve health care through the political process. As the political action arm of the ANA since 1974, N-CAP has functioned to educate nurses politically, to encourage their participation in the political process, and to provide financial support and endorsements for political candidates who support issues of consequence to nursing and good health care. Nurses themselves are encouraged to run for elective office and to work for political campaigns. To date, few nurses are visible as legislators.

As the Kalisches put it, "Nurses belong to one of the largest and most neglected groups in our voting population" (1976, p 29). Many nurses have yet to learn the importance of political action as a strategy for advancing nursing and changing health-care policy. Obviously, nurses do not have to become legislators themselves to influence policy, but they must participate in local politics in some meaningful way. At the federal level, nurses have been noticeably absent from key decision-making positions related to health policy and allocations of health-care funds. An outstanding exception is Carolyne K. Davis, Ph.D., a nurse who admirably served a term of unprecedented length (1981–1985) as administrator for the federal Health Care Financing Administration (HCFA), which controlled a multi–billion dollar Medicare budget.

Nurses' failure to participate in local and state politics has meant that federal monies shared locally seldom come to nursing. One congressman suggested that if 1000 nurses entered a national congressional office seeking support for a legislative issue, they would get results (Pursell, 1980, p 107). His congressional district in Michigan has some 5000 registered nurses. In 1979, the Carter administration attempted virtually to eliminate national funding for nursing education and research. Nurses, working with supportive congressional members, were successful in reversing this cutback attempt. One politically involved nurse's fascinating diary of this effort is presented in "It Could Happen Again" (Rinke, 1980).

Nurses do not have to wait for legislation that relates to their issues to be introduced. What nurses need to realize is that they can form bipartisan coalitions of their colleagues to draft legislation and then seek congressional sponsors. If nurses expect to influence health-care policy, they need to be informed, visible, and vocal in the local, state, and federal arenas. Political action should be seen as a group strategy that uses all the individual and group techniques presented. As nurses come to a new awareness and involvement regarding political action, they do not need to be the most neglected group of our voting populations.

In the keynote address to the Biennial ANA Meeting in June 1980, Rhetaugh Dumas proclaimed, "In a cost-conscious era, good intentions and unassuming, capable nursing work are essential, but no substitute for data, assertiveness, and political skill." Her words are equally true today. Political nurses use power, control, and decision making. They trust themselves to say, "I think, I believe, and I accept the challenges." They are active persons whose mode of functioning is to create action rather than merely to react. They also recognize that there has been, within recent years, a trend away form *consumers* — who merely use resources — to *prosumers*, who create resources. Just as the nurse encourages the client to assume control over his or her health by developing strengths, the nurse needs to openly assume control of nursing and its services. By individual and group action, the political nurse demonstrates that personal and professional power and freedom are created by nurses, not given by others. As Mundinger reminded us, "Not to distinguish nursing's contribution is to lose it" (1980, p 151).

CONCLUSION

This chapter has presented nursing today as the health science of caring. Nursing theory and research were explained as essential to both science and professionalization. The major purpose of both nursing theory and nursing research was seen as answering puzzling questions from nursing practice. Selected nursing theorists were highlighted.

Contemporary nursing issues were introduced in the context of problems common to nursing and other professions. Specialty areas of practice and traditional and nontraditional practice options were described along with nursing's independent, interdependent, and dependent functions. Educational opportunities and requirements related to various nursing functions were indicated. Leadership by nurses was noted as needed for both nursing and health care. Individual and group strategies for increasing nurse self-actualization, leadership, and influence were emphasized.

STUDY QUESTIONS

1 How has your personal concept changed of nursing:
   a As art?
   b As science?
   c As profession?
2 How do you see yourself contributing to nursing's:
   a Art?
   b Science?
   c Professionalism?
3 Explain how the problems and issues identified in this chapter have the potential to stimulate the growth of nursing as a profession.
4 How might new practice options for nurses affect other health professionals and the health-care delivery system?
5 How does the independent functioning of nurses facilitate collegial relationships with other health-care professionals?
6 Describe what actions you as an individual nurse might take to improve nursing's public image.
7 How could the nature and potential of nursing receive more attention in your community?
8 Describe additional group strategies for increasing nursing's influence on health care.

REFERENCES

American Nurses' Association: A Social Policy Statement. Kansas City, MO, American Nurses' Association Pub. Code NP-63 35M, December 1980

American Nurses' Association, Commission on Nursing Education: A Case for Baccalaureate Preparation in Nursing. Kansas City, MO, American Nurses' Association, 1979

Backscheider JE: Self-care requirements, self-care capabilities and nursing systems in the diabetic nurse management clinic. Am J Pub Health 64:1138–1146, 1974

Boodley C: A Nursing Study of the Experience of Having a Health Examination. Ph.D. Dissertation, University of Michigan, 1986

Brooten D, Kumar S, Brown LP, et al: A randomized clinical trial of early hospital discharge and home follow-up of very-low birth-weight infants. N Engl J Med 315:934–939, 1986

Butler PM: Hospital Embedding–Diffusion Mechanisms and Nurses' Knowledge of a Diffused Innovation. Ph.D. Dissertation, University of Michigan, 1987

Chinn PL, Jacobs MK: Theory and Nursing: A Systematic Approach, 2nd ed. St. Louis, CV Mosby, 1987

de Bono E: Lateral Thinking: Creativity Step by Step. New York, Harper & Row, 1970

Denyes MJ: Measurement of self-care agency in adolescents (abstr). Nurs Res 31:63, 1982

Dumas RG: Challenges to Nursing in the 1980's. Biennial American Nurses Association, June 1980

Dumas RG, Leonard RC: The effect of nursing on the incidence of postoperative vomiting. Nurs Res 63:52–59, 1963

Engel G: Grief and grieving. Am J Nurs 64:93–98, 1964

Erickson HC, Tomlin EM, Swain MA: Modeling and Role Modeling: A Theory and Paradigm for Nursing. Englewood Cliffs, NJ, Prentice-Hall, 1983

Fagin C: Nursing's pivotal role in achieving competition in health care. Paper presented at American Academy of Nursing meeting. Washington, DC, September 1981

Fawcett J: Assessing and understanding the cesarean father. In Kehoe CF (ed): The Cesarean Experience: Theoretical and Clinical Perspectives for Nurses, pp 143–156. New York, Appleton-Century-Crofts, 1981

Fawcett J: Analysis and Evaluation of Conceptual Models of Nursing. Philadelphia, FA Davis, 1984

Galligan AC: Using Roy's concept of adaptation to care for young children. Am J Maternal Child Nurs 4:24–28, 1979

Glaser B, Strauss A: Awareness of Dying. Chicago, Aldine, 1966

Harmer B (revised by Henderson V): Textbook of Principles and Practice of Nursing, 5th ed. New York, Macmillan, 1955

Hein P: Grooks 1. Garden City, NY, Doubleday, 1966

Henderson V: The Nature of Nursing. New York, Macmillan, 1966

Henning M, Jardin A: The Managerial Woman. New York, Pocket Books, 1978

Horsley J, Crane J, Crabtree MK, et al: Using Research to Improve Nursing Practice: A Guide. New York, Grune & Stratton, 1983

International Council of Nurses: ICN Basic Principles of Nursing Care. London, Association, 1961

Kalisch BJ, Kalisch PA: A discourse on the politics of nursing. J Nurs Admin 6:29–34, 1976

Kalisch BJ, Kalisch PA: Politics of Nursing. Philadelphia, JB Lippincott, 1982

Kalisch PA, Kalisch BJ: How the public sees nurse-midwives: 1978 news coverage of nurse-midwifery in the nation's press. J Nurse-Midwifery 25:31–39, 1980

Kalisch PA, Kalisch BJ: When nurses were national heroines: Images of nursing in American film, 1942–1945. Nurs Forum 20:15–61, 1981

Kelley LY: Dimensions of Professional Nursing, 5th ed. New York, Macmillan, 1985

King IM: Toward a Theory of Nursing: General Concepts of Human Behavior. New York, John Wiley & Sons, 1971

King IM: A Theory for Nursing: Systems, Concepts, Process. New York, John Wiley & Sons, 1981

Leininger MM: Transcultural Nursing: Concepts, Theories and Practices. New York, John Wiley & Sons, 1978

Leininger MM: Caring: A Central focus of nursing and health care services. Nurs Health Care 176:135–143, 1980.

Leininger MM: The phenomenon of caring: Importance, research questions and theoretical considerations. In Caring: An Essential Human Need (Proceedings of the three national caring conferences.) Thorofare, NJ, Charles B Slack, 1981, pp 3–15

Levine ME: The four conservation principles of nursing. Nurs Forum 6:45–59, 1967

Levine ME: Introduction to Clinical Nursing, 2nd ed. Philadelphia, FA Davis, 1973

Lysaught J: Action in affirmation: Toward an unambiguous profession of nursing. Paper presented at ANA Biennial Convention, Houston, June 1980

Maslow AH: Motivation and Personality, 2nd ed. New York, Harper & Row, 1970

Mauksch I: Nursing Practice and Education for the '80s. Paper presented at ANA Biennial Convention, Houston, June 1980

Merton R: The functions of the professional association. Am J Nurs 1:50–54, 1958

Mundinger M: Autonomy in Nursing. Germantown, MD, Aspen Systems, 1980

National Council of State Boards of Nursing: The Model Practice Act. London, Association, 1982

Neuman B: The Betty Neuman health-care systems model: A total person approach to patient problems. In JP Riehl, C Roy (eds): Conceptual Models for Nursing Practice, pp 99–114. New York, Appleton-Century-Crofts, 1974

Neuman B: The Neuman's Systems Model: Application to Nursing Education and Practice. New York, Appleton-Century-Crofts, 1982

Newman MA: Theory Development in Nursing. Philadelphia, FA Davis, 1979

Nightingale F: Notes on Nursing: What It Is and What It Is Not. London, Harrison, 1859. Facsimile edition: Philadelphia, JB Lippincott, 1966

Nursing case management, p 5. Am Nurse June 1988

Orem DE: Guides for Developing Curricula for the Education of Practical Nurses. Washington, DC, U.S. Government Printing Office, 1959

Orem DE: Concepts of Practice, 3rd ed. New York, McGraw-Hill, 1985

Orlando I: The Dynamic Nurse-Patient Relationship. New York, GP Putnams Sons, 1961

Parse RR: Man-Living-Health: A Theory of Nursing. New York, John Wiley & Sons, 1981

Peplau H: Interpersonal Relations in Nursing. New York, GP Putnams Sons, 1952

Piaget J: The Psychology of Intelligence. Totowa, NJ, Littlefield, Adams, 1973

Polit DF, Hungler BP: Essentials of Nursing Research: Methods and Applications. Philadelphia, JB Lippincott, 1985

Pursell C: Congressman urges greater nursing role in health policy formation. Nurs Health Care 2:107, 1980

Reiter F: The nurse clinician. Am J Nurs 2:274–280, 1966

Rinke LT: It could happen again. Nurs Outlook 7:449–451, 1980

Rogers CR: Carl Rogers on Personal Power. New York, Dell, 1977

Rogers ME: An Introduction to the Theoretical Basis of Nursing. Philadelphia, FA Davis, 1970

Rogers ME: Nursing: A science of unitary man. In JP Riehl, C Roy (eds): Conceptual Models for Nursing Practice, 2nd ed. New York, Appleton-Century-Crofts, 1980

Rosenfeld P: Nursing education in crisis—a look at recruitment and retention. Nurs Health Care 8:283–286, 1987

Roy C: Adaptation: A conceptual framework for nursing. Nurs Outlook 18:42–45, March, 1970

Roy C: Introduction to Nursing: An Adaptation Model, 2nd ed. Englewood Cliffs, NJ, Prentice-Hall, 1984

Selye H: The Stress of Life. New York, McGraw-Hill, 1956

Stevens BJ: Nursing Theory: Analysis, Application, Evaluation. Boston, Little, Brown, 1984

Swanson JM, Chenitz WC: Why qualitative research in nursing? Nurs Outlook 30:241–245, 1982

Torres G: The place of concepts and theories within nursing. In The Nursing Theories: The Base for Professional Nursing Practice, pp 1–10. Englewood Cliffs, NJ Prentice-Hall, 1980

Utz SW: Applying the Neuman model to nursing practice with hypertensive clients. Cardio-Vasc Nurs 16:29–34, 1980

Watson J: Nursing: The Philosophy and Science of Caring. Boston, Little, Brown, 1979

Watson J: Nursing: Human Science and Human Care. Norwalk, CT, Appleton-Century-Crofts, 1985

4 | PERSON

KEY WORDS	After completing this chapter, students will be able to:
Accommodation	**State how the concept of holism applies to nursing.**
Adaptation	**Describe how the concept of system applies to nursing.**
Assimilation	**Relate the concept of the person's view of self to one's own self.**
Body image	
Development	**Describe several principles of growth and development.**
Holism	**Apply ideas from the theories of Maslow, Erikson, Piaget, and**
Identity crisis	**Carl Rogers to real-life situations.**
Operation	
Self	
Spirit	
System	
Value	
Variable	

Each person is a unique and complex human being consisting of biological, psychological, and sociological components. These components include unique characteristics as well as characteristics held in common with other persons. As an open system, the components of the person are in constant interaction internally and with the environment. Inherent in this interaction is a unifying element, called the **spirit**. This component, although not necessarily religious in nature, may be viewed as such and is the inspiring or animating principle that pervades thought, feeling, and action. Nurses view the person as a complete, holistic being who is greater than the sum of his or her individual parts, with a spirit that makes him or her unique from fellow creatures.

Each person in his or her uniqueness has the ability to grow and develop throughout the life span. Knowing this, nurses apply growth and development theories to the delivery of relevant and effective nursing care. In this chapter, we cite several prominent theorists to provide background and resource material for understanding skills that nurses use in practice. For example, understanding how persons think assists health teaching. Being aware of psychosocial development provides nurses with guidelines for counseling. An appreciation of the physical growth patterns that take place in persons at different ages and stages helps nurses concentrate on pertinent areas when performing physical assessment. An appreciation of how these components of the person interact sets the tone for holistic care and demonstrates the unending potential of the human being throughout life.

The subjects and theories introduced in this chapter are vast. Students are expected to use the basic ideas presented here to understand aspects both common and unique to all persons. For a more thorough exploration, the reader is referred to publications cited at the end of this chapter.

THE PERSON AS A SYSTEM

Holism

The words *holistic* and *holism* are derived from the Greek word meaning whole. **Holism** is basically a theory that the universe, and especially living nature, is seen in terms of interacting wholes that are more than the mere sum of their parts. Smuts (1926) indicated that holism is a theory that describes the parts of a person as dependent on each other and coordinated in a systematic fashion. According to this theory, studying one part of a person indicates the need to consider how that part interrelates with all other parts of the person. An appreciation for the parts as a whole suggests the purpose and function of each individual part. The interrelationships also contribute to making the whole greater than the sum of its parts. This interrelation further increases the complexity of each of us as unique individuals. Figure 4–1 is a typical representation of the holistic person. Note the following points:

1 The subsystems represent interacting wholes that are greater than the sum of the parts.
2 The broken lines between the subsystems indicate the passage of energy among the subsystems.
3 Inherent throughout the whole are the genetic base and spiritual drive that make all persons unique.

General Systems Theory

As stated previously, the human being is an open system. In discussing the meaning of system, Abbey stated that a **system** is "an organized unit with a set of components that mutually react. The system acts as a whole; the dysfunction of a part causes a system disturbance rather than the loss of a single function" (1978, pp 20–21). Systems are found everywhere.

For example, a car is a mechanical system with many parts, all of which must function with reasonable precision for the car to move. A plant is a living system with interacting parts consisting of leaves, stems, roots, and many smaller structures. All of the parts function together to promote life and growth. These two systems—car and plant—have definite boundaries that are readily apparent.

Other systems within our social structure have less apparent boundaries. The public school system, as a social system, might exemplify this idea. Certainly each individual school has visible boundaries in the form of its building, teachers, students, books, and desks. However, each school district has its own school board, and each state has certain legislation relating to its particular school system. Financial support comes from a variety of sources. Philosophies of education, which may vary considerably across the nation, permeate each component of the system. In this large and unwieldy system, the interrelationships of the components are less evident. Consideration of each individual school and its parts in the system makes the functioning of the larger system more understandable. Thus, the public school system is made up of thousands of smaller systems that can be called subsystems. A

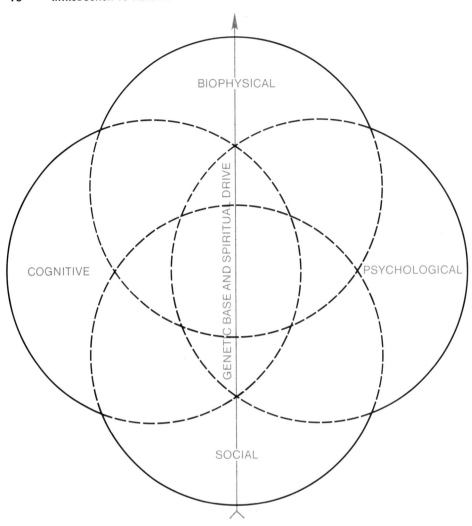

Figure 4–1   A holistic model. (Erickson H, Tomlin E, Swain MA: Modeling and Role-Modeling: A Theory and Paradigm for Nursing, p 45. Englewood Cliffs, NJ, Prentice-Hall, 1983)

subsystem has the same characteristics as a system but is considered a part of the larger system as well.

General systems theory is a formalized means of describing the interplay of many systems. The idea of general systems theory was proposed by Ludwig von Bertalanffy in the 1950s. He wrote, "General systems theory then consists of the scientific exploration of 'wholes and wholeness' . . . the interdisciplinary nature of concepts, models, and principles applying to 'systems' provides a possible approach toward the unification of science" (1968, p 30). Klir suggested the following definition: "General Systems Theory in the broadest sense refers to a collection of general concepts, principles, tools, problems, methods, and techniques associated with systems" (1972, p 1).

Open and Closed Systems

Systems are essentially of two types: open and closed. The distinguishing difference is the extent to which a system can exchange matter, energy, and information with its environment. The environment of the system has been defined by Hall and Fagan as all factors that affect the system and also all factors that are affected by the system (1968). The *open system* is one that can exchange matter, energy, and information with its environment; a *closed system* cannot. Because nearly all systems contain many subsystems, it is possible to have an open system that contains several closed subsystems. Systems that are essentially open include living, social, behavioral, and environmental systems. All of these contain closed subsystems.

As examples of open systems, persons constantly exchange matter, energy, and information with the environment. We hear, see, and process information that is given to us and then disseminate it to others. We adapt to the weather by changing clothes. We absorb energy from the sun, from food, and from other sources. As living systems, we are capable of self-regulation and growth.

Chemical reactions are examples of closed systems. Some compounds, when dissolved in water, dissociate reversibility to produce negatively charged ions (anions) and hydrogen ions, for example,

$$\text{Lactic acid} \longrightarrow H^+ + \text{lactate}$$
$$\text{Carbonic acid} \longrightarrow H^+ + \text{bicarbonate}$$

These systems will remain the same forever and be unaffected by their environments unless new variables are added. Persons have closed systems within them; for instance, the chemical reaction shown here occurs continuously within the body and helps to maintain an internal stability. Another example of a closed system is the withdrawal reflex that protects a person from painful stimuli. This reflex is an autonomic reaction within the system of the person in response to an outside stimulus.

Systems Theory Applied to the Person

The human being contains many systems and subsystems that interrelate in an integrated fashion to become one total system. We have already mentioned the biological, psychological, social, spiritual, and genetic components that constitute this interaction. Each of these could be considered a system having subsystems. For instance, the biological system contains subsystems such as the neurological, circulatory, and gastrointestinal systems. The neurological system in turn consists of the brain, the spinal cord, and the peripheral nerves throughout the body. Each of these parts is a subsystem in itself. The circulatory system consists of the heart and the blood vessels. The two systems interrelate as the brain sends messages to the heart that regulate its pumping. The heart, however, must pump to keep the brain functioning so that it can send signals.

The psychological system contains subsystems that include thinking and feeling. Our feeling states also affect the autonomic nervous system, which signals the heart to beat faster or slower.

As indicated earlier, systems are open when they exchange energy with other systems. Consider another important example of this notion: the systems of the person constantly exchange energy not only among themselves—the internal systems—but also with the outside environment.

TABLE 4–1
SELECTED VARIABLES OF THE PERSON

Biological	Psychological	Sociological	Spiritual
Age	Attitudes	Basic needs	Beliefs
Genetic structure	Basic needs	Culture	Philosophy of life
Sex	Body image	Family	Religion
Race	Communication	Group membership	Values
Biological rhythms	Coping mechanisms	Language	
Basic needs	Defense mechanisms	Life-style	
Growth	Feeling states	Relationships with	
Acid–base balance	Level of develop-	others	
Circulation	mental task	Roles	
Digestion	resolution	Role prescriptions	
Electrolyte balance	Perception	School systems	
Immune response	Self-concept		
Mobility	Values		
Reproduction	Cognition		
Respiration	Consciousness		
Temperature	Knowledge		
regulation	Memory		
Physical health	Thought process		
Past illnesses			

Each system contains many variables. Polit and Hungler defined a variable as "a characteristic or attribute of a person or object that varies (i.e., takes on different values) within the population under study (e.g., body temperature, age, heart rate)" (1987, p 538). Systems and variables are both components of a larger whole. In many instances, both terms apply to the same object or event. Table 4–1 lists some of the variables that are part of the complex biopsychosocial system called the person.

Many of these variables, although associated primarily with the stated classification, may also be associated appropriately with another heading under certain circumstances. The concept of role, for example, is generally thought of as a sociological variable. However, there are many psychological components to this notion and some might consider it as classified with those variables.

Exchange of Energy Among the Subsystems of a Person

Systems have a certain amount of energy that can be exchanged within the subsystems and with the environment. If the person—a being greater than the whole of his or her combined parts—uses coping mechanisms that help achieve a successful growth and development throughout his or her life, each subsystem will retain its maximum potential health. However, if one component—such as the psychological subsystem—becomes stressed, the person may be unable to cope effectively. At that point energy may be drawn from another subsystem, which in turn may become less healthy.

To apply this idea to everyday situations, consider two kinds of examples: those that represent a temporary breakdown in a system, and those that reflect more far-reaching implications. Note the interactions of several subsystems in the brief but difficult common cold:

- A stuffed nose often causes a headache, difficult breathing, and unclear thinking.
- Constant nose blowing causes soreness to the skin of the nose.
- Muscles and joints often ache.
- One may act irritably, causing others to stay away.
- Often during a cold, persons have feelings of low self-esteem and inadequacy.

Mercifully, a cold is brief. Our natural recuperative powers quickly reassert themselves and the brief unpleasantness is forgotten. The example, however, demonstrates the many effects that a "simple cold" can have. Although it most specifically affects the upper respiratory system, it can also affect our general physical state and how we think, act, and respond to others. Energy is used to cope with the physical aspects and we are often left drained psychologically and socially as well. Moreover, the cold is an event that may have been precipitated by other factors in our lives. For example, students who feel overburdened with course work and examinations may be more susceptible to contracting a cold.

Sometimes persons with severe illnesses such as heart disease or cancer can point to events that they relate to their problems. One woman stated that her blood sugar had gone way up (900 mg/dl; norm, 90 to 110 mg/dl) when her son died. Furthermore, she indicated that it would not come down until she finally began to resolve her grief. This clinical example suggests that in trying to cope with severe psychological stress, the woman drew on her physical energy as well. Others might not connect two events this closely, but nurses often note that patients develop illness 6 months to a year after a loss. Research into the mind-body connection is not conclusive at this time but the relationships are often noted. Consider how often we connect physical and psychological subsystems in our common language: we talk of aching or broken hearts, cold feet, a pain in the neck, eyes as the windows of the soul, and so forth. These examples suggest that one component of a person has an effect on the person as a whole.

| BASIC NEEDS OF PERSONS

Maslow's Hierarchy of Needs

The extensive work of Abraham Maslow on the theory of motivation and the basic needs of humans has provided a framework through which nurses can understand both themselves and their clients. Maslow's basic belief was that each person wants to be the most self-actualized person he or she possibly can be. In other words, the person wishes to reach the fullest potential and to become all he or she is capable of becoming.

This notion led Maslow to study how and why some persons become self-actualized and others do not. He stated,

> If I had had to condense the thesis of this book [*Motivation and Personality*] into a single sentence, I would have said that, in *addition* to what the psychologies of the time had to say about human nature, man also had a higher nature and that this was

instinctoid, i.e., part of his essence. And if I could have had a second sentence I would have stressed the profoundly holistic nature of human nature. (1970, p ix)

Maslow pointed out that if we are truly to understand persons we must consider their highest aspirations: growth, self-actualization, the striving toward health, the quest for identity and autonomy, and the yearning for excellence. He believed that the "instinctoid nature of basic needs" constitutes a system of intrinsic human values that are not only wanted and desired by all human beings, but also needed, in the sense that they are necessary to avoid illness and psychopathology (1970, p xiii). This statement is suggestive or the previous discussion on exchange of energy among the subsystems of the person.

Figure 4–2 is a representation of the hierarchy of human needs as identified by Maslow, beginning with the basic physiological needs and progressing to the need for safety and security, the need for love and belonging, the need for self-esteem, and finally, the need for self-actualization.

The following ideas are extracted and adapted from Maslow (1970). Nurses may use these ideas to apply basic need theory to practice:

1   The basic needs are present in all of us all of the time but if met, do not motivate our behavior.
2   Persons function from a state of deficit or a state of being. When one experiences a deficit state (associated with unmet physiological, safety and security, love and belonging, or self-esteem needs), one's behavior is motivated by those needs. When one is experiencing a being state, behavior is motivated by the growth needs which are self-actualization and the quest for knowledge, truth, and beauty.
3   The basic needs can be regarded as rights as well as needs.
4   As one group of needs is gratified, another of a higher order will appear.

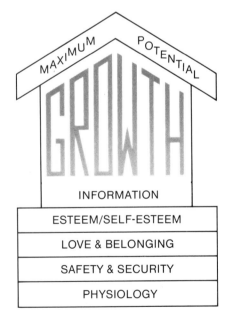

Figure 4–2   Maslow's hierarchy of needs.
(Erickson H, Tomlin E, Swain MA: Modeling and Role-Modeling: A Theory and Paradigm for Nursing, p 57. Englewood Cliffs, NJ, Prentice-Hall, 1983)

5   Although all persons have the same basic needs, the means by which they meet those needs will vary considerably among individuals.

6   The gratification of needs is not an absolute state. Rather, one level of needs may be gratified to a certain point and then another group will begin to appear.

7   The physiological needs serve as channels for many other needs as well. The person who thinks he or she is hungry may actually be seeking comfort or dependence rather than nutrition.

8   A conscious desire or motivated behavior may serve as a kind of channel through which other purposes may express themselves. The person who seeks sexual encounters may be searching for a sense of belonging.

9   Although a person may be quite capable of meeting his or her basic needs and be generally physically healthy, safe, loving, and self-actualized, stress may occur in this individual's life and cause a reappearance of a basic need, which the person will again strive to gratify.

10   Needs may be either conscious or unconscious.

11   The gratification of needs may be determined in some measure by one's cultural expression.

12   There are multiple motivations for and determinants of behavior. Thus, to say that a person would respond in any exact manner to this hierarchy of needs would be to oversimplify human nature.

If we accept the general premise that all human beings strive for health and excellence, it makes sense for nurses to plan accordingly. This statement seems to be reasonable when we consider the many persons who certainly behave as if they were striving as suggested. We also encounter persons in a helpless, hopeless state, and some individuals whose behavior is antisocial or criminal. These persons may cause us to question the general premise. A further consideration of the basic needs may shed light on the meaning of certain behavior.

Physiological Needs

A list of basic **physiological needs** might include oxygen and gas exchange, fluids, food, elimination, rest, avoidance of pain, and sexual fulfillment. In translating these needs to our everyday existence, we remember instances when we were somewhat hungry, tired, or had a slight headache, and yet could continue with our usual activities. As the needs became greater, however, the urgency to gratify them became stronger. Usual activities were performed less effectively because the needs dominated our thoughts. For most persons, it is a simple matter to obtain food or rest, and to cope with a headache.

Persons on strict diets, however, who often feel quite hungry, report that they have such a heightened awareness of food, that they notice every picture of it, smell every aroma, and think and even dream about it constantly. As food is denied to a greater and greater extent, all other wishes and desires may be lost and the quest for food will dominate totally.

An extremely fatigued person, however, may find that the need for rest dominates even though he or she has not eaten recently. Generally, persons respond to basic needs according to a number of variables. These may include life style, cultural values, general health, and that which they have come to know is attainable. Other responses to the hunger state are also interesting. For example, consider the need to create, as expressed by the artist or the poet. These persons may avoid a steady-paying job and endure hunger so that they can continue to meet their self-actualization needs. The scholar may have the means by which to take care of his or her physiological needs, but the scholar's work dominates this person's whole being. As long as life can be sustained, these persons may give little attention to gratification of the physiological needs. Consider the clinical example in the box.

One nurse told of an elderly gentleman brought to the hospital by concerned neighbors. He was obviously starving, inadequately clothed, and confused. The neighbors said that there had been no food or heat in the house and that the fuel tank was empty. The nurse assumed that the man was poverty stricken. However, as she helped him to undress, she discovered wads of money in his pockets. Later, the authorities went to his home and found piles of money in drawers and canisters. What prevented this man from using his money or accepting the assistance of neighbors is not clear. Consideration of the next level of needs may suggest some ideas.

Safety and Security Needs

Safety and security needs might be listed as follows: security; stability; dependence; protection; freedom from fear, anxiety, and chaos; the need for structure, order, law, limits; strength in the protector; and so forth (Maslow, 1970, p 39).

Children frequently demonstrate these needs as they "test" their parents to determine whether limits will be set on their behavior. If children are permitted to throw temper

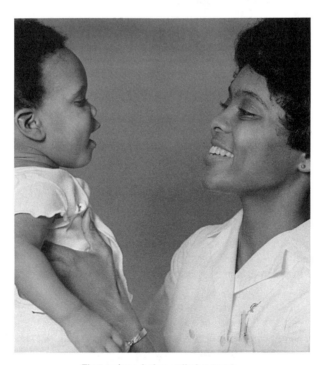

That unique being called *person*.

tantrums, they may eventually feel unsafe: they may feel that adults will not stop them from behaving badly and thereby protect them from themselves. Maslow believed that when safety and security needs are met in childhood, they are less likely to surface in later years. However, when a severe stress occurs, an adult may feel unsafe. If the stress becomes overwhelming, and if safety is severely threatened — as may have been the case with the elderly man mentioned in the example — the safety needs will dominate even the physiological ones.

Nurses often see the safety of a relatively secure adult threatened when illness and hospitalization are experienced. At times, the safety need may be conscious and the person may express his or her fears. However, if the need is unconscious and fears are not expressed, we often see what is termed the "difficult patient." This is the person who cannot participate well in his or her care. This individual may exhibit anger and hostility toward the nurses, yet call them constantly with requests. Consideration of underlying factors associated with such behavior helps nurses to plan interventions related to the development of trust and the meeting of safety needs.

Love and Belonging Needs

Love and belonging needs include the following: affectionate relationships; a place in the family and in other social groups; the need for a spouse, sweetheart, lover, children, friends; the need for roots in a particular neighborhood or place. Maslow clearly pointed out that these needs include the need to give as well as to receive love, warmth, affection, and friendship. Persons who cannot meet these needs feel rejected, abandoned, and without roots. As they feel more and more that no one cares about them, they develop a sense of helpless hopelessness and diminished self-esteem (1970, p 43).

The sexual drive, mentioned earlier as a physiological need, can be considered as purely biological in that context. Beyond that, however, sexual expression may be a channel through which love and belonging needs are met. Sexuality is usually considered an aspect of most intimate relationships. However, persons seeking gratification of love and belonging needs may engage in sexual activity that they afterwards regret. They may say they did it because, at least for a little while, it helped them feel as if they belonged to someone.

Nurses often discover that persons whose love and belonging needs are met can respond readily to help, and can mobilize their health resources with ease. They have a support system of family and friends in which they feel both a sense of belonging and a sense of security.

Esteem Needs

Esteem needs include a high evaluation of the self, self-respect, self-esteem, and the esteem of others. Maslow suggested that these needs can be divided into two subsets: those related to self-esteem (desire for strength, achievement, adequacy, mastery, competence, and independence) and those related to respect and esteem from others (reputation, prestige, status, fame, glory, dominance, recognition, attention, importance, dignity, and appreciation).

Those who can meet their needs for self-esteem will face the world with confidence and a sense of self-worth, capability, adequacy, and usefulness or purpose in the scheme of things. Those whose needs are thwarted will often demonstrate helplessness, inferiority, and weakness. They will be discouraged and nonassertive, demonstrating a diminished sense of the confidence they need to face their daily activities. Maslow also pointed out the danger that persons face if they gratify their esteem needs primarily from the opinions of others: to have the deserved respect of others is rewarding, but true esteem comes from within (1970, pp 45–46).

Self-Actualization Needs

The self-actualization need is the impulse to reach one's fullest potential, the need to become that which one is capable of becoming, the desire for self-fulfillment (Maslow, 1970, p 46). Self actualization needs, emerge when the physiological, safety, love, and esteem needs have been basically met.

Maslow described the self-actualized person as having a variety of characteristics, some of which are spontaneity, centering on problems rather than self, enjoying solitude and privacy, autonomy (independence from culture and environment), continued fresh appreciation for the basic goods of life, creativity, and the ability to develop deep and profound interpersonal relationships. These persons are not perfect, however. Maslow also described some of their shortcomings: they can be silly, wasteful, thoughtless, boring, stubborn, and irritating; they may be somewhat vain and given to outbursts of temper (1970, p 175).

Maslow also discussed two other higher levels of basic needs: the desire to know and understand, which is satisfied by acquiring knowledge through curiosity, learning, philosophizing, and experimenting; and the aesthetic need, the need for beauty and specifically for beauty in one's environment.

Erickson and colleagues (1983) described the self-actualization, knowing-understanding, and aesthetic needs as the growth needs. They indicated that persons who can generally meet their lower-level basic needs will begin to have a recurrence of these needs if they are thwarted in attempts to meet the growth needs. For example, professionals who perceive themselves as stagnant in the growth of their knowledge and development regarding their particular field may feel unsafe, inadequate, and without a group.

Spiritual Needs

Basic needs have been identified that flow from the biopsychosocial spheres of the person. Because persons have also been described as spiritual beings, it follows that there are needs associated with the spiritual sphere. Although Maslow himself did not deal directly with this issue, some authors have attempted to describe the notion. It might be suggested that spiritual needs include the following: the need to believe in a Supreme Being or in a special order for the universe, the need to believe that one has a place in that Being or order and that life has meaning and the need to feel hopeful about one's destiny.

We can speculate where spiritual needs might be placed on the hierarchy. Some might consider them a higher order of need arising after others have been gratified. Others might suggest that they are present even prior to the physiological needs as described by Maslow. We might also consider that the spiritual needs are inherent in all the other needs and therefore are not appropriately defined as a separate category. However we choose to look at this notion, we will want to be aware that most persons have a philosophy or a system of faith that directs their lives and serves as a refuge in times of need.

The Freedoms

Maslow indicated that, to meet any of the basic needs, certain conditions must exist. He listed those conditions as a series of freedoms. The freedoms include freedom to speak, to do what one wishes so long as it does not harm others, to express oneself, to seek justice, to find fairness, honesty, and orderliness in the group (1970, p 47). Nurses will be more effective if they are aware of clients' basic needs and how they can be met by facilitating expression of thought and by protecting the freedoms.

THE PERSON'S PERCEPTION OF SELF

View of Self

As nurses work to help clients meet their basic needs, they learn how persons view themselves. Our **self-concept** is a collection of notions, feelings, and beliefs about ourselves with which we identify and through which we relate and communicate with others and interact with the environment. The ideas of self-concept are developed from many of the variables inherent in the biopsychosocial systems of the person (previously listed in Table 4–1). Persons generally have a self-ideal that might be considered the superego. The *self-ideal* refers to how we believe we ought to function and behave given a personal value system and a set of personal standards. We develop this ideal through influences derived from family structure, cultural values, teachers, and our own talents, strengths, and goals for the future.

Self-Esteem and Body Image

An important aspect of self-concept is our sense of self-esteem — the personal judgment we make about our own self-worth. People may arrive at this perception by considering how they compare to their self-ideal and how often they attain personal goals. The ability to set and attain goals provides the person with a sense of control over his or her life as well as with a hopeful feeling about the future.

Another component of self-concept is body image. The body is the structural, functional, substantive, and visible part of the self. It is the packaging in which the self is enclosed and through which individuals interact with other persons and the environment. Our *body image* is how we view or think of that physical part of ourselves. Nurses often note that persons who are comfortable with their appearance generally have a high sense of self-esteem. Tolstoy said, "I am convinced that nothing has so marked an influence on the direction of a man's mind as his appearance, and not his appearance in itself so much as his conviction that it is attractive or unattractive" (1904).

When the view of the self does not correspond with what we actually see, a decrease of self-esteem may result. This has been noted in persons who have had surgery, whether or not the surgical alteration is visible to others. Some theorists believe that *phantom pain* — the pain that occurs in an absent body part such as an amputated limb — is the result of nerve activity. Others, however, suggest that the pain may also be associated with the alteration in one's body image or view of the physical self.

Some persons feel a disruption in their body image when they must wear glasses or a hearing aid. Others describe difficulty in communicating or in projecting themselves effectively when, in their view, their hair or clothes are not right. Daphne du Maurier described the feelings of her hero in *Scapegoat* when he first notices the man who resembles him exactly.

> The resemblance made me slightly sick, reminding me of moments when, passing a shop window, I had suddenly seen my reflection, and the man in the mirror had been a grotesque caricature of what, conceitedly, I had believed myself to be. Such incidents left me chastened, sore, with ego deflated. (1957, p 17)

Inner Versus Outward Feelings

Our total self-concept consists not only of how we believe we appear but also of the expectations we have of our behavior and achievements. Sometimes we are unsure of who that self is and how that person ought to be expressed. The expression *identity crisis* is common in our current Western culture; it refers to difficulty we sometimes have in grasping the meaning of our inner workings (thinking and feeling) or outward behavior. How we present ourselves to others may be vastly different from how we actually feel about ourselves.

Again we turn to du Maurier's hero as he talks of his struggle to understand his real self as opposed to the self he presents to others. He appears to be a quiet, law-abiding professor, aged 38, but he wonders about the self, the man within.

> Who he was and whence he sprang, what urges and what longings he might possess, I could not tell. I was so used to denying him expression that his ways were unknown to me; but he might have had a mocking laugh, a casual heart, a swift-roused temper and a ribald tongue. . . . Perhaps, if I had not kept him locked within me, he might have laughed, roistered, fought and lied. Perhaps he suffered, perhaps he hated, perhaps he lived by cruelty alone. He might have murdered, stolen or spent himself in lost causes, loved humanity, embraced a faith that believed in the divinity of both God and Man. Whatever his nature, he always hovered beneath the insignificant facade of that pale self who now sat in the church. . . . The question was, how to unlock the door? What lever would set the other free? (1957, pp 14–15)

It is essential that nurses understand themselves. As they become more comfortable with their own self-concept, they are better able to understand the strivings of their clients. As nurses are aware of their own inner workings, they can more readily accept the inner workings of others as well as the facade persons present to the world, an acceptance that will enable nurses to find the uniqueness of each person and to use that uniqueness to facilitate growth.

Values

The particular value system a person espouses is another way in which that individual is unique and yet shares features in common with others. Our values help us to view ourselves in relation to others.

A **value** is a belief or a custom that frequently arises from cultural or ethnic backgrounds, from family tradition, from peer group ideas and practices, from political philosophies in one's country, and from educational and religious philosophies with which one identifies. Some values are unique to the individual; other values are more readily identified as arising from a particular group, philosophy, or culture.

Because we all form values and value systems, we also engage in a practice called *value judgment*. This practice refers to a personal decision about whether something is right or wrong. These decisions are usually affected by the society, the culture, and the period of history in which we live. We generally hold these decisions to be true and right and find support for them from others around us who agree and will support our claim to righteousness.

Because we are nurses as well as persons, we also have another set of values under which we operate. We are expected to provide care for others who often feel or believe differently from ourselves. The professional value system, as well as a personal one, often dictates that nurses must not abandon the person who has sought their care. Nurses can handle this situation in two different ways. First nurses may decide to continue care. To maintain their own integrity, however, nurses may not become involved in the process but merely support the person as he or she carries through the plan himself or herself. The notion of empathy and techniques in problem solving are discussed in succeeding chapters and will be of use to the nurse involved in this kind of situation. Second, if values are seriously threatened, the nurse may decide to find another nurse or agencies to assist the client.

We might consider the example of a person who wishes to terminate his or her chemotherapy for cancer. The nurse may know, given certain statistics, that chemotherapy offers a chance for long-term survival, while termination may result in less than a year of life. The nurse may believe that stopping therapy is an inappropriate decision, but can remain objective and act as a listener so the person can explore his or her ideas. However, the nurse whose values are seriously threatened may want to engage another nurse who is comfortable with this person's decision to assist the person with planning and problem solving.

GENERAL PRINCIPLES OF GROWTH AND DEVELOPMENT

The purpose of this next section is to suggest an application of several growth and development theories to the delivery of effective nursing care. Growth and development are variables in the biopsychosocial functioning of the person. We wish to acquaint students with several prominent theorists to provide background and resource material for understanding skills nurses use in practice. This knowledge increases our awareness of the total person concept. For example, knowledge about psychosocial development helps the nurse work with the teenager whose lagging physical development contributes to poor school work. The most exciting reason for considering growth and development, however, is that it demonstrates the unending potential of the human being throughout life.

The subject and theories of growth and development are far more lengthy than can be described here. A brief discussion is included in this text for the purposes stated above. We expect that students will use the ideas presented to understand aspects that are both common and unique to clients. For a more thorough examination of the subject, refer to the publications cited at the end of this chapter.

Growth

The term **growth** refers to an actual biological or quantitative increase in physical size, that is, the enlargement of any body components by an increase in the number of cells.

Maturation means development of those cells until they can be completely used by the organism (Turner and Helms, 1979, p 7).

Some key ideas related to growth are as follows.

- Physical growth occurs at different rates among individuals.
- Growth of the body parts and systems of a person occurs at different rates; for example, a child may be within normal height and weight ranges for age 5 years but have a less mature urinary elimination system that causes bed wetting. During adolescence, a person's features may appear too large for the face but will eventually be in proper proportion as the size of the head increases.
- A wide range of normal values exists for height, weight, muscle development, and physical abilities at all ages and stages of development. Charts that describe physical characteristics of different ages should be used only as guidelines.

Development

"**Development** is the patterned, orderly, lifelong changes in structure, thought, or behavior that evolve as a result of maturation of physical and mental capacity, experiences, and learning and result in a new level of maturity and integration" (Murray and Zentner, 1985, p 33). A developmental task is a growth responsibility that arises at a certain time in the course of development. If resolution of the task occurs, satisfaction and success with later tasks will probably result. Failure to resolve the tasks in a satisfactory manner leads to unhappiness, disapproval by society, and difficulty with later developmental tasks and functions.

Some principles of development to consider are listed below:

1 Development that occurs in childhood provides a base for the rest of life.
2 Development proceeds in a predictable and sequential way throughout life.
3 The developing person acquires competency in four major areas across the life span.
   a Physical: gaining motor and neurological capacities.
   b Cognitive: learning how to perceive, think, and communicate thoughts and feelings.
   c Emotional: developing awareness and acceptance of self as a unique individual, reacting to the environment, coping with stresses, assuming responsibility for personal behavior.
   d Social: learning to interrelate first with the family and later with different persons in many situations
   (Murray and Zentner, 1985, p 37)

When performing a nursing assessment (see discussion of the nursing process, Chapter 8), it is especially useful to consider those aspects of development that are most pertinent to the client's age. For example, the 6-year-old child will be learning to write in school. Thus, an assessment of his or her fine motor development would be useful. The adolescent person who is struggling with identity and change in body image may benefit from assessment and care planning related to secondary sex characteristics and the condition of the skin. Older adults experiencing changes in body structure will be helped if planning centers on their motor ability.

The discussion in the following sections of this chapter will describe the theories of Erik Erikson, a major theorist in psychosocial development, and Jean Piaget, a major theorist in cognitive development. These two men are well known and accepted in their fields. Their work provides nurses with a base for understanding the development of the psychological and social components of the person.

PSYCHOSOCIAL DEVELOPMENT: ERIKSON

Our discussion of Erikson begins with his enumeration of developmental tasks as outlined in Table 4–2. The following ideas from Erikson's classic work, *Childhood and Society* (1963), can be used by nurses to apply concepts from psychosocial developmental theory to practice:

1   At each stage of development, a nuclear conflict arises (e.g., trust versus mistrust). The negative senses (mistrust, shame, guilt, etc.) of each stage are the dynamic counterparts of the positive ones throughout life. Aspects of these counterparts are present in all of us at one time or another.

2   Developmental levels are resolved, not achieved.

3   At each stage of development, a ratio—preferably a favorable one—develops between the positive and negative senses of each nuclear conflict such that skills are formed throughout life for coping with stress. For example, trust is learned in infancy through satisfaction of basic needs.

4   Stressors have an impact on our lives and new inner conflicts develop throughout the life span. Our ability to cope is closely associated with the ratio of resolution that has occurred during work on previous tasks.

5   At each age, all the developmental tasks are present in us at some level.

6   Each task exists from birth in some form before its critical time for resolution normally arrives.

7   Theorists have suggested that the first two tasks (trust versus mistrust and autonomy versus shame and doubt) lay the groundwork for the person's future. Many conflicts that occur in later life may well be a reflection of the ratio of resolution that has occurred in those early tasks. For example, Erikson believes that in society at large, the resolution of basic trust is reflected in faith (religion, social action, or scientific pursuit). The resolution of autonomy is reflected in the principles of law and order.

8   Evidence suggests that persons become ill—physically and psychologically—if the impact of stressors is overwhelming. This phenomenon is influenced by the achievement of coping skills through developmental task resolution.

9   The strength acquired at any stage is tested by the necessity to transcend it in such a way that the individual can take chances in the next stage with what was most vulnerably precious in the last one. For example, as the child resolves autonomy versus shame and doubt, he or she can move on to the next task and not need to demand his or her own way unreasonably.

10   Erikson believed these stages of development are present in all of the human species. The realization and demonstration of resolution may be reflected in the particular customs and style of many different ethnic, cultural, and national groups. The essence of development, however, is the same for us all.

We continue to work on resolution of all the tasks throughout life. Erikson described the outcome potential of the favorable ratios of each stage of development. He called the words italicized below the *basic virtues*. He

(Text continues on page 97)

TABLE 4–2
DEVELOPMENTAL TASKS ACCORDING TO ERIKSON

Age	Task	Favorable Outcome	Unfavorable Outcome
Birth–1 year	Basic trust versus mistrust	Lets mother out of sight without undue anxiety or rage.	Senses an inner division; feels deprived or divided: feels abandoned.
		Learns that mother has become an inner certainty and an outer predictability.	Develops defense mechanisms, projection and introjection against anticipated loss or disappointment. Projection: "Attributing one's own thoughts or impulses to another person" (Stuart, 1979, p 84). Introjection: "Intense type of identification in which a person incorporates qualities or values of another person or group into his own ego structure" (p 84)
		Correlates inner remembrances and anticipation of sensation with outer sameness of experience; this leads to familiarity and prediction. Engages in constant testing of relationships both inside and outside.	
		Begins not only to trust the outer provider but also to trust oneself and the capacity of one's own organs to cope with urges.	
1–3 years	Autonomy versus shame and doubt	Develops a set of social modalities associated with holding on and letting go.	Develops a set of social modalities associated with holding on and letting go.

(*TABLE* 4–2 continued)

Age	Task	Favorable Outcome	Unfavorable Outcome
		Benign expectations: letting go (to let be); holding on (to have and to hold).	Hostile expectations: letting go (letting loose of detructive forces); holding on (destructive or cruel restraining forces).
		Experiences definite wish to have a choice, begins to stand on own two feet, begins to develop a sense of self-control without loss of self-esteem; this can develop into a lasting sense of good will and pride.	Shame: becomes conscious of being upright and exposed; tries to get away with things unseen; could become defiant and shameless. Doubt: senses that one is dominated by the will of others; senses a loss of control and of foreign overcontrol; develops a lasting propensity for doubt and shame.
		Develops basic faith in existence. Autonomy fostered in childhood helps develop a sense of justice later in life.	
4–5 years	Initiative versus guilt	Senses hope and new responsibility; a vigorous unfolding. Learns quickly and avidly.	Superego becomes cruel and uncompromising, causing repression in some persons (who becomes inhibited or impotent) and exhibitionism ("showing off") in others.
		Develops judgment; is active, energetic; develops direction; can undertake, plan, and attack a task.	
		Cooperates, works with other children for a purpose, constructs and plans cooperatively.	

(Table 4–2 continues)

(*TABLE 4–2 continued*)

Age	Task	Favorable Outcome	Unfavorable Outcome
		Establishes a moral sense that restricts the horizon of the permissible.	Submerges rage, which causes self-righteousness. Often psychosomatic disease is noted in the adult who fails to resolve this developmental task.
6–11 years	Industry versus inferiority	Wins recognition by producing things, because this is the age of formal and systematic instruction, whether the school is the classroom, field, or jungle.	
		Begins readiness to move beyond or outside the family.	Remains unsure of status with peers and partners.
		Begins to handle tools and develops skills with them.	
		Applies self to skills and tasks.	Feels unsure of skills and tools.
		Directs attention and perseveres; goes beyond desire to plan and develops a sense of satisfaction in work completion.	
		Senses a division of labor and differential opportunity.	Restricts self and horizons to include only own work; becomes a conformist and thoughtless slave of the technology.
		Senses the characteristics of the culture.	Begins to feel the color of skin and background of parents and to feel judged by it.
12–20 years	Identity versus role confusion	Questions continuity and sameness from past; searches for a new continuity and sameness.	Confuses sex roles because of doubt regarding sexual identity.

(TABLE 4–2 continued)

Age	Task	Favorable Outcome	Unfavorable Outcome
		Concerns self with appearance to others versus what one feels oneself to be.	Overidentifies with heroes, cliques, and crowds (to the loss of individual identity). Behaves in a clannish and cruel manner to all those who are different (a defense against a sense of identity confusion).
		Develops a confidence that the inner sameness and continuity prepared in the past are matched by the sameness and continuity of one's meaning for others, as evidenced in the tangible promise of a career.	
		Senses an ideology and a commitment to it; finds self in the stage between the morality learned by the child and the ethics developed by the adult.	Becomes an easy prey to cruel totalitarian doctrines and ideology.
20–40 years, early adulthood	Intimary versus isolation	Becomes eager and willing to fuse one's identity with others; ready for intimacy; has capacity to commit oneself to concrete affiliations and partnerships.	Avoids intimate relationships and commitment for fear of ego loss. This leads to a deep sense of isolation and self-absorption.
		Develops the ethical strength to abide by one's commitments.	Develops prejudice.

(Table 4–2 continues)

(TABLE 4–2 continued)

Age	Task	Favorable Outcome	Unfavorable Outcome
		Welcomes situations that require self-abandonment: solidarity of close affiliations, sexual unions, close friendships, physical combat, and experiences of inspiration from teachers, institutions, and the recesses of the self.	Fears others' encroachment on one's territory.
41–60 years, middle adulthood.	Generativity versus stagnation	Concerns self with establishing and guiding the next generation. Mature persons need to be needed.	Experiences a pervasive sense of stagnation and personal impoverishment; needs pseudointimacy.
		Produces and creates.	
		Believes in and has faith in the species, sees the child or the younger generation as a welcome trust.	Indulges self; early invalidism, physical or psychological disorders becomes a vehicle of self-concern.
64 years and on, late adulthood	Ego integrity versus despair	Sees self as the originator of others or a generator of products and ideas. In this person, the fruits of other stages of development gradually ripen: hope, willpower, purpose, competence, fidelity, love, care, and wisdom.	Feels despair: time is too short to start over.
		Senses an assurance that there is order and meaning in the sense of the world and of the spirit.	

(TABLE 4–2 continued)

Age	Task	Favorable Outcome	Unfavorable Outcome
		Accepts one's own life cycle as the way it had to be. Experiences a sense of comradeship with the past.	Does not accept one's only life cycle as the ultimate of life.
		Defends the dignity of one's own life style.	
		Experiences a final consolation and emotional integration.	Behaves with disgust, which hides despair and the fear of death.
		Acceptance of death.	

(Adapted from Erikson E: Childhood and Society, 2nd ed, pp 247–274. New York, WW Norton, 1963)

pointed out that these basic virtues are those that reemerge from generation to generation and constitute the spirit and relevance of human systems:

- Basic trust versus mistrust: drive and *hope*
- Autonomy versus shame and doubt: self-control and *willpower*
- Initiative versus guilt: direction and *purpose*
- Industry versus inferiority: method and *competence*
- Identity versus role confusion: devotion and *fidelity*
- Intimacy versus isolation: affiliation and *love*
- Generativity versus stagnation: production and *care*
- Ego integrity versus despair: renunciation and *wisdom*

The boxed anecdotes are entries from the logs of two nursing students. Both students have recorded their experiences with persons representing two of the age groups discussed by Erikson. They have described these persons appropriately and with insight.

Example 1. According to Erikson, these children are working on the tasks of initiative versus guilt. Today the children were working with sponge painting, making pumpkin faces. Julie was acting silly like 4-year-olds do and just colored the whole piece of paper (pumpkin) while watching others make eyes, nose, and mouth. Christopher was soaking up lots of paint in his sponge, then pressing it down hard so it made a big pool of paint. Even after he was told not to press so hard, he went ahead and did it anyway. Sometimes (probably a lot of the time) children of this age do not listen very well; they just go ahead with what they are doing. The rest of the children, from what I observed, did a good job of making two eyes, a nose, and a mouth on their pumpkins, showing their ability to be creative. Kevin did better in this aspect than some of the others but he observed for a while before he started to draw.

When the children were having their snack they were acting silly, which is normal for this age group. They were grabbing each others' arms and shaking them. Kevin would do this to Carey, but he wouldn't let her do it to him. Maybe this was Kevin's way of protecting his body, which children of this age are now learning to do (A. Keskey, personal communication, November 1980).

Example 2. According to Erikson, Mrs. Holden is facing integrity versus disgust and despair. I feel Mrs. Holden has resolved this task. She was telling me about the "old Ann Arbor," the way it was when she was young. Some of what she liked then included such things as no cars on campus. She explained how things have changed so much, especially for women (i.e., athletics, females in the band, cheerleading). Even so, as she looks at it, she always has had the philosophy that she was only young once and that it was her opportune time to have fun, and she did. Granted, things maybe did not turn out exactly the way she had planned (she did not get into medical school), yet she became a med. tech. and worked in that field for many years. She also became a teacher. Mrs. Holden adjusted to her life as she went along and had fun in the process. Now, when she looks back, she doesn't regret any of it or hopelessly long for the past. She accepts it as a good part of her life, which she enjoys remembering and talking about with people like me.

Mrs. Holden has pursued new interests in order to gain status, recognition, and a feeling of being needed. She also uses her nurturing qualities to help others (myself, her friends) and in so doing feels needed and feels good about herself (K. O'Shea, personal communication, November, 1980).

The theories of Maslow and Erikson blend well together. One might note that a person's ability to meet his or her basic needs is reflected by the degree to which the person has resolved the developmental tasks of trust and autonomy. When stress seriously affects one's sense of safety, adaptive coping can occur if the person has a sense of trust, self-control, direction, purpose, and competence. In other words, the ability to meet our basic needs on a daily basis is directly related to the amount of skill we have developed through resolution of the developmental tasks.

Maslow emphasized that the basic needs are satisfied not only by receiving but also by giving. In fact, giving is essential to satisfaction. We provide a safe atmosphere and protect the safety needs of small children and others who are unable to do this for themselves. We wish to give love and friendship, as well as to receive it. Erikson pointed out the need to be trusted as well as to trust, to develop a sense of devotion and intimacy toward others, and to produce or care for the next generation. He maintained that the mature person needs to be needed, and that the older adult develops wisdom that he or she wishes to pass on to the younger generation.

If, as persons ourselves, or as persons who are nurses, we consider our own development and ability to meet our basic needs, we can be more effective in helping others move toward the basic virtues and self-actualization.

| COGNITIVE DEVELOPMENT: PIAGET

Piaget described cognitive development as a continuous progression from the spontaneous movements and reflexes of the newborn, to acquired habits of the infant, to the beginning of the development of intelligence which becomes apparent toward the end of the first year of life. Cognitive development is cumulative; understanding of new experiences evolves from what was learned during earlier ones. Piaget (1973) identified four major levels in the development of cognition or growth of thought, which follow.

Sensoriomotor Level: Birth to 2 Years

The following discussion describes the mechanism of progression toward the development of intelligence.

Assimilation

Reality data (i.e., input from the real world) are treated or modified in such a way as to become incorporated into the structure of the person. Piaget used *structure* to describe how information is organized within the person to make a simple mental image or pattern of action. Although the necessary mental structures are genetically destined, these structures mature with age. The organizing activity of the person is as important as the interrelationships inherent in the external stimuli. This idea might be represented in the following way.

$$\text{Stimulus} \longleftrightarrow \text{Response}$$
$$\text{Person}$$

The input stimulus is filtered through a person who develops action-schemes or, at a higher level, the operations of thought, which in turn are modified and enriched when the person's behavioral repertoire increases to meet the demands of reality. **Assimilation** then is the process of taking novel information and making it fit a preconceived notion about objects or the world. Later, the child will be able to find new ways of looking at things.

Accommodation

Accommodation is the alteration of internal schemes to fit reality: reconciling new experiences or objects by revising the old plan to fit the new input. Singer and Revenson (1978) provide us with an example of this process in the infant. Initially, the child attempts to understand something new by using old solutions, that is, by assimilation. When this method does not work, the youngster is forced to modify his or her existing view of the world to interpret the experience. The baby who attempts to drink milk from a rattle (assimilation) quickly learns that rattles make noise but do not yield milk. The rattle no longer substitutes for feeding (accommodation).

This dual process of assimilation-accommodation leads to **adaptation**, which is a continuing process of learning from the environment and learning to adjust to alterations in the environment. Adaptation allows the child to form a *schema*, a more complex mental image, an action organization that a person uses to explain what he or she sees and hears (Singer and Revenson, 1978, pp 13–15).

During the period from birth to 2 years, the infant relies on the senses and his or her motor activity for information about the world. Reflex actions occur during this period. The infant recognizes them as successful actions but has no knowledge about them. The infant's understanding of the world involves only perceptions and objects with which he or she has direct experience. As language appears, usually at about 1.5 to 2 years, the development of symbolic or preconceptual thought begins. Toward the end of the sensorimotor phase, the child begins to understand the concept of *object permanence*: the child begins to realize that objects can exist apart from himself or herself. When the child cannot see an object, he or she begins to understand that it is still there. The child can accept the mother leaving his or her sight because the child knows she is near and will return.

Preoperational Level: Age 2 to 7 Years

The preoperational level is the period of curiosity, questioning, and investigation. Children take an interest in their environment but still interpret it according to their own point of view. This approach is called **egocentrism**. The child uses explanations of the world he or she knows and makes up others to answer his or her questions. An especially descriptive example of preoperational thinking found in literature is the following discussion between Scout (Jean Louise Finch) and Miss Maudie Atkinson in Harper Lee's novel To Kill a Mockingbird. Scout at age 6 is asking questions about Boo Radley, a reclusive man who lives in her neighborhood, and whom Scout has never seen.

> "Miss Maudie," I said one evening, "do you think Boo Radley's still alive?"
> "His name's Arthur and he's alive," she said. . . .
> "Yessum. How do you know?". . . .
> "What a morbid question. But I suppose it's a morbid subject. I know he's alive,
> Jean Louise, because I haven't seen him carried out yet."
> "Maybe he died and they stuffed him up the chimney."
> (1960, p 48)

In this conversation, both Scout and Miss Maudie deal with object permanence and preoperational thinking. Scout worries that if she cannot see the man, he does not exist. However, if he has died they must have done something with him because no one was seen carrying him out. Thus, the solution of stuffing him up the chimney satisfies her to some extent. Miss Maudie believes that if she has not seen him carried out, his death has not occurred. However, she is more concrete than is Scout and does not create a silly explanation to satisfy her curiosity. Still, we can make the observation that even adults may revert to earlier thinking when things become too confusing or overwhelming.

Concrete Operations Level: Age 7 to 11 Years

Piaget defines an **operation** as an interiorized action or an action performed in the mind (Singer and Revenson, 1978, p 20). Several qualities characterize the concrete operations level:

- *Reversibility*. The direction of thought can be reversed mentally. When children learn addition, they can then learn subtraction. The child knows how to find the way to school and how to turn around and find the way home again.
- *Seriation*. The child has the ability to arrange objects mentally according to a quantitative dimension such as size or weight.
- *Conservation*. The person has the ability to see that objects or quantities remain the same despite a change in their physical appearance. The child understands such quantities as number, substance (mass), area, weight, volume. The child can understand that a quantity of liquid is the same whether it fills a short, fat container or a tall, thin one.

The child applies his or her concrete operations to objects that are physically present. As adults, we often use concrete operations when we first learn a new skill. We wish to be told how to proceed step by step. Later, we can think more broadly and develop our own process while continuing to follow the basic principles. Some people learn more quickly than others, depending on background knowledge, skill, and general abilities.

Formal Operations Level: Age 11 to 16 Years

The child can now consider objects that are not present and perform formal operations by considering the future and the abstract. As the child reaches adolescence, he or she can problem solve using more rational and scientific processes. The child's thinking is more flexible and he or she can consider various ways to solve a problem or view an experience. The child can make relationships among several pieces of information and draw rational conclusions. Piaget hypothesized that we do not develop any new mental structures after the stage of formal operations. He believed that intellectual development from this point on consists of an increase of knowledge and depth of understanding.

Nursing Implications

The theory of cognitive development as described by Piaget helps nurses recognize how children develop intelligence and learn to think. The theory suggests that certain approaches to teaching are more effective at different times. For example, we recognize that stress also affects how our adult clients think and learn and may cause them to revert to earlier ways of processing information. Moreover, the response to learning under stress may vary according to the individual. Some persons learn when alarmed or aroused because of a critical need for information, whereas others are unable to concentrate on the task at hand. The nurse will want to assess how stress affects a particular person's ability to learn.

Piaget described intelligence as the indispensable instrument for interaction between the subject and the universe. Feeling directs behavior by assigning a value to its end; feeling provides the energy necessary for action and knowledge gives a structure to it. Piaget stated that every action involves an energetic or affective aspect and a structural or cognitive aspect (Piaget 1973, pp 4–5).

It is wise to take note of the fact that the ages stated for each level are somewhat arbitrary. That is, a child may be either slower or faster than suggested in reaching a new level; the range of normal is very broad.

Nurses also note that adults demonstrate great variance in the ability to use formal operations of thought. This quality becomes apparent when we assist adult clients to learn about their health needs. Those who are more comfortable with concrete thought operations may take longer to understand and apply new information; those who have used formal thought processes may understand more quickly. Therefore, nurses contemplating health teaching and care planning will need to assess both age level and the client's ability to grasp and apply information.

In summary, we might reconsider how nurses can use the theories of Erikson, Piaget, and Maslow together when planning nursing care. For example, we know that persons use their intelligence as well as their feeling states to solve problems and to develop skills toward the resolution of developmental tasks. Infants learn to trust, in part, because they use their beginning cognitive skills of recognition and memory to know who mother is. The adolescent or young adult uses the ability to think conceptually and to make relationships among the pieces of information he or she receives. This assists the individual to make good decisions about how to take care of himself or herself and how to plan the direction he or she wishes his or her life to take. If we consider Maslow's theories, we know that a person's ability to meet the basic needs may also influence the decisions the person makes about self and his or her life.

FROM DEVELOPMENTAL THEORY TO CLINICAL APPLICATION

We have drawn from the works of Maslow and Erikson to talk about the control persons have in realizing their potential. Nurses view persons as individuals with the potential to take care of themselves and achieve a high level of health. Carl Rogers provided us with several important "learnings" — as he called them — which give support to the concepts of person-centered nursing care and self-care as discussed in Chapter 6. He developed a person-centered therapy throughout his many years as a counselor and psychotherapist. He stated,

> It is the *client* who knows what hurts, what directions to go, what problems are crucial, what experiences have been deeply buried. It began to occur to me that unless I had a need to demonstrate my own cleverness and learning, I would do better to rely upon the client for the direction of movement in the process. (1961, pp 11–12)

Rogers described how he learned to listen to and accept himself and his own feelings about a particular person or a situation. He believed that to act one way on the surface while feeling another way underneath becomes more of a hindrance than a help in developing a therapeutic (healing) relationship. According to Rogers, it is important for a person not to try to be something he or she is not.

Although Carl Rogers did not use the word *empathy* (which the student will find in Chapter 9), he nevertheless described it when he gave us another of his learnings: "I have found it of enormous value when I can permit myself to understand another person" (1961, p 18). He used the word *permit* because he believed that too often we respond immediately to another person's ideas as right or wrong, good or bad, moral or immoral. We respond because of our own value system and out of fear that if we really understand the person, it might somehow change us or our way of thinking, a distressing notion. We do not want to lose a part of ourselves in response to another person. He went on to point out, however, that rather than changing, we become enriched and can grow when we truly understand the ideas and feelings of others.

Rogers believed strongly in learning from his own experience and in trusting what he had learned. He stated, "I can only try to live by *my* interpretation of the current meaning of *my* experience, and try to give others the permission and freedom to develop their own inward freedom and thus their own meaningful interpretation of their own experience. If there is such a thing as truth, this free individual process of search should, I believe, converge toward it" (1961, p 27). These words provide for nurses the essence of the person-centered approach to nursing care and can, if we return to them again and again, assist us in developing and delivering effective and relevant care to the persons nurses seek to help toward the healthy state.

OTHER THEORETICAL VIEWS
OF PERSON

The material presented so far in this chapter offers humanistic and varied views of person that are not exclusive to the discipline of nursing: the view is generic and applicable to all persons as suggested earlier in the Erikson discussion. Nursing, however, is unique among the health professions in claiming the holistic biopsychosocial person as the client of its care. Also, there are other theorists — nurse-theorists — who present a somewhat different view of the concept of person. Selected views of *person* as described by nurse-theorists are briefly mentioned here to illustrate how the basic concept can be enriched or modified in its application to nursing.

Within the science of nursing, various theorists have suggested refinements of the concept *person* based on their particular conceptual models. According to Fawcett (1984), each conceptual model provides a "distinctive" frame of reference regarding how an important phenomenon like person is defined and described. The following selected examples provide brief illustrations of this point.

Orem defined a person as "a unity that can be viewed as functioning biologically, symbolically, and socially" (1980, p 120). In her model, persons who are healthy are able to care for themselves. Individual people have a need for nursing care when they are unable to care for themselves. Self-care needs are of three kinds: universal, developmental, or health-deviation. Ability to meet personal needs is "self-care agency." The universal self-care needs are comparable to Maslow's basic needs. Developmental needs relate to points in the life cycle (as in Erikson or Piaget stages), whereas health-deviation needs relate to alterations in both human structure and function. "Functioning symbolically," as Orem suggests, might encompass both the psychological and spiritual elements of person-centered care.

Martha Rogers described *person* — that is, the unitary man (1970) and the human being (1983) — as synergistic: a whole greater and different than the sum of its parts. Man (1970) was explicitly defined as an energy field, as was his or her environment which Martha Rogers viewed as all the universe external to unitary man. In later writing, Rogers regarded person and environment as "integral [belonging as a part of the whole] with each other" (1980, p. 232). Clearly, person as an energy field was conceptualized as more than the visible physical being and also a whole greater than the sum of its parts.

According to Martha Rogers, other characteristics of person are wholeness and unidirectionality in moving through time-space and the powers of perception and thought. "Abstraction and imagery, language and thought, sensation and emotion are fundamental attributes of man's humanness" (1970, p 67). These qualities take on importance as persons make choices about interaction with the environment and also convey to nurses their thoughts and emotions about changes in their health status. Rogers's distinctive theoretical characteristic of person, however, is the notion of person as energy field. This unique notion of person offers interesting appeal for high-technology, space age health care.

Sister Callista Roy described *person* as a biopsychosocial being and also as an adaptive system as evident in the following explanation:

> The nature of man includes the biological level with components such as anatomical parts which function physiologically. . . . These anatomical parts function as a whole to contribute to the biological constancy of man. At the same time, man has a psychological

nature. His various biological systems, headed by the complex nervous system, together produce meaningful behavior. This behavior is organized in such a way that man has constancy in his life of perceiving, learning, and acting. Lastly, man is a social being, and his behavior is related to the behavior of others on group levels such as family, community, and work groups. (1976, p. 11)

Roy also noted that a person has "two major internal processor subsystems, the regulator and the cognator" (Roy and Roberts, 1981, p. 43). The *regulator subsystem* is concerned mostly with physiological needs. The *cognator subsystem* assists with coping related not only to physiologic needs but also self-concept, role function, and interdependence, that is, the other adaptive "modes" of Roy's model. Work is ongoing to make her mechanistic model more holistic.

As these and other theoretical views of person are refined, they will undoubtedly influence both future nursing research and care delivery. Many aspiring professionals are strongly attracted to nursing because of the opportunity to work closely with persons in all aspects of their beings: biological, psychological, social, cultural, and spiritual.

THIS INCREDIBLE BEING: THE PERSON

We have briefly explored the essence of this incredible being called the person whose subsystems interrelate and produce a being greater than the sum of his parts. What causes the person to be strong in the face of weakness, healthy in the face of illness, brave in the face of grief? How is it that the person can continue to grow and flourish through a lifetime, and even during periods of great strife? The very nature of the unique person is perplexing and our understanding, though developing, is still limited. In her book, *Heartsounds* (1980), Lear described her husband who lived through a cardiac crisis despite medical expectations to the contrary.

> An intern recalled, "We got a guy with an infiltrated intravenous. So he wasn't getting dopamine, the drug to maintain blood pressure. He had no palpable blood pressure and yet he was able to talk to us. This in itself was unusual. He was in cardiac shock: blood pressure too low to maintain life; no urine; decreased mentation; clammy extremities. I would have thought his chances of coming through were very, very small."

And after Mrs. Lear's husband had improved the cardiologist came out to tell the family.

> "He's better. He wants to know every detail of treatment. He's driving them all crazy in there. It's unbelievable. It's something spiritual, that fight, that fight that keeps him alive."

When Mrs. Lear goes in to see her husband she describes it like this.

> He lay still panting, his eyes closed, his face remote behind the [oxygen] mask, and I wondered *Better?* but surely they are wrong. How can anyone who looks like this be *better?* And I bent down again . . . and whispered, "Darling, you're much *better*. You've got to *fight*. You're going to *make it*. You're going to *make it*."
>
> And with one sudden swift move he ripped the mask off his face and turned to confront me directly. His eyes consumed me. *"I've already made it"* he said. (1980, pp 338–339)

| CONCLUSION

This chapter presented a holistic perspective of the person based on Maslow's hierarchy of basic human needs. Each person shares basic needs and aspirations with other persons but is also unique in heritage, particular needs, and striving. Values and perceptions of self contribute another dimension to a person. The self-actualizing tendency of man motivates the person to fulfill individual potential. Using this holistic perspective, the nurse considers clients' strengths and needs, not in isolation but in relation to other needs and strengths. The holistic person is the recipient of nursing care. Person-centered care is the essence of professional nursing.

This chapter also introduced some of the basic understandings of growth and development that apply to person-centered nursing care. The resolution of developmental tasks is a lifelong process, as is self-actualization. Both illustrate that life itself is a dynamic process of becoming. The cognitive skills that are uniquely human cannot be separated from other aspects of the holistic person. If a person experiences an alteration in any component of the holistic system, it may be reflected in functioning that is characteristic of an earlier stage of growth and development.

| STUDY QUESTIONS

1   Consider the following situation: a 45-year-old man is in the hospital recovering from a heart attack. His wife divorced him a year ago, leaving their three teenage children in his care. The children are alone while he is in the hospital. Consider the biopsychosocial needs of this man and discuss how the concept of holism applies in this situation.

2   Explain the terms *open system* and *closed system* and discuss how they occur within the person.

3   Describe the notion of energy movement between systems and subsystems.

4   Discuss the categories of basic needs on Maslow's hierarchy and give an example of each.

5   Consider yourself as a person. How do such terms as self-concept, self-ideal, self-esteem, and body image apply to you?

6   Consider the following situation: A 40-year-old woman is hospitalized for a radical mastectomy (surgical removal of the breast). Throughout her recovery period she wears a large heavy robe, even though it is summer. She is aloof to the female nurses and openly rude to her male doctor. She stares out the window when her husband visits and shows little interest in the activities of her children. Analyze this woman's response using the concepts discussed in the section on the person's view of self.

7   Discuss the notions of *value* and *value judgment*. What kinds of experiences influence how we develop value systems? How would you feel about a person who refuses chemotherapy for cancer? If you were unable to assist such a person, how would you feel about yourself?

8   Discuss how the terms *growth*, *maturation*, and *development* are pertinent to each person.

9   State the age, the developmental task, and the basic virtue of each age of man

according to Erikson. Describe how these factors would influence the nursing care of a variety of persons.

10 Consider several persons in different stages and assess their resolution of the Erikson developmental tasks. Describe the balance they have attained between the favorable and unfavorable outcomes for their particular level.

11 Define the terms associated with Piaget's theory of cognitive development. Describe how you would use this theory when giving safety tips to first-graders.

12 Identify "learnings" according to Carl Rogers and suggest an application for such ideas.

| REFERENCES

Abbey JC: General systems theory: A framework for nursing. In Putt A (ed): General Systems Theory Applied to Nursing, pp 9–16. Boston, Little, Brown, 1978

du Maurier D: The Scapegoat. Garden City, NY, Doubleday, 1957

Erickson HC, Tomlin EM, Swain MA: Modeling and Role-Modeling: A Theory and Paradigm for Nursing. Englewood Cliffs, NJ, Prentice-Hall, 1983

Erikson EH: Childhood and Society, 2nd ed. New York, WW Norton, 1963

Fawcett J: Analysis and Evaluation of Conceptual Models of Nursing. Philadelphia, FA Davis, 1984

Hall AD, Fagen RE: Definitions of Systems. In Buckley W (ed): Modern Systems Research for the Behavioral Scientist, pp 81–92. Chicago, Aldine, 1968

Klir GJ: Preview: The polyphonic general systems theory. In Klir GJ (ed): Trends in General Systems Theory. New York, John Wiley & Sons, 1972

Lear MW: Heartsounds. New York, Simon & Schuster, 1980

Lee H: To Kill a Mockingbird. Philadelphia, JB Lippincott, 1960

Maslow A: Motivation and Personality, 2nd ed. New York, Harper & Row, 1970

Murray RB, Zentner JP: Nursing Assessment and Health Promotion Through the Life Span, 3rd ed. Englewood Cliffs, NJ, Prentice-Hall, 1985

Orem DE: Nursing: Concepts of Practice, 2nd ed. New York, McGraw-Hill, 1980

Piaget J: The Psychology of Intelligence. Totowa, NJ, Littlefield, Adams & Co, 1973

Polit D, Hungler B: Nursing Research: Principles and Methods, 3rd ed. Philadelphia, JB Lippincott, 1987

Rogers CR: On Becoming a Person. Boston, Houghton Mifflin, 1961

Rogers ME: An Introduction to the Theoretical Basis of Nursing. Philadelphia, FA Davis, 1970

Rogers ME: Nursing: A science of unitary man. In Riehl JP, Roy C (eds): Conceptual Models for Nursing Practice, 2nd ed, pp 329–337. New York, Appleton-Century-Crofts, 1980

Rogers ME: Science of Unitary Human Being: A Paradigm for Nursing. In Clements EW, Roberts FB (eds): Family Health: A Theoretical Approach to Nursing Care, pp 390–391. New York, John Wiley & Sons, 1983

Roy C: Introduction to Nursing: An Adaptational Model. Englewood Cliffs, NJ, Prentice-Hall, 1976

Roy C, Roberts SL: Theory Construction in Nursing: An Adaptation Model. Englewood Cliffs, NJ, Prentice-Hall, 1981

Singer DG, Revenson TA: A Piaget Primer: How a Child Thinks. New York, New American Library, 1978

Smuts JC: Holism and Evolution. New York, Macmillan, 1926

Tolstoy L: Childhood. In Tolstoy L: The Complete Works of Count Tolstoy, vol I. Dana Estes, 1904. Reissued by Colonial Press

Turner JS, Helms DB: Life Span Development. Philadelphia, WB Saunders, 1979

von Bertalanffy L: General systems theory: A critical review. In Buckley W (ed): Modern Systems Research for the Behavioral Scientist, pp 11–30. Chicago, Aldine, 1968

5 | ENVIRONMENT

KEY WORDS	After completing this chapter, students will be able to:
Boundary	**Define the environment.**
Communication	**Identify the relationship of person–environment interaction to**
Culture	**health.**
Ecology	
Environment	**Describe several nurse-theorists' concepts of environment.**
Ethnicity	**Discuss factors within the immediate physical environment and**
Family	**the physical environment of the community that affect health.**
Group	
Norm	**Discuss how the social environment affects health.**
Person–environment fit	**Identify the relevance of cultural factors to health care.**
Position	
Role	
Social support	
Society	
Value orientation	

The relationship of the environment to health has been recognized by nurses since the time of Florence Nightingale. Nightingale was one of the first health professionals to emphasize the importance of a healthy environment in the prevention of illness and maintenance of wellness. During the last several decades, chronic disease and pollution have become significant threats to health. Thus, we have seen increased investigation of environmental influences on health within a variety of disciplines including medicine, public health, and sociology.

Nursing, with its emphasis on the care of holistic persons, continues to be concerned with the phenomena of the human being's interaction with the environment in clinical practice, research, and theory development. This chapter examines the interaction between persons and their environment from the perspectives of systems theory and several nurse-theorists. Physical, social, and cultural aspects of the environment as well as their relevance for nursing are also described. Throughout the chapter, the role of nursing in providing an optimum environment for the maintenance of wellness is emphasized.

THE CONCEPT OF ENVIRONMENT

Systems Theory

Environment has been defined in many ways. "Environment refers to the social and physical world outside the system, boundaries, or the community in which the system exists" (Murray and Zentner, 1985, p 7). Systems theory identifies the concepts of external and internal environments. Internal environment includes everything internal to a system's boundaries. The internal environment of a human system includes a variety of subsystems; among these are biological, psychological, sociological, and spiritual systems. This concept was discussed previously in Chapter 4. The external environment includes anything external to a system's boundaries. While most people usually think of environment as consisting of physical surroundings — such as air, climate, water, or buildings — the external environment includes such intangibles as social, cultural, political, and economic systems. Murray and Zentner have stated that "the external environment includes all stimuli, objects, and people impinging on a person" (1985, p 13). In this chapter, we will limit discussion to physical, social, and cultural environments. Political and economic systems affecting health care are discussed in Chapter 7.

Because persons and environment are both open systems, both are constantly interacting, each affecting and being affected by the other. Thus, while we would like to think of ourselves as masters over the environment, we are changed by our surroundings even as we try to alter them. For example, while we use pesticides to kill disease-bearing insects, those chemicals have entered the food chain and may predispose us to cancer. Humans have changed the courses of rivers and restructured the land, yet we are prone to the effects of barometric pressure changes and lunar cycles as evidenced by fluctuations in crime rates (Moos, 1973).

Nurses use systems theory to describe environmental influences on health. Several nurse-theorists have described the relationship of the concept of environment to health in their models of nursing. The theories of Nightingale, Roy, and Rogers are particularly useful in examining the concept of environment.

Nursing Theories

Nightingale

Florence Nightingale was the first nurse to recognize the importance of environmental factors in relation to health. In the mid-1800s, little was known about principles of sanitation: Louis Pasteur's bacteriological studies and Joseph Lister's research on antisepsis were in their early stages. Communicable diseases were the most common cause of death. Contaminated food and water and stale air contributed to the high incidence of bacteria-caused illness. Nightingale believed that fresh air, sunlight, and attention to cleanliness were essential to the recovery of the sick (Nightingale, 1859, p 15). Indeed, by employing these sanitation principles, she was able to reduce the mortality rate of wounded soldiers in the Crimean War from an appalling 42% to just 2.2% (Kalisch and Kalisch, 1986, p 51).

Nightingale believed that the human body had natural healing powers and that the nurse's job was to put persons in the best possible condition for nature to act (Nightingale, 1859, p 75). Given the general medical treatments at the time (bizarre herbs, heavy metals, fomentations), she was correct in her belief that the physician's care often did more harm than good. Her concept of nursing care focused heavily on modifying the physical environment and included the following "five essential points":

- Pure air
- Pure water
- Efficient drainage
- Cleanliness
- Light
  (Nightingale, 1859, p 15)

Nightingale also discussed other environmental factors such as elimination of unnecessary noise, provision of appropriate environmental stimuli, quality of diet, and bedding. Although current concepts of health and the environment are more complex than Nightingale's, most of her writing continues to be relevant for today's nurses.

Roy

Because Roy's nursing model is based on systems theory, it includes environment as an essential component. Roy defined the environment as all of the internal and external conditions, circumstances, and influences surrounding or affecting the development and behavior of persons or groups (Roy, 1987, p 42). Roy acknowledged both an internal and an external environment. Roy classified environmental stimuli as the following:

Focal stimulus. The degree of change or stimulus most immediately confronting the person and the one to which the person must make an adaptive response, that is, the factor that precipitates the behavior.

Contextual stimuli. All other stimuli present that contribute to the behavior caused or precipitated by the focal stimulus.

Residual stimuli. Factors that may be affecting behavior but whose effects are not validated. (1987, p 42)

Changes in the environment provoke coping responses; the human's positive response to a changing environment is adaptation (Roy, 1987, p 42). Nursing's goal is to promote adaptation (or a positive response to environmental change) by removing the focal stimulus or changing the contextual or residual stimuli. The box contains an example of nursing care using the Roy model.

Mrs. Miller is a 28-year-old pregnant woman who is experiencing constipation. In her situation, the physiological changes of pregnancy are the focal stimuli causing constipation. Because the nurse cannot alter this state until Mrs. Miller delivers, the nurse concentrates on contextual stimuli, such as Mrs. Miller's poor fluid intake and low-fiber diet, and the residual stimulus of this client's poor bowel habits prior to pregnancy. The nurse develops a teaching plan that includes increasing fluid and fiber intake as well as information on the hazards of chronic laxative use. By changing contextual and residual stimuli, the nurse hopes to help Mrs. Miller to achieve normal elimination.

Rogers

Martha Rogers's concepts of persons and the environment were influenced by Einstein's physical theories. Rogers believed that both persons and the environment are open systems consisting of energy fields. As energy fields, persons extend beyond their skin and thus are continuous with the environment. The boundaries between persons and the environment are arbitrary because it is difficult to identify where the energy system of a person ends and the environment begins. Thus, persons and environment are constantly interacting to affect and be affected by each other. Nursing seeks to promote a "symphonic interaction between man and environment, to strengthen the adherence and integrity of the human field, and to direct and redirect patterning of the human and environmental fields" (Rogers, 1970, p 122).

| THE PHYSICAL ENVIRONMENT

The physical environment refers to factors that exist in the external environment, such as air, water, food, furnishings, noise, and lighting. The physical environment consists of natural phenomena—such as climate and geography—and human-made phenomena— such as buildings and industry.

The effect of human-made phenomena on the natural environment is currently of great concern. Environmental pollution caused by human activities is becoming increasingly significant as a health hazard. **Ecology** is the study of the relationship between humans and the external environment. An intimate interdependency exists between living things and the environment which the field of ecology seeks to explain.

Ecology is an important science for nurses because it provides insight into factors that affect the health and adaptation of persons. For example, ecological studies might examine the high incidence of malignancy in areas of heavy toxic waste discharge by an industry. Obviously, such health hazards are of concern to nurses, particularly those in community and occupational health nursing. The following discussion first considers the physical environment of the community and then the immediate physical environment, examining factors that influence health.

Physical Environment of the Community

Physical environment of the community is composed of many factors both natural and human-made. They include climate, geography, air quality, water quality, soil quality, and food purity.

Climate

Climate refers to the average weather conditions at a place over a period of years, including factors such as average temperature, humidity, precipitation, and wind velocity. Climate is related to the incidence of particular health problems. For example, malaria and encephalitis are serious health problems in tropical climates which support the breeding of disease-bearing mosquitoes. Climate can exacerbate or relieve chronic health problems. You may have known someone with chronic respiratory disease who moved to Arizona because the dry, pollen-free climate helped relieve symptoms. The weather has also been shown to affect people's behavior: studies have found an increased incidence of violent behavior when temperatures are high (Moos, 1973).

Geography

Geography describes the features of an area: the physical components of land, sea, and air, and the plant and animal life which are supported by these physical features. Like climate, the geography of a region is related to the health status of the population residing there. For example, the Japanese and the Eskimos have a low incidence of cardiac disease. Both groups live in oceanic regions and eat a diet rich in seafood. It is believed that this diet, which is rich in fish oil, may confer protection against heart disease.

Mountainous regions such as the Appalachians and the Rockies make access to health care difficult. Health-care providers need to be creative in assisting people in these areas to reach their services. Mobile health centers and helicopter transportation for emergency victims are used in providing health care.

Air Quality

The quality of air, particularly in urban areas, is deteriorating rapidly. Air pollution, the introduction of impurities into the air, is a major problem in many urban areas. Air pollutants can be classified as particulate matter, organic gases, and inorganic gases. Two major sources of air pollution are automobile emissions — which contain nitrous oxides — and industrial smoke discharge — which emit sulfur oxides (Jarvis, 1985, p 811). Coal-burning factories are significant sources of sulfur oxides which are converted to sulfuric acid in the atmosphere. The resultant "acid rain" has caused incalculable losses to crops and forests. Fossil fuels are predicted to cause a "greenhouse effect" which will warm our climates with unknown effects on agriculture and health.

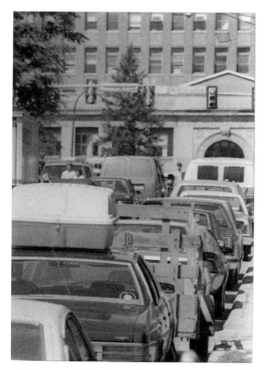

Environment includes social, natural, and human-made variables.

Air pollution can exacerbate symptoms in persons with respiratory disease and allergies. In addition, industries may release noxious chemicals into the atmosphere as by-products of manufacturing. Substances such as asbestos and vinyl chlorides (by-products of plastics manufacturing) are carcinogenic and are suspected to be a factor in the increased incidence of malignancy in communities where these chemicals are produced.

Water Quality

Water quality is a major concern of communities. Pollution is becoming more difficult to combat as industrialization increases and population spreads into new regions, creating new demands for water. Local water treatment plants are responsible for purifying the water supply for their communities. Residential and commercial growth may strain the ability of treatment plants to adequately treat water and inadequate treatment facilities are a source of pollution. Industries that discharge toxic wastes are another source of pollution. Among the growing list of hazardous wastes are radioactive substances. Agriculture is also responsible for pollution due to runoff of pesticides and fertilizers into the water supply.

Water pollution may be responsible for illness related to bacterial contamination (e.g., hepatitis). Industrial contaminants such as mercury may enter the food chain, tainting fish and causing illness in humans who consume them.

Soil Quality

Soil quality is a recent issue of concern as the effects of careless dumping of toxic wastes are being discovered. Radioactive materials, by-products of plastics manufacturing, or pesticides have been implicated in increased incidence of birth defects, miscarriage, and cancer.

A well-publicized example of these problems occurred in 1978 at Love Canal in New York. One hundred homes were built over a former toxic dump site. The miscarriage rate in the area was 30%, a number of cancer deaths occurred, and children and animals were burned by contact with the toxic ooze from the soil. In other instances, inadequately disposed substances have seeped into the ground water, making the drinking water in entire communities unsafe.

Food Purity

The safety of the food supply is of great concern to health professionals. The food chain may be contaminated when pesticides are inappropriately used in agriculture, when animals ingest contaminated water, or when air or soil pollutants come into contact with crops, livestock, or fishing grounds. A disastrous example occurred in Michigan in the mid-1970s when polybrominated biphenyls were accidentally mixed with livestock feed during production. The contaminated feed was ingested by cattle which were in turn consumed by Michigan residents before the accident was discovered. The contamination was so widespread that polybrominated biphenyls could be found in human breast milk. It may be decades before all of this accident's effects on human health can be identified.

Food can also be contaminated by bacteria or other organisms. Salmonella, Staphylococcus, and Shigella are common culprits in illnesses caused by ingesting contaminated food. Poultry and seafood products are especially susceptible to bacterial contamination. *Clostridium Botulinum* (botulism) is a microorganism that produces a deadly toxin. Because it survives in anaerobic environments — that is, those without free oxygen — it is a dangerous contaminant of canned foods.

Nursing Implications

Community health nurses are actively involved in identifying or intervening with environmentally caused health problems. Epidemiology is the study of the incidence, distribution, and control of disease in a human population. Nurses in the community may be involved in case finding or health screening programs that produce data for epidemiologic studies. As an example, nurses may identify a large number of cases of giardiasis, a waterborne gastrointestinal disease. They report their findings to the local water treatment authorities who test the community's water supply and confirm the presence of the parasite. The nurses implement a program of preventive education in the area to curb further incidence of the disease.

The Environmental Protection Agency (EPA), established in 1970, is the federal body responsible for establishing standards and regulations related to air and water purity, noise, solid waste disposal, and control of toxic substances (Table 5–1). In addition, local and state governments may also have authority in matters of water treatment, solid waste disposal, and air purity. Since government agencies are involved in environmental pollution controls, political activity can be a useful tool for nurses. For instance, nurses may serve on community boards, be involved in lobbying efforts, or even achieve political office in order to affect public policy related to environmental health. A growing number of nurse-researchers are studying environmentally related health problems. The opportunities and challenges of maintaining a healthful physical environment in the community are limitless. See the box for environmental health resources of interest to nurses.

Environmental Health Resources

The American Association of Occupational Health Nurses, Inc.
3500 Piedmont Road, NE
Atlanta, GA 30305-1513

The Cancer Information Clearing House
National Cancer Institute
Building 31, Room 10A18
9000 Rockville Pike
Bethesda, MD 20205
(Request information on occupational and environmental cancer.)

The Center for Devices and Radiological Health
Public Health Service
Food and Drug Administration
Division of Professional Practices (HZ-250)
1901 Chapman Avenue
Rockville, MD 20857
(Request information on the safe use of medical devices, x-rays, and radioactive materials.)

The Department of Health and Human Services
Public Health Service
Centers for Disease Control
National Institute for Occupational Safety and Health
4676 Columbia Parkway
Cincinnati, OH 45226

Environmental Action
Suite 731
1346 Connecticut Avenue, NW
Washington, DC 20036

Environmental Defense Fund
444 Park Avenue South
New York, NY 10016

The Environmental Protection Agency
401 M Street, SW Washington, DC 20460
(Provides information on many environmental subjects including water pollution, hazardous and solid waste disposal, air and noise pollution, pesticides, and radiation.)

Friends of the Earth
530 7th Street, SE
Washington, DC 20003
(A nonprofit environmental
    organization involved with
    issues such as clean water,
    clean air, pesticides, and the
    ozone layer.)
**The National Network to Prevent
Birth Defects**
Box 15309 Southeast Station
Washington, DC 20003
The National Wildlife Federation
1412 16th Street, NW
Washington, DC 20036
(A nonprofit organization encouraging
    wise use and management of
    the earth's resources on which
    human life and welfare depend.)
**Nurses' Environmental Health
Watch**
RCU P.O. Box 1277
New York, NY 10185
(Nursing organization dedicated to
    educating nurses and the public
    about environmental health
    hazards.)

Office on Smoking and Health
United States Department of
    Health and Human Services
110 Park Building
5600 Fishers Lane
Rockville, MD 20857
(The leading government agency that
    collects and disseminates all
    materials related to smoking and
    tobacco use.)
The Sierra Club
330 Pennsylvania Avenue, SE
Washington, DC 20033
(202) 547-1144
(Citizens interest group that
    promotes preservation of natural
    resources.)
**United States Environmental
Protection Agency**
Office of Water Regulations and
    Standards
Washington, DC 20460
(Request information on water
    resources and water pollution.)
**The United States Government
Printing Office**
Superintendent of Documents
Washington, DC 20402
(Request selected bibliography on
    specific environmental pollution
    areas such as air and water
    pollution.)

(Mancino D: The future and environmental health nursing. Imprint 32:44, 1985)

The Immediate Physical Environment

The immediate environment may involve a variety of settings. The most important of these for health status are the home and work environments, and for the ill individual, the hospital. Nurses often can influence the health of the immediate environment in all of these settings. Of particular relevance to health are safety factors, temperature, lighting, noise, and room arrangement.

Safety Factors

One of the biggest health-related concerns for nurses is safety of the environment. Many safety factors can be directly influenced by nurses. Accidents are ranked as the third cause of death in the United States for all ages and the leading cause of death up to age 45 years

TABLE 5 – 1
SELECTED EXAMPLES OF MAJOR ENVIRONMENTAL LEGISLATIVE ACTS INVOLVING THE ENVIRONMENTAL PROTECTION AGENCY

Subject	Legislative Act	Purposes
Air pollution	Air Quality Control Act, 1970; amended, 1977	The act grants EPA authority to establish national air quality standards to protect community health and welfare. The act also calls for states to examine air quality more closely and, if standards are not being met, to revise state plans.
Water quality	Water Pollution Control Act Amendments, 1972	The act imposes on EPA the task of restoring and maintaining the chemical, physical, and biological integrity of the nation's waters.
Water quality	Safe Drinking Water Act, 1974; amended, 1977	The act requires that EPA issue regulations that set national standards to protect drinking water.
Ocean dumping	Marine Protection Research and Sanctuaries Act, 1972	The act authorizes EPA to establish a dumping permit program and site for dumping. The Army Corps of Engineers is authorized to control dredged material.
Noise	Noise Control Act, 1972; amended, 1978	The act calls for EPA to establish standards and promulgate regulations concerning major sources of noise. The act further requires EPA to conduct research into the effects and control of noise and to help states and local assistance programs.
Solid waste	Solid Waste Disposal Act, 1965; Resource Conservation and Recovery Act, 1976	The acts provide for the establishment of regulations and devise EPA programs to ensure safe disposal of wastes, that is, toxic substances, pesticides, explosives. They also require states to look at existing waste disposal sites and develop plans.
Toxic substances	Toxic Substances Control Act, 1976	The Act compels industry to develop adequate data on the effect of chemical substances on health and the environments and to regulate and ban substances when necessary.

(Stanhope M, Lancaster J: Community Health Nursing, 2nd ed, p 324. St. Louis, CV Mosby, 1988)

(Walker, 1986, p 1547). Injuries are often classified according to their source and include mechanical, thermal, electrical, radiation, and chemical injuries.

Mechanical Injury.   Falls are one of the most common injuries in the home and hospital. In the client, factors such as poor eyesight, dizziness, confusion, and weakness may be involved and the elderly are at particularly high risk for falls. Physical hazards in the environment may also contribute to falls: standing water on floors, loose rugs, objects cluttering stairs and floors, and electrical cords in pathways. Infants and toddlers are another group at high risk for falls. These children should never be left unattended on high places — such as changing tables — and stairways should be blocked. Mechanical injury in the workplace may include lacerations, back injury, and eye trauma. Motor vehicle accidents are a significant health risk, particularly in adolescents and young adults.

Thermal Injury.   Burns are another common source of injury in the home, workplace, and hospital. Burns in the hospital can be caused by improper use of therapeutic heat — such as hot water bottles or heating pads — or from faulty electrical devices. In the home, fires are a dangerous source of thermal injury and are associated with a death rate of 2.7% (U.S. Department of Commerce, 1982 – 1983). Scalding liquids, improper use of flammables such as gasoline, as well as woodstoves, kerosene heaters, and faulty electrical appliances are all potential sources of burns in the home. Children and elderly persons are the age groups at high risk for injury from burns.

Electrical Injury.   Hospitals use a wide variety of electrical devices for diagnostic and therapeutic purposes. Electrocardiographs, mechanical ventilators, defibrillators (devices that use electric current to restore normal cardiac rhythm), and bovies (electrical devices used to coagulate small areas of bleeding during surgery) are just some of the electrical devices which are used in patient care. Because the hazards of electrical shock are always present, nurses must carefully protect themselves and their clients from injury. Although electrical devices are housed in insulating material that reduces the flow of leakage current, a small amount of leakage does occur. When a nurse touches an appliance and a client simultaneously, a small amount of current flows from the electrical device, through the nurse, and into the client. Although this current is usually harmless, certain clients — such as those who have abraded skin or are attached to monitors — may sustain injury. Other hazards include frayed electrical cords, overloaded circuits, and improperly grounded equipment (Meth, 1980).

In the home, electricity can be a hazard if circuits are overloaded, electrical cords become frayed — thus losing their protective insulation — three-pronged plugs are bypassed causing loss of grounding, or electrical devices are used near water sources (such as hair dryers being used while bathing). Uncovered electrical outlets can be hazards to toddlers who may try to insert fingers, keys, pencils, and the like into them.

Radiation.   Like electricity, radiation has many diagnostic and therapeutic uses in the hospital. X-rays are a common tool used in diagnosis, particularly now that computer technology has increased the range of information which can be obtained. Radioactive cobalt or cesium is used in the treatment of cancer. However, this invaluable tool may be a hazard to all who are exposed to it. The effects of radiation depend on the length of exposure, the proximity to exposure, the adequacy of shielding, and the sensitivity of organs to radiation effects. Side effects of radiation exposure include radiation sickness, change in bone marrow function, burns, sterility, and skin ulcers. Long-term exposure to radiation can be carcinogenic. Unborn babies are at high risk from radiation, particularly during the first 3 months of development. Effects of fetal exposure include abortion, birth defects, and childhood leukemia. Pregnant women should be extremely cautious about exposure to sources of radioactivity. Pregnant nurses need to take careful precautions against exposure to radiation at work.

Radiation is becoming an important hazard in the home and workplace as well. Industrial uses of radiation include electric power generation, lasers, and radioisotopes used for measuring, testing, and processing (Stanhope and Lancaster, 1988, p 313). In the home, electronic devices such as microwave ovens may yield exposure to radiation, although this is minimal. Nurses in occupational and community health have the important task of reviewing home and work environments for radiation hazards and implementing safety programs.

Chemical Hazards.   In the hospital, the most significant source of chemical injury is also one of the most important therapeutic agents: medications. Because nurses are responsible for most medication administration in the hospital, they have a responsibility to protect their clients from harmful effects of medications. Nurses monitor their clients for undesired effects (side effects) and signs of drug toxicity. Nurses are also responsible for administering drugs cautiously so medication errors are avoided. Poisoning can also occur when substances are not labeled or labels are not read carefully. For example, liquid soap may look like medicine and be mistakenly swallowed if left unlabeled at the client's bedside.

Chemical injuries are also a concern in the home and at work. Workers in many industries come into contact with chemicals which may be hazardous if inhaled or if prolonged skin contact occurs. For instance, anesthetic gases are an occupational hazard for health-care workers in the operating room. Poisoning is a potential danger in households with small children. Cleaning agents, medications, and paint supplies are just some of the hazardous materials that should be stored safely out of reach.

Infection Control

Infections are a serious source of concern for hospitalized persons. Nosocomial infections (those acquired in the hospital) can add much time and expense to a person's hospital stay. For infections to develop, the following components must exist:

- A significant number of microorganisms entering the host
- A virulent microorganism (one that is efficient at causing disease)
- A susceptible host

Hospitals, by their nature, house many pathogenic (infection-causing) microorganisms. Hospitalized persons have increased susceptibility to infection because of weakened natural defenses, such as breaks in the skin and decreased or altered immune system. Prevention of infection requires knowledge of principles of asepsis. Asepsis means freedom from infectious agents. One of the most important techniques in asepsis is handwashing. This is one of the first skills that nursing students learn and the technique that is most often neglected in practice.

Day care centers are another type of institution where infections are likely to spread. Both children and workers need to be careful to wash hands when preparing food or eating, when toileting or changing diapers, and after sneezing. Much opportunity exists for nurses to do health teaching related to infection control in these agencies.

Other Factors in the Immediate Environment

Temperature and Humidity.   Comfortable room temperature ranges from 68°F to 74°F; comfortable humidity is about 30% to 60%. In illness, many factors — such as presence of fever, joint disease, and respiratory symptoms — may require adjustments in room temperature and humidity for clients to feel comfortable. Elderly persons often prefer higher room temperatures.

Lighting.   Lighting contributes to clients' safety in the hospital. Lighting should be adequate to allow persons to navigate safely, particularly at night. Lighting should follow natural cycles, that is, brighter in the day hours, dimmer at night. Constant exposure to bright lights is uncomfortable, inhibits sleep, and can be disorienting. This possibility is a concern in intensive care units, which often use bright lighting day and night.

Elderly persons may experience visual change that make them susceptible to discomfort from glare. They may also need greater illumination. Nurses need to provide indirect but sufficient lighting when the elderly are reading or learning self-care skills in the home or the hospital.

Noise and Odors.   Noise is defined as unwanted sound (Jarvis, 1985, p 818). It is a problem that is becoming increasingly significant as a health hazard, particularly on the job. Noise exposure can lead to permanent hearing loss, interference with job performance, sleep interference, and psychological stress. Noise-induced hearing loss affects 10 to 20 million workers in the United States alone (Jarvis, 1985, p 822). The Occupational Safety and Health Administration (OSHA) has set standards for the level of noise and length of exposure at the workplace. Nurses may be involved in case finding for auditory problems by conducting hearing tests at the workplace. Occupational health nurses may see other noise-related problems such as stress and interference with job performance. These nurses are often responsible for assisting with noise abatement programs as well as caring for individual workers.

Although the fictional television hospitals all bear signs proclaiming, "Quiet! Hospital Zone," real life hospitals are notoriously noisy. Sleep interference is a common complaint of hospitalized persons. Sources of noise in the hospital include transportation and handling of equipment, beeps and alarms of monitoring devices, telephones and paging systems, and noise generated by patients and hospital staff. Hospital noise can also induce stress in ill persons and can contribute to sensory overload, a perceptual disturbance caused by excessive sensory stimulation (Lindenmuth et al, 1980).

Hospitals can also contain many sources of unpleasant odors such as drainage, excreta, and cleaning agents. Sick persons are often quite sensitive to odors. Even pleasant smells such as food, fragrant flowers, or the nurse's perfume can be very offensive to the ill individual.

Layout and Decor.   Many health problems are associated with changes in functional ability. Fatigue, shortness of breath, cardiac problems, and neurological and bone or joint changes all can affect the person's ability to function in his or her environment. Nurses, along with other health team members such as occupational or physical therapists, assist persons to adapt their living quarters to suit their altered abilities. An example can be found in the box.

Mrs. Rush is a 72-year-old woman who had a leg amputated. While she was recovering from surgery, the nurses and physical therapists noted her abilities to walk with her walker and the occupational therapist obtained a description of her home environment. Mrs. Rush, her husband, and the health team decided on changes that would accommodate her current level of mobility. Because Mrs. Rush could not negotiate stairs, they decided to move her sleeping quarters to the first floor. After Mrs. Rush was discharged, the community health nurse assisted her to arrange her cooking supplies and furniture so that she could perform her usual activities with her walker. These environmental adaptations helped her to maintain optimum independence in spite of her mobility changes.

Decor is a factor that can affect mood. A variety of colors, art work, display of gifts, and family photographs are all sources of sensory stimulation and can uplift mood in the hospitalized person. Children respond best to bright colors; use of strong patterns can help infants develop visual tracking skills.

Health-care institutions have found that homelike environments can reduce psychological stress and have positive effects on clients' health. In psychiatric units, the use of homelike furnishings and layout diminish the sense of institutionalization and ease the transition between hospital and home when the client is discharged. In obstetrics, birthing centers have become a popular choice for prospective parents. A birthing room resembles a hotel suite as contrasted with the typical labor room with its hospital bed, hard, straight-backed chairs, and display of technical equipment. Some practitioners believe that a homelike environment can actually encourage the normal progress of labor and contribute to healthier mothers and babies. Other settings where the environments are becoming more homelike include hospices (where dying persons are cared for) and pediatric units.

Whether the setting is the home or the hospital, decor is a matter of personal preference and nurses should not alter the clients' immediate environments without consulting them. In the hospital, clients' bedsides become their personal space at a time when many possessions and routines have been given up (e.g., privacy, usual clothing, personal furnishings, decisions about mealtimes). Thus, it is particularly important to arrange bedside articles according to clients' preferences to the fullest extent possible.

Nursing Implications

Nursing care in relation to the immediate physical environment has four major goals:

1 Safety promotion
2 Control of communicable disease
3 Provision of comfort and appropriate sensory stimuli
4 Maximizing the person-environment fit

Nurses have the knowledge and ability to implement a wide range of actions that promote healthy environments. These actions include manipulation of environmental factors and client teachings.

Safety Promotion. Provision of a safe environment is a primary nursing responsibility. In the hospital, nurses constantly observe the environment for hazards such as malfunctioning electrical equipment, cords or items on the floor (which could be tripped over), inadequate lighting, or improperly labeled medications. Table 5 – 2 lists categories of hazards in the hospital environment and nursing actions to prevent client injury.

Accidents are a frequent cause of injury in the home and workplace. Nurses can be instrumental in helping clients to survey the home and work environments and plan appropriate protective measures. Occupational health nurses have a key role in identifying health hazards in the workplace, assessment and nursing care for work-related injuries, and safety programs for employees. These nurses also assist with implementing standards and record keeping for federal programs, particularly OSHA regulations.

Accidents are the leading killers of children (Pillitteri, 1987, p 1289). Community health, pediatric, and school nurses can help to prevent such tragedies by implementing safety teaching for children and parents. Nurses also assist parents to survey their homes for possible safety hazards and make appropriate changes. A summary of actions to promote childhood safety is found in Table 5 – 3.

Accidents continue to be a leading cause of death in adulthood. Here again, health teaching and environmental alterations can prevent many accidents from occurring. Teaching clients how to establish environments that promote motor vehicle safety, prevent fires, promote electrical safety, and — especially for the elderly — prevent falls is an important nursing activity. Specific suggestions include the following:

1   Avoid overloading electrical circuits or outlets.
2   Use caution with hot liquids, particularly oils.
3   Label hazardous substances clearly and leave in their original containers.
4   Store flammable substances away from heat sources.
5   Never smoke in bed.
6   Discard all unused medications and always leave medications in their original containers.
7   Keep pathways clear from toys, slippery rugs, etc.
8   Use caution when climbing ladders.
9   Keep stairways well lighted and uncluttered.
10   Check electrical cords for fraying.
11   Use grounded plugs correctly; avoid adapters.

Control of Communicable Disease. Pathogens are transmitted through several modes, including:

- Contact route — direct (person to person) or indirect (through inanimate objects)
- Vehicle route (contaminated foods, water, medications, serum)
- Airborne route (droplets or dust)
- Vector-borne route (insects, vermin)

Interruption of these routes of transmission is one means of infection control. Handwashing is the most important measure that prevents the transmission of microorganisms. Use of running water, soap, and friction for at least 30 seconds is essential to good hand washing. In the hospital, hands should be washed before and after any direct patient contact, before handling food or medications, and after handling used equipment and supplies. Teaching

TABLE 5-2
POTENTIAL INJURIES IN THE HOSPITAL AND PREVENTIVE ACTIONS

Potential Injury	Prevention
Falls	Wipe up spilled liquids promptly
	Remove objects in clients' pathways
	Use siderails and place call lights within reach
	Never leave infants unattended
	Keep beds in lowest position
	Avoid dangling electrical cords and drainage tubing
	Use brakes on beds and wheelchairs
	Accompany clients who are susceptible to dizziness, confusion, weakness when they are ambulating
	Use safe transferring techniques when moving clients
Electrical shock	Check line cords and plugs for defects
	Remove cords from sockets by grasping the plug
	Be sure that clients who are attached to electrical devices are properly grounded
	Check electrical equipment for proper functioning
Poisoning or medication-related injuries	Remove harmful substances from clients' bedsides when not in use (e.g., disinfectants, antiseptics, liquid soaps)
	Never put hazardous substances in drinking or medication cups
	Never leave medications at bedside
	Carefully check labels on medications and verify correct dosage before administering
	Identify clients correctly before administering medications
	Watch for side effects; check for drug allergies
	Chart medications promptly after administering
	Keep medication supplies out of reach (especially in pediatric units)
Burns	Check temperature of bath water or hot compresses before client use
	Use heating pads, heat lamps cautiously (pay attention to length of time used, distance from heat source, and temperature of device)
	Caution clients from smoking in bed (particularly confused or drowsy clients)
	Avoid smoking near oxygen sources
	Know agency policy regarding fire procedures
	Avoid overloading electrical sockets
Radiation	Watch for signs of radiation injury for clients receiving radiation therapy
	Use proper shielding; limit exposure time near clients who have radioactive implants
	Know hospital policy regarding radiation therapy

TABLE 5–3
POTENTIAL CHILDHOOD INJURIES AND PREVENTIVE ACTIONS

Potential Injury	Prevention
Burns	Teach child the meaning of "hot"
	Lock up matches
	Keep hot liquids, electric cords from hot appliances out of reach
	Turn pot handles away from reach when cooking
	Place guards around heat sources (e.g., fireplaces, barbecue grills, portable heaters)
Falls	Block stairways safely
	Never leave children unattended on high surfaces
	Keep crib rails up
Drowning, suffocation	Never leave child unattended in bathroom (can drown in bathtub or toilet)
	Never leave child unattended in swimming or wading pools
	Toys should be too large to swallow; small parts should be securely fastened
	Keep buttons, coins, small candies, etc., off floor and out of reach
	Avoid toys or objects with long cords
	Keep plastic bags out of reach
Poisoning	Keep medications, household cleaners, other hazardous substances properly labeled and out of reach
Vehicle accidents	Use approved car seats for young children
	Use safety belts for older children
	Teach traffic safety to children
	Use approved helmets when riding motorcycles, snowmobiles
	Teach bicycle safety
General Safety Precautions	
	Keep emergency numbers for fire, police, medical care, and poison control posted in a conspicuous place
	Teach older children what to do in emergency situations.

good hand-washing technique to clients can control the transmission of pathogens in the home, workplace, schools, and day care centers. Even toddlers are capable of learning to wash hands at mealtime and after toileting. Along with hand washing, personal hygiene measures interrupt the transmission of infection. Years ago, maintaining personal hygiene was as uncomplicated as bathing, covering the mouth when sneezing, and disposing of body wastes appropriately. In today's era of sexually transmitted diseases and AIDS (acquired immune deficiency syndrome), teaching personal hygiene measures includes discussion of the dangers of sharing drug paraphernalia and indiscriminate sexual intercourse. Fear of AIDS is a national concern and nurses can do much to relieve anxiety by discussing how the disease is spread and how to protect against contracting it.

Sanitation measures are a second means of preventing communicable diseases. Community health nurses can do much in terms of educating people about proper disposal of trash and wastes. Nurses may teach home care of the person with a communicable disease, including measures for cleaning dishes and bedding and disposal of contaminated supplies. Nurses are also involved with water and food purity issues and may be the first to identify outbreaks of illness caused by contaminated food or water. In the hospital, nurses are responsible for proper disposal of used supplies such as contaminated dressings, hypodermic equipment, and linens. Isolation technique — which involves special precautions such as private rooms, gowns, masks, and gloves — may be implemented when caring for persons with certain communicable diseases.

Modification of the environment is a third means of infection control. Pathogens, microorganisms that are capable of causing disease, prefer warm, moist, dark environments. Overcrowding and high temperature and humidity are housing conditions which increase the incidence of infection. Community health nurses are often involved in reducing these environmental conditions. Two special means of altering the environment for microorganisms are disinfection and sterilization. Disinfection removes all pathogenic organisms from an object. An example is disinfection of a hospital room after a client is discharged. Sterilization removes all microorganisms and their spores. Heat, chemicals, and radiation are methods used for disinfecting and sterilizing equipment and supplies.

A fourth means of reducing communicable disease is altering factors related to host susceptibility. One important method is immunization, a process whereby antibodies or weakened antigens are administered to produce immunity to specific diseases. Nurses are responsible for planning and implementing community immunization programs. Nurses also maintain persons' resistance to disease by good nutrition, skin care that prevents breaks in the integument, and promoting adequate rest. Certain persons are particularly susceptible to infection and require careful protection from microorganisms. The elderly and newborns, persons receiving immunosuppressive drugs (e.g., following organ transplants), persons receiving chemotherapy for cancer, and persons who have wounds (which includes postoperative patients) are among those who require careful precautions against infection.

Provision of Comfort and Sensory Stimulation. Maintaining a comfortable environment is an important nursing responsibility, particularly for ill or hospitalized persons. These individuals often lack control over stressful environmental factors such as noise, bright lights, and odors. Thus, it is up to nurses to identify and control these variables. It is useful to obtain a description of the client's preferred level of lighting, privacy, temperature, and humidity. Illness may change the ability to tolerate environmental factors. For instance, during high fevers, persons may find bright lights and warm room temperatures to be uncomfortable. Some examples of nursing actions to promote a comfortable environment are the following:

- Turn off bright task lighting after completing nursing procedures.
- Adjust curtains or doors to provide the desired level of privacy.

- Reduce irritating noise sources such as monitor sounds, staff conversations, radio or television noise.
- Provide clients with controls for lighting, television, and radio so that they can adjust these to their preference.
- Mask undesirable odors with room deodorants; remove odor sources such as soiled dressings or bedpans promptly.

In addition to factors of lighting, temperature, noise, odor, and privacy, decor can enhance the comfort of an environment. As mentioned earlier, homelike decor is becoming more evident in health-care institutions. Displaying photographs, gifts, or meaningful items from home is one means of providing a more individualized environment for the hospitalized person.

Appropriate sensory stimulation in the environment is essential to health. Lack of appropriate stimuli can cause boredom and depression. At the extremes, too much or too little environmental stimulation can lead to sensory overload and sensory deprivation, syndromes that are characterized by altered perception and disorientation. Provision of normal day-to-night patterns of lighting, clocks, calendars, opportunities for socializing, and reduction of noise are nursing actions which provide appropriate sensory stimulation for clients. For infants and children, adequate stimuli are essential to normal development. In the hospital, nurses provide stimuli by talking and playing with children and using mobiles, music boxes, or favorite toys from home. Nurses can influence sensory environment in the home by teaching parents about child care, nurturing, and play activities that stimulate normal development. Much of this education can take place when the child comes to the health-care setting for checkups.

Maximizing Person – Environment Fit.   A basic premise of this chapter is that persons are constantly interacting with their environment and this interaction influences health. Nurses are concerned with the nature of this interaction, a concept that Killien (1985) called **person – environment fit**. Killien defined *fit* as the match between needs and resources of the individual and demands and resources of the environment (p 268). Fit is unique for each person – environment system and can be maximized by modifying the needs or demands and the resources of either the person or the environment.

The example of Mrs. Rush that was presented earlier shows how health-care professionals can assist clients to modify their environment to fit altered functional ability following an illness. Another example is the nurse who is caring for a client with newly diagnosed emphysema. The nurse counsels the client regarding his or her cigarette smoking and teaches breathing techniques. These actions modify the needs and resources of the client. In addition, the nurse discusses ways of adding humidity to the home and explores means of obtaining an air filter for the furnace. The focus of these interventions is modification of the environment. By examining the client's situation in the context of his or her environment, the nurse can provide broader and more individualized strategies that are more likely to be successful in optimizing health.

| THE SOCIAL ENVIRONMENT

Societies are groups of people sufficiently organized to carry out the conditions necessary to live together (Hall, 1985, p 30). The social environment consists of the social systems with which a person interacts. These social systems may include the person's family, school, neighborhood, social or hobby club, or community. The interaction of a person with the social environment is becoming increasingly recognized as a factor affecting his health. Likewise, a social system such as a family or community may be the "client" for whom nurses care. For these reasons, it is essential for nurses to have an understanding of the various social systems and the structures and processes that comprise them.

The Structure of Social Systems

Social systems are characterized by structural components, among which are boundaries, norms, roles, and positions.

Boundaries separate the members of a social system from the environment. They distinguish members from nonmembers. Boundaries may be rigid and highly defined — such as those of a nuclear family — or flexible — such as those of a drop-in support group for new mothers. Boundaries of social systems vary in their permeability. Some are relatively impermeable, meaning that the system interacts minimally with its environment. An example might be an alcoholic family whose members keep to themselves and are not accepting of outside assistance.

Norms are expected behaviors. They provide rules about standards of appropriate behavior in particular situations. Norms flow from cultural values about what is important in various situations. Church attendance on Sunday may be a norm for a religious group.

Roles are sets of expected behaviors which are normatively defined. Roles serve to make behavior predictable and role enactment — the carrying out of a role — makes social interactions run smoothly. The role of motherhood in the United States is associated with nurturing and child-rearing behaviors. A mother who relegates these behaviors to her husband or a baby sitter might run the risk of being labeled an "oddball" or a "deviant." Some roles are explicit and formal; others are implicit (not readily apparent) or informal. For example, in a family, a man could have a formal role of "breadwinner" and an informal role of "dominator." Inability to perform one's role — that is, role deprivation — leads to diminished self-esteem, anxiety, or depression. Nurses often deal with these concerns when they care for ill persons.

Positions are syntheses of related roles and represent the location of persons in a social system (Hall, 1985, p 40). Positions have many roles associated with them. For example, the position of staff nurse in a hospital may involve roles of bedside care-giver, hospital employee, patient advocate, committee member, and mentor to inexperienced nurses.

Processes of Social Systems

Three major processes of social systems are input, throughput, and output. Input is the process of taking energy, information, or matter into the system. Throughput involves using this energy, information, or matter to fulfill its functions and produce output, or the products of the social system. A family might take in information on child-rearing and use it to raise a child who can become a productive member of society. To carry out these processes, social systems need a communication system, a decision-making system, and a means of allocating power.

Types of Social Systems

As discussed earlier, social systems are of many types, from informal recreational groups to defined communities. The social systems with which nurses are most concerned are families, groups, and communities.

Families

The basic unit of organization in every society is the **family**. The concept of family is changing rapidly in this country. Whereas earlier, a definition would have specified the nuclear family (mother, father, and dependent children), such a description would not allow for some arrangements that are encountered today: unmarried couples and their unrelated children, homosexual families, the person who lives alone, and extended families are a few examples. Friedman defined family as "a group of people emotionally joined together who live in close geographical proximity" (1986, p 8). Yet even this definition does not accommodate all of the types of families just mentioned. Because the definition of family is so variable, it is important to ascertain whom the client identifies as significant family members.

The health of individuals is heavily dependent on family influences. The family socializes individuals, that is, influences them to take on the norms and values of society. Acquisition of attitudes, beliefs, and behaviors related to health is part of this process. Families also nurture individuals, enabling them to grow and develop normally. Persons who have healthy physical and psychosocial development are more able to withstand stressors and maintain wellness. The economic status of one's family also influences health status; it affects ability to obtain health care, good nutrition, safe living conditions, and so forth. Family structures and processes such as norms, roles, decision making, and communication all affect the health of the family and its individual members.

Family structures that have importance for nurses include boundaries, positions, roles, and norms. Boundaries that are too rigid may inhibit a family that needs help from accepting it. The roles and norms associated with family positions are changing rapidly. Many mothers now hold jobs, assuming a "breadwinner" role, and fathers are taking on child-rearing roles by becoming more involved in caretaking activities. Nurses cannot assume that family roles are assigned in a traditional manner and should identify which roles are threatened by health problems of a family member.

Many functions of the family have been identified, including the following.

- Physical functions, for example, providing food, shelter, and health care
- Affectional functions, for example, generating affection, providing a sense of security, and companionship
- Social functions, for example, developing sense of responsibility for behavior and social values, preparing members to assume productive societal roles (Murray and Zentner, 1985, pp 524–525)

Processes of communication, decision making, and power allocation are essential to fulfilling these functions. Nurses who are working with families evaluate these processes as they affect the health status of family members. For example, in Arab families, the male members assume power and make decisions for females. If a nurse were teaching an Arab woman about a health problem, it would be essential to include her husband.

Groups

A **group** is an assembly of people who share specific functions or goals and who interact over a period of time. Health-related groups are a relatively recent phenomenon, but it is possible to find an appropriate resource group for almost every health concern. Nurses have opportunities to work with groups such as childbirth preparation classes, cancer support groups, bereavement support groups, postmastectomy groups, or psychotherapy groups. It is obvious that groups are a component of the social environment with potential to influence health.

Groups possess structure consisting of boundaries, roles, norms, and positions and are characterized by processes of communication, decision making, and power allocation. In examining a group's boundaries, a nurse might identify who the members are and how the group defines its membership. For example, a support group for women who are having infertility problems might feel uncomfortable or angry with a group member who becomes pregnant. The members may ask her to leave the group despite her continued need for emotional support.

The relationship of group members to each other in terms of roles, duties, and responsibilities is another important consideration. Roles may be formal—such as that of notetaker—or informal—such as mediator or scapegoat. The position of leader may be formal; in "leaderless" groups, informal leaders develop. When a group is having difficulty performing its functions, the difficulty may be related to conflicting roles within the group.

A group's communication process affects its ability to fulfill its functions. For example, a formal, structured communication process such as going from one member to another for ideas is unlikely to encourage spontaneous expression of thoughts and feelings in a new mothers' support group. Power and decision-making processes also affect a group's ability to achieve its goals. Leadership styles are related to how a group makes decisions. Autocratic group leaders determine their groups' functions and roles with little input from members. Democratic leaders share power and facilitate decision making with group members.

Nurses often function as leaders of health-related groups and need to develop effective leadership styles that suit the purposes of the group. Some characteristics of an effective group leader include the following:

1   Conveys security and acceptance of own limits; in turn, accepts others and helps them feel safe.
2   Demonstrates friendliness, empathy, and concern for others.
3   Listens carefully for unspoken as well as verbal messages.
4   Insists on freedom rather than perfection within the group.
5   Is capable of using humor kindly and appropriately.
6   Permits dissent from group members.
7   Does not resort to and does not permit blaming or persecution of members.
8   Does not anticipate immediate release from conflict but strives to cope with and gain meaning from the conflict as part of the resolving process.
9   Does not permit self to be used as a means to an end and does not use others in this manner (manipulation).
10 Does not assume superiority over others
    (Murray and Zentner, 1985, p 208)

Communities

A **community** can be defined as a group of people living in the same locality and under the same government; having common norms and cultures, health interests, and needs (Jarvis, 1985, p 18). A community has enormous impact on the health status of individuals by providing and allocating health-care resources, influencing access to health care, and affecting living conditions that are related to health. Nurses can learn much about the wellness of a community by examining its structures and processes, including those related to decision making, information sharing, power allocation, production and distribution of goods and services, and social control. Examples of factors that influence a community's health are the following:

- The economic climate — unemployment affects ability to pay for health care and poverty is related to poor health status
- Cultural, racial, and ethnic backgrounds of residents — cultural variations affect health beliefs and racial and ethnic backgrounds affect susceptibility to specific health problems
- Types of industries within the community's boundaries — industrial pollutants and occupational-related injuries are significant health hazards.
- Crowding and adequacy of housing — substandard housing and crowding are associated with increased incidence of communicable disease and accidents; crowding is also linked to high incidence of mental illness
- The type and variety of health-care agencies present — availability of major hospitals, emergency and specialty care (such as obstetrics, mental health, or rehabilitation), services of physicians, nurses, and other health-care professionals all affect the quality of health care in a community
- The presence and adequacy of government programs for financing personal health care — ability to obtain Medicare or Medicaid affects access to health care for the poor and elderly

Nurses can do much to affect the community environment. Community health is a nursing specialty concerned with the well-being of populations, or the community at large. One tool used by community health nurses is the community assessment, which is an examination of variables such as statistics about residents, physical size and characteristics, medical services and facilities, economic status, and health status (Jarvis, 1985, p 21). Such information provides insights into the health needs of the community. On the basis of these findings, nurses engage in health promotion and health maintenance programs, health education activities, program planning, and political activity.

Some specific nursing actions were described above when the physical environment was discussed. Other examples include providing a screening program for hypertension, health education for high risk mothers and infants, or a rural clinic for a medically under served community.

Political activity is an important tool for influencing the health of the community environment. Although nurses cannot directly relieve problems such as crowding, lack of funding for health care, or a depressed community economy, they can take indirect action through politics. For instance, nurses can lobby local political leaders for development of community housing or drug abuse programs. Nurses can support political candidates who are sympathetic to the community's health needs by working on election campaigns and voting for these individuals.

Social Support

An important function of the systems that comprise the social environment is social support. **Social support** has been defined as

- Information leading the subject to believe he is cared for and loved, esteemed and valued, belongs to a network of communication and mutual obligation (Cobb, 1976, p 300)
- Support accessible to an individual through social ties to other individuals, groups, and the larger community (Lin et al, 1979, p 109)
- A flow of emotional concern, instrumental aid, information, and/or appraisal . . . between people (House, 1981, p 26)

The notion that social support is related to health is relatively recent; publications related to this topic began to appear in the early 1970s. Earlier work—such as Cannon's (1929) studies of neuroendocrine responses to emotions and Wolff's (1953) identification of psychosocial factors leading to specific diseases—led social researchers to identify a possible link between social phenomena and health.

In 1967, Holmes and Rahe published their classic study on the relationship of social change (caused by stressful life events) to the development of illness. This study was followed by an investigation by Nuckolls and colleagues (1972) of the effect of social support on pregnant women who had a high degree of social change. Women who had high social support were found to have fewer medical complications than those with low social support. De Araujo (1973) identified a similar effect when he found that asthmatic persons with high life changes and low social support needed higher doses of steroid medication to control their disease. Gore (1978) identified that the presence of social support had a favorable effect on serum cholesterol levels and the mental health of men who experienced the life change of job loss.

Cassel (1974, 1976) summarized the findings of a variety of research studies, stating that a stressful social environment increases susceptibility to illness and that social support confers resistance to disease. Broadhead and associates (1983) reviewed more than 90 studies on social support, finding evidence to suggest that: (1) support acts as a buffer or effect modifier against life stress, and (2) support has a causal relationship with health. However, the authors caution that more research is needed before conclusions can be made.

Functions and Sources of Social Support

Pender (1982) identified two ways that social support may positively affect health (p 335). Social networks may "buffer" the effects of life change, as identified by the work of Nuckolls and colleagues, De Araujo, and Gore. Or, supportive social systems can offer stability to the person by decreasing the likelihood of life change and resultant stress. These explanations are depicted in Figure 5–1. Social support groups decrease or buffer stress by (1) modifying interpersonal or environmental conditions, (2) controlling how persons perceive the meaning of an experience, and (3) promoting appropriate emotional arousal (Pender, 1982, p 336).

Social support has many sources. If you consider persons whom you feel close to, share confidences with, or can rely on during difficult times, you will have identified your personal support network. Sources of support that have been identified in the literature include family, neighbors, friends, coworkers, religious organizations, self-help groups, and helping professionals (e.g., social workers, physicians, nurses). For many individuals, the

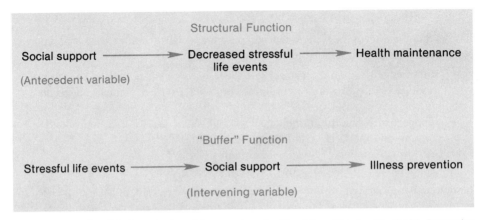

Figure 5–1   Possible impact of social support on health status. (Pender NJ: Health Promotion in Nursing Practice, p 336. Norwalk, CT, Appleton-Century-Crofts, 1982)

family provides the most significant source of support. The informal sources (family, peers, recreational groups, and so forth) are often identified as the most important by individuals. This may be related to mutual sharing and spontaneity that characterize informal helping relationships.

Nursing Implications

Since social support is clearly related to the person's health status, this concept is an important nursing concern. Nurses find it useful to identify the significant sources of support in the client's social environment and enhance the effectiveness of the support systems. An examination of the client's support systems includes the following factors:

- Who provides support: Does the client have a confidant? Are the spouse, family, friends supportive? Does the client participate in organizations or activities?
- What helping behaviors are important to the client: financial assistance, emotional support, information sources, etc.?
- Is the support system adequate from the client's perspective: Is there enough support of the kind desired by the client?

Once the support system has been identified, nurses help to maintain its adequacy or to alleviate deficits, which may involve working directly with the support persons as in the following example.

Mr. Young has been housebound since a stroke 6 months ago that left him partially paralyzed and emotionally depressed. His wife has been providing much of his physical care as well as emotional support. The home care nurse has located relief care for Mr. Young so that Mrs. Young can go out occasionally with a friend. The nurse also listens to Mrs. Young's concerns and encourages her to care well for herself. By caring for Mrs. Young, the nurse hopes to ensure that she will continue to be a healthy source of support for her husband.

Nurses can also assist persons to extend their sources of support or make better use of those which are currently available. Some possible ways of developing or strengthening social support include the following:

- Developing effective parenting skills
- Improving marital relationships
- Increasing assertiveness
- Becoming active in religious groups,
- Joining interest groups (e.g., leisure activities, political work)
- Seeking out lay or professional help (e.g., self-help groups, social workers)

Each person's need for social support is unique; what one person finds helpful might not be useful for another. Studies indicate that the need for social support varies with personal differences and the degree and type of crisis (Norbeck, 1981). Remember that the *person's* — not the nurse's — appraisal of the adequacy of available support is critical. Refrain from making personal judgments about clients' social support without validating these impressions with them.

In summary, social support is a phenomenon that has only recently been studied, but that appears to have a significant relationship to health. Because nurses focus their care on the whole person, they have a unique ability to assist clients to maximize the support available from the social environment. Using this holistic approach, nurses can aid in the prevention of illness and the achievement of optimum health.

| THE CULTURAL ENVIRONMENT

Like the social environment, cultural influences have an enormous effect on health. Culture affects how we define health, how illness is manifested, and the way in which we deal with health problems. In the last two decades, the nursing profession has become acutely aware of cultural variations and their impact on providing person-centered care. Official statements have been published, recognizing nursing's contribution toward meeting the "health needs of a diverse and multicultural society" (National League for Nursing, 1977, p 13) and toward considering "individual value systems and lifestyles" (American Nurses' Association, 1976, p 4).

To meet the needs of clients from various cultural backgrounds, it is necessary to gain some insight into culture as a component of the person's environment and its influence on adaptation through health and illness.

Definition and Characteristics of Culture

There are numerous theories and definitions of the anthropological concept of **culture**. Downs defined culture as "a system of symbols shared by a group of humans and transmitted by them to upcoming generations" (1975, p 45).

Murray and Zentner defined culture as "a group's design for living . . . (including shared) assumptions about the nature of the physical and social world, goals in life, attitudes, roles and values" (1985, p 415). How persons resolve problems related to basic human needs is strongly influenced by their cultural backgrounds.

Three major characteristics of culture have been identified by Murray and Zentner (1985).

1   Culture is learned.
2   Culture is capable of change, but remains stable.
3   There are components or patterns present in every culture.

As a small child, a person learns behaviors, values, attitudes, and beliefs within his or her cultural family system, a major teaching and supportive unit. This learning is largely influenced by the person's social status within a society and how he or she adapts to experiences in the environment. These values are learned and accepted for a time but then are modified or rejected as the person is exposed to subgroups within a culture (Frances and Munjas, 1976).

The second cultural characteristic relates to language, traditions, and norms or customs that may act as stabilizers for a culture. But time, events, and location can have a great impact on these stabilizing factors of culture. For instance, Hirabayashi (1975) discussed the variations between three generations of Japanese migrants and their style of adaptation to America. The deferent behavioral traits of the first generation were detrimental to the second generation when negative stereotypes of Japanese-Americans prevailed during World War II. Thus there evolved a third, more radical, generation in the 1960s.

The third characteristics of culture is the cultural components or cultural patterns that are generally evident among all societies. These include communication systems, means of economic and physical survival, transportation systems, family systems, social customs and mores, and religious systems. These cultural components form the basis for cultural variables of the person.

Cultural Variables of the Person

The phrase *cultural variables of the person* refers to those characteristics that a person exhibits or identifies with from a particular cultural group. These variables may or may not be exhibited by every person from a cultural group. Any individual, depending on his or her personal experience, may have all, none, or any combination of these variables.

Ethnic and Racial Identity

Ethnic origin and racial background have a great influence on how a person reacts and is reacted to by others in the health-care environment. Werner defined **ethnicity** as a group's affiliation due to shared linguistic, racial, (religious), and/or cultural background" (1979, p 343).

A person's ethnicity can be identified by any of the following.

- Language and communication process — for example, Spanish, Chinese, or Tagalog (Filipino)
- Racial background — for example, tribe, people, nation of same stock or human type such as blacks, whites
- Cultural background — for example, art, customs, laws, morals

Thus, if a nurse were caring for a person from a Hispanic background, a distinction among Mexican-American, Cuban, or Puerto Rican would be important. Likewise, the nurse would need to distinguish between Iroquois or Navajo Native American. These individual groups would have very different ethnic backgrounds affecting their health and illness beliefs, health behaviors, value systems, and language and communication process.

Because the melting pot concept is now less popular, the importance of accepting and appreciating culturally diverse people is receiving more attention. There has been a tremendous upsurge in trying to find one's ancestral "roots."

Value Orientations

Values are "intrinsic beliefs about the worth of an entity or concept" (Frances and Munjas, 1976, p 59). As such, they provide the basis for each person's attitudes and behaviors and they assist in establishing hierarchies of needs and goals. Kluckholn and Strodtbeck (1961) defined **value orientations** as principles that assist in the solution of common human problems. Among the value orientations that may differ across cultures are those concerning human nature, human-to-nature and human-to-human relationships, and time.

Staples (1976) compared time orientations between blacks and the white dominant American culture.

- Black value orientation — schedules are flexible; activities happening now are important, as is adapting to ranges in time rather than fixed periods
- White value orientation — society dictates how a person regulates his or her life; punctuality is a high priority

The white nurse who adheres to fixed schedules for baths, meals, medications, and sleep may find conflict with a black person who is very flexible in his or her time orientation. Similarly, precise clinic appointments may have different meanings to white nurses and black clients. Conflict and frustration can frequently be lessened with insight into value orientations different from the nurse's own.

Language and Intercultural Communication

Samovar and Porter described **communication** as a "dynamic process whereby human behavior, both verbal and nonverbal, is perceived and responded to" (1976, p 5). They further stated that intercultural communicating "occurs whenever a message producer is a member of one culture and a message receiver is a member of another" (p 4). Persons from two different cultural groups will attempt to understand each other from their own cultural frameworks. Persons' cultural frameworks greatly influence their social perception, which involves attaching meaning to an object or event in their environment. For instance, perceptions of pain, complaints of symptoms of illness, reactions to death and dying, and meanings attached to messages are all influenced by a person's cultural perception.

Samovar and Porter further emphasized that cultural differences are often responsible for communication problems. For example, eye contact and a friendly handshake are acceptable in the dominant American culture, indicating understanding and attentiveness, but they have very different meanings for the Native American. In many tribes, looking one in the eye is considered disrespectful and an intrusion on a person's private soul that results in "soul loss" (Primeaux, 1977, p 94). Nurses may think Native Americans are not listening or comprehending any conversation if there is no eye contact, but this assumption is not necessarily true.

Differences in word connotations affect our ability to communicate interculturally. For example, a nurse may associate *hospital* with health care. On the other hand, a Chinese-American may associate *hospital* with uncleanliness and death because in the Chinese belief system, a patient's spirit may get lost in a hospital and be unable to find its way home (Campbell and Chang, 1973).

Denotative meanings of words can also result in cultural communication problems.

For instance, a black youth may say, "I heard his house was really bad," which actually means, "I heard his house was really nice, good, or fantastic." Such a statement may confuse those who are not of this racial or cultural group.

Family System

Traditionally the family in American society has functioned as a group for the allocation, accumulation, and consumption of material resources. The family also plays a major role in personality development, identity formation, status assignment, and value orientation (Smith et al, 1978).

One might assess the family by looking at its structural patterns: Is it *matrilineal* or *patrilineal* with family descent determined through women or men? These structural patterns, along with family roles, are culturally determined. For example, the strong feeling for family among Filipinos is derived from Chinese influence in which old traditional patterns are imposed by the family patriarch or a similarly authoritative matriarch. Respect and deference are shown for decisions made by elders (DeGarcia, 1979). Nurses may be concerned about families who hover over Filipino patients, but this can be an added asset in promoting family-centered nursing. The nurse may also find it helpful to seek out the Filipino elders when decisions are being made about patient care of an ill family member.

Psychological well-being depends on adaptation to the social and human environment. Because of racial attitudes toward these minority groups in America, the main function of the family is to promote survival. Many ethnic minority families have shown tremendous adaptability and flexibility. Otto (1962) indicated that this resilience is due to family loyalty and intrafamily cooperation, ability of family self-help, flexibility in performing family roles, and providing for physical and spiritual needs of the family.

Nursing Implications. If a nurse is assessing ethnic-minority families, it would be helpful to capitalize on these strengths in meeting the client's health-care needs. When nurses are interviewing ethnic minority persons, it is important to consider the impact of the family on decisions related to nursing care. For example, in Mexican-American families, the "family" comes first and the "self" is second. The family is sought first in meeting health-care needs and others are sought when no other alternatives exist (White, 1977). One may conclude that the family unit among ethnic minority groups is a major source of stability.

Cultural Healing Beliefs and Practices

Cultural healing beliefs are beliefs that reflect a specific cultural orientation towards health and illness. They include cause of illness, treatment measures, illness prevention, and health promotion. According to Moore and associates, "Beliefs reflect perceived relationships between culture and environment . . . [and] beliefs (may) pertain directly to cause-effect relationships" (1980, p 199). In many instances, these beliefs contrast greatly with the traditional scientific medical theories about health and illness. Several authors (Snow, 1974; Holland, 1978) have discovered through research that these cultural health belief systems exist and indeed are prevalent among ethnic and cultural groups.

Holland (1978) studied the health-illness concepts of Mexican-Americans in Arizona. He found, especially among poor peasant populations, a strong adherence to a "miracle-oriented" system of magicoreligious beliefs and rituals for controlling stressful life events. Disease concepts are based on this magicoreligious belief system: Good health and prosperity are maintained when there is a balance between good and evil forces. Ill health and life's difficulties occur when this equilibrium is disturbed, and then a person will suffer a host of consequences. An example of one of the traditional Mexican illnesses is the emotional disease called *susto*, which refers to any disturbing or unstabilizing experience such as accidents or fearful events that cause "fright sickness" in which the "spirit" is separated from the body. The person afflicted may experience diarrhea, elevated temperature, anorexia, listlessness, or withdrawal. Treatment is done by a curer who calls the spirit back to the person's body with prayers and candle burning before saints (Holland, 1978).

Prior to Holland's study, Snow (1974) examined the cultural healing systems of low-income black Americans in Tucson, Arizona. Themes indicated that this cultural group perceives the world as a hostile and dangerous place and people were perceived as helpless and dependent on outside help. Good health was associated with success in life and bad luck with illness. Treatment of illness was done by using home remedies and preventatives, such as turpentine and kerosene and not letting cold air enter a menstruating or pregnant woman's body. Cultural healers were used who had special powers to cure natural and unnatural illnesses. Powers to cure were thought to be healing gifts from God, inborn, or learned from others.

Nursing Implications.   It is not the intent of these examples to give in-depth information but to encourage awareness of these cultural belief systems. Although these beliefs and practices may seem unusual, they are understandable in their cultural context. The nurse must be aware of how these beliefs affect a person's response to the health-care system. A person may reject the health-care environment due to vast differences in cultural belief systems.

According to Scott (1974), health professionals should, when feasible, use a treatment plan that demonstrates respect for and reflects a person's cultural healing system. For instance, on a person's admission to the hospital, assess what healing remedies have been helpful and incorporate them into the treatment plan. If a person believes he or she has been "hexed," try to alleviate his fears by combining orthodox treatment of symptoms with a cultural healer to remove the spell.

Religious Beliefs and Practices

A person's religion may also influence his concept of health and illness, treatment programs, and recovery. Religion can also act as a resource in facing crises related to critical illnesses or death. However, it must not be assumed that all persons from certain ethnic or cultural backgrounds have the same or similar religious belief systems. Pumphrey (1977) described several religious belief systems and their characteristics as related to birth, death, health crisis, diet, and special beliefs. The nurse should assess these characteristics in a person's religious belief system and determine their influence on the health state.

A thin line exists between religious and cultural beliefs that makes it difficult to separate the two. For example, Filipinos have a strong sense of destiny related to their Asian background and a deep faith in God drawn from the Spanish influence in their culture. This may account for why some Filipinos resign themselves and suffer in silence, attributing their illness state to God's will (DeGarcia, 1979). Some religious groups may object to medical interventions as shown by the refusal of Jehovah's Witnesses to allow blood transfusions or the avoidance of drugs by Seventh Day Adventists unless they are absolutely necessary (Pumphrey, 1977).

Nursing Implications.   Again, the intent of this chapter is to alert nurses to the importance of understanding religious cultural belief systems and to encourage them to be supportive of beliefs that promote comfort and adaptation.

Nutritional Behavior and Cultural Influences

The kinds of foods eaten, the way they are prepared, and the manner in which they are consumed are practices that are embedded strongly in the behavioral systems of each culture. When a person enters the health-care system, he or she brings all of his or her cultural beliefs and practices about food with him. Frequently, the person's food preferences and manner of consumption conflict with those of the health-care system, which may cause some distress if there is no means of meeting his cultural needs. For example, Schubin (1980) described the incident of a Mexican-American patient who disappeared from his hospital room soon after undergoing major surgery. He had gone home to obtain specific cultural foods — tacos, tortillas, and beans. Later he returned, believing that these foods would speed his recovery.

Niehoff (1969) and Lee (1957) both described "proper" and "improper" foods according to the food values characteristic of a cultural system. Such foods stir positive or negative feelings depending on how the culture views the food. For example, while North Americans are strongly adverse to insects in their diet (improper food), the Ifugaons of the Philippines regard dragon flies as a human (proper) food (Lee, 1957). Similarly, North Americans regard milk as a good food, but Southeast Asians do not. North Americans may consider ice water to be refreshing, but a Chinese person believes that it shocks the system and is harmful to health. Historically, water was boiled in China because of inadequate sanitation (Campbell and Chang, 1973).

Religious beliefs and practices may strongly influence nutritional behavior. For example, Black Muslim doctrine prohibits intake of alcoholic beverages, pork, and foods such as cornbread and collards that are traditionally eaten by black Americans. Orthodox Jews who observe strict kosher dietary laws will not eat pork, and shellfish or combine meat and milk at the same meal (Pumphrey, 1977).

Finally, the influence of food in the cause and treatment of disease is related to one's cultural background. The Chinese believe that foods have "hot" (yang), or "cold" (yin) properties and can influence recovery from disease. Hot or "yang" diseases such as ear infections are treated with cold foods such as wintermelon. Some black persons believe that blood volume increases or decreases related to the consumption of certain foods. For example "high blood" (which may be confused with "high blood pressure") is believed to result from excessive ingestion of rich foods and is treated with astringent foods. Vinegar, pickles, or epsom salts may be eaten to open the pores, allowing sweating and bringing down the "high blood."

Nursing Implications.   When assessing a person's nutritional status, the nurse may gain clues to cultural patterns of food intake and the possible implications these patterns may have on diet teaching and illness. Although it would be difficult to have a vast knowledge of all existing food habits, nurses should be aware of the cultural food preferences of the people living in close proximity to the hospital or clinic. Whatever their own personal preferences, nurses must be careful not to impose their values about food consumption and preparation on those whose cultural nutrition patterns differ.

Cultural Influences on the Person

Chapter 4 described the social, psychological, and biophysical subsystems of the person. Each of these subsystems is influenced by the person's cultural environment. Let us examine the relationship between persons and their cultural environment.

Cultural Influences on Sociological Variables of Persons

Previous discussion centered on the family as the basic socializing unit that introduces a person to the values, attitudes, customs, and social habits of a particular cultural group. The nurse must assess other social variables among ethnic-minority persons: economic status, educational status, social network, and valued social institutions. The relationship between cultural variables and sociological variables is best seen in the consideration of socioeconomic influences on health care.

According to Kosa and Zola (1975), American society is classified into three socioeconomic levels: middle and upper class, blue-collar working class, and the poverty population. These authors contended that a large number of ethnic minorities (i.e., blacks, Hispanics, Native Americans, and other poor ethnic minorities) are part of the lowest of the three strata, characterized by high unemployment, low income, poor housing and living conditions, and low educational standards.

Many literature sources (Irvine, 1970; Bullough and Bullough, 1972; Ruffin, 1979) state that these socioeconomic problems have a profound effect on levels of health among ethnic minorities. Ruffin (1979) concluded that the effects of poverty as a social environment result in a higher degree and more serious kinds of morbidity. A second conclusion was that poverty hampers the poor in maintaining or regaining their health; that is, they are less likely to seek preventive or diagnostic services without symptoms.

For example, the statistics reported by Irvine depict the percentage of Native American infants born on reservations who die annually (32.3 per 1000) as higher than that of the general United States population (23.7 per 1000). The mortality rate for Native American infants in the first year of life is 25 per 1000 versus 7 per 1000 nationally (1970, p 453).

Nursing Implications.   What should be the nurse's approach to incorporating into care both variables of poverty and ethnicity? When the nurse is from a different cultural group than the client, differences in behavioral expectations will exist.

Watts (1967) discussed these issues in her article, "Social Class, Ethnic Background, and Patient Care." Watts stated that nurses have difficulty in caring for patients from lower socioeconomic classes because their expectations of patient behavior contrast with actual behavior, and they have problems understanding these patients' attitudes and their expectations of nurses.

For instance, if a black person who is poor and unemployed fails to return for a follow-up visit for chronic leg ulcers, this may be interpreted by the nurse as a lack of interest in his or her well-being. To this black person the value of "time" and of meeting economic needs may be more important than a return clinic visit.

Nurses should be aware of the dynamics of poverty and available resources. They cannot always remedy the immediate factors relative to poverty, but genuine interest and understanding of behavior and attitudes of poor ethnic minority persons will help to resolve conflicts in dealing with this dilemma.

Cultural Influences on Psychological Variables of Persons

A major psychological variable that is influenced by the cultural environment is self-concept. How family, peers, external environment, and society characterize behavior strongly influences the development of self-concept. The labeling of a characteristic as either "good" or "bad" is the evaluative component of self-concept known as "self-esteem" or one's worth on a scale from very low to very high (Frances and Munjas, 1976).

Smith and associates (1978) defined the self-concept of minorities as follows:

- The way minority persons see themselves from their viewpoint
- The way (nonminority) "others" view them and prescribe what minority persons should be
- The way they "wish" to be known to others and to themselves
- Combination of the three definitions

Nursing Implications.   The nurse's perception of the ethnic minority person and how the person relates to the nurse's perception (based on his or her self-concept) determines the outcome of the nurse-person relationship. Hein (1980) reinforced this statement, saying that if the nurse's role of helper is based on superiority due to negative feelings about a person, the person may not believe the nurse is sincerely interested in his or her needs and welfare.

The nurse should assess how the ethnic minority person responded to psychological stress in the clinical setting. For example, how does this person respond to the psychological distress of physical pain? Davitz and colleagues (1976) did an excellent cross-cultural study on nurses' beliefs about patient suffering. They found 554 nurses from 6 different cultures varied in their interpretations and attitudes about suffering associated with illness and injury (i.e., cancer, trauma, infection, etc.).

A nurse should be aware of both differences and similarities cross-culturally as a way of developing sensitivity to persons with varied cultural backgrounds and avoiding stereotypic approaches in relieving psychological and physical distress.

Cultural Influences on Biophysical Variables of Persons

Biophysical variations among ethnic minority groups influence the findings from physical assessments. Findings that would indicate disease in white persons may be normal in blacks, Asians, or Native Americans. For example, Mongolian spots, which are areas of bluish-black pigmentation of no clinical significance, are common in these ethnic groups. They may be mistaken for bruises by inexperienced health-care practitioners. Also, skin color changes that signify disease such as jaundice and cyanosis may be difficult to detect in dark-skinned individuals.

Certain ethnic groups are at higher risk for development of specific diseases. Some reasons include environmental influences, genetic factors, and inadequate health-care resources. As examples: there is a high incidence of hypertension in black males, and Jews of Eastern European descent are at risk for Tay-Sachs disease. This information is significant for nurses who are involved in health screening programs.

A final factor related to physical differences is growth and development patterns. For example, studies have shown black children to be taller and heavier than white children between ages of 5 to 14. Also, a study by Malina (1971) showed that black children have thinner skinfolds than white children regardless of socioeconomic level, indicating that nutrition is not a factor. Malina suggested "that criteria for evaluating nutritional status via skin folds should be different for American Negro and white samples" (p 37). All of these variations would be very important for the school nurse or pediatric nurse practitioner doing physical assessments of children.

Nursing Approaches to Cultural Differences

Throughout this section, the need for nurses' awareness of cultural patterns has been emphasized. Knowledgeable nurses can greatly assist clients who are struggling with differences between their own cultural norms and those of the health-care system.

Nurses also need to develop an openness to beliefs and behaviors that differ from theirs. Nurses are often unintentionally guilty of ethnocentrism, the belief that one's own cultural or ethnic group is superior to others. Whenever a nurse labels a client's food practices as "strange" or his or her beliefs about folk remedies as "worthless," the nurse is acting from ethnocentrism.

Nursing students may find it hard to accept that the client's health beliefs and behaviors have as much validity as their own. It is helpful to think of belief systems as different colored eyeglasses that one can try on to temporarily view the world from the client's perspective. Flexibility, open-mindedness, willingness to learn, and the ability to establish trust are all important attributes when caring for clients from different cultural groups.

I CONCLUSION

This chapter has examined the physical, social, and cultural aspects of the environment. Environment can be described as the social and physical world outside the system (the person). Persons and their environments are constantly interacting, each changing and being changed by the other. The physical environment is conceptualized as consisting of the community environment with related ecological issues and the immediate environment with concomitant concerns of safety, function, and comfort. The social environment is comprised of the social systems of family, group, and community. One important function of the social environment—social support—has been shown to be positively related to health. Culture, a concept that is related to the social environment, has multiple relationships to health. Cultural differences between clients and health professionals in health and illness beliefs, language, nutrition, and so forth affect clients' experiences as they seek health care.

Nurses view persons as holistic beings who interact continuously with their environments. Thus, nurses have considerable knowledge and skills for analyzing how the interaction between persons and their environment affects their health. With this analysis, nurses are capable of making appropriate environmental alterations. Specific examples of how nurses can improve health through environmental changes were presented throughout the chapter.

| STUDY QUESTIONS

1 Review the newspaper or a news magazine for one week. What environmental issues are receiving media attention? What action could you take to affect these problems?

2 Examine your home environment for safety hazards. Now look again and identify hazards if the following people came to visit your home:
   a A toddler
   b A person who uses a cane or a walker
   c An elderly person with poor vision

3 How can nurses control infection in the following situations?
   a A day-care center
   b Caring for a person in the home
   c Caring for clients in the hospital

4 Ask several people to define their family. How do their responses differ from the definitions presented in this chapter?

5 Examine a group to which you belong for the following factors:
   a Roles of group members
   b Communication patterns,
   c Decision-making processes.

   What changes would strengthen the functioning of your group?

6 Examine the community where you live for the following factors:
   a Do most employers provide health insurance for their employees? What is the level of unemployment?
   b Is there a hospital in your community? What kinds of services does it provide? Where do people go for specialty care?
   c What kinds of industries are present in your community? Do any present health hazards?
   d What health-care services are provided by the local government?

   How do these factors in the community system affect health care?

7 What is social support? Why is it important for nurses to identify the adequacy of social support for their clients?

8 Mr. Chin, a native of Taiwan, has been diagnosed with high blood pressure. He eats a great deal of soy sauce (which has high sodium content) and his physician has prescribed a low-sodium diet. What factors in the cultural environment must be considered in caring for this client?

| REFERENCES

American Nurses' Association: Code for Nurses with Interpretive Statements. Kansas City, MO, American Nurses' Association, 1976, 1985

Broadhead WE, Kaplan BH, et al: The epidemiologic evidence for a relationship between social support and health. Am J Epidemiol 117:521–531, 1983

Bullough B, Bullough VL: Poverty, Ethnic Identity and Health Care. New York, Appleton-Century-Crofts, 1972

Campbell T, Chang B: Health care of the Chinese in America. Nurs Outlook 21:245–239, 1973

Cannon WB: Bodily Changes In Pain, Hunger, Fear, and Rage, 2nd ed. New York, Appleton, 1929

Cassel J: Psychosocial processes and stress: Theoretical formulations. Int J Health Serv 4(3):471–482, 1974

Cassel J: The contribution of the social environment to host resistance. Am J Epidemiol 104:107–123, 1976

Cobb S: Social support as a moderator of life stress. Psychosom Med 38:300–314, 1976

Davitz LJ, Sameshima Y, Davitz J: Suffering as viewed in six different cultures. Am J Nurs 76:1296–1297, 1976

De Araujo G, van Arsdel PP, Holmes TH, et al: Life change, coping ability, and chronic intrinsic asthma. J Psychosomat Res 17:359–363, 1973

DeGarcia RT: Cultural influences on Filipino patients. Am J Nurs 79:1412–1414, 1979

Downs JF: Cultures in Crisis, 2nd ed. Beverly Hills, CA, Glencoe, 1975

Frances GM, Munjas BD: Manual of Social Psychologic Assessment. New York, Appleton-Century-Crofts, 1976

Friedman M: Family Nursing: Theory and Assessment, 2nd ed. Norwalk, CT, Appleton-Century-Crofts, 1986

Gore S: The effect of social support in moderating the health consequences of unemployment. J Health Soc Behav 19:157–165, 1978

Hall J: Social organization. In Hall J, Weaver BR (eds): Distributive Nursing Practice: A Systems Approach to Community Health, 2nd ed, pp 30–43. Philadelphia, JB Lippincott, 1985

Hein EC: Communication in Nursing Practice, 2nd ed. Boston, Little, Brown, 1980

Hirabayashi JN: The quiet American? A re-evaluation. Amerasia J 3(1):114–127, 1975

Holland WR: Mexican American medical beliefs: Science or magic? In Martinez RA (ed): Hispanic Culture and Health Care (Fact, Fiction, Folklore), pp 99–119. St. Louis, CV Mosby, 1978

Holmes TH, Rahe RH: The social readjustment rating scale. J Psychosom Res 11:213–218, 1967

House JS: Work Stress and Social Support. Reading, MA, Addison-Wesley, 1981

Irvine J: On not being upper-class. N Engl J Med 282:453, 1970

Jarvis LL: Community Health Nursing, 2nd ed. Philadelphia, FA Davis, 1985

Kalisch PA, Kalisch BJ: The Advance of American Nursing, 2nd ed. Boston, Little, Brown, 1986

Killien MG: An environmental approach to nursing practice. In Hall JE, Weaver BR: Distributive Nursing Practice: A Systems Approach to Community Health, 2nd ed, pp 259–277. Philadelphia, JB Lippincott, 1985

Kluckholn FR, Strodtbeck FL: Variations in Value Orientations, Evanston, IL, Row, Peterson, 1961

Kosa J, Zola I (eds): Poverty and Health: A Sociological Analysis. Cambridge, MA, Harvard University Press, 1975

Lee D: Cultural factors in dietary choice. Am J Clin Nutr 5(2):166–170, 1957

Lin N, Ensel WM, Simeone RS, et al: Social support, stressful life events and illness: A model and an empirical test. J Health Soc Behav 20:109–119, 1979

Lindenmuth JE, Breu CS, Malooley JA: Sensory overload. Am J Nurs 80:1456–1458, 1980

Malina RM: Skinfolds in American negro and white children. J Am Diet Assoc 59:34–40, 1971

Mancino D: The future and environmental health nursing. Imprint 32(3):42–45, 1985

Meth IM: Electrical safety in the hospital. Am J Nurs 80:1344–1348, 1980

Moore LG, Van Arsdale PW, Glittenberg JE, et al: The Biocultural Basis of Health. St. Louis, CV Mosby, 1980

Moos R: Conceptualizations of human environments. Am Psychologist 28:652–665, 1973

Murray RB, Zentner JP: Nursing Concepts for Health Promotion, 3rd ed. Englewood Cliffs, NJ, Prentice-Hall, 1985

National League for Nursing, Department of Baccalaureate and Higher Degree Programs: Criteria for the Appraisal of Baccalaureate and Higher Degree Programs in Nursing. Publication No. 15-1251, 4th ed. New York, National League for Nursing, 1977

Neihoff A: Changing food habits. J Nutr Edu 1(1):10–11, 1969

Nightingale F: Notes on Nursing: What It Is and What It Is Not. London, Harrison, 1859. Facsimile edition: Philadelphia, JB Lippincott, 1966

Norbeck J: Social support: A model for clinical research and application. Adv Nurs Sci 3(4):43–59, 1981

Nuckolls KB, Cassel J, Kaplan BH: Psychosocial assets, life crisis, and the prognosis of pregnancy. Am J Epidemiology 95:431–441, 1972

Otto H: What is a strong family? Marriage Fam Living 24:72–80, 1962

Pender NJ: Health Promotion in Nursing Practice. Norwalk, CT, Appleton-Century-Crofts, 1982

Pillitteri A: Child Health Nursing, 3rd ed. Boston, Little, Brown, 1987

Primeaux M: Caring for the American Indian patient. Am J Nurs 77(1):91–96, 1977

Pumphrey JB: Recognizing your patient's spiritual needs. Nursing '77 7(12):64–70, 1977

Rogers M: An Introduction to the Theoretical Basis of Nursing. Philadelphia, FA Davis, 1970

Roy SC: Roy's adaptation model. In Parse RR (ed): Nursing Science: Major Paradigms, Theories, and Critiques, pp 35–45. Philadelphia, WB Saunders, 1987

Ruffin JE: Changing Perspectives in Ethnicity and Health, A Strategy for Change. Kansas City, MO, American Nurses' Association, 1979

Samovar LA, Porter RE (eds): Intercultural Communication: A Reader, 2nd ed. Belmont, CA, Wadsworth, 1976

Schubin S: Nursing patients from different cultures. Nursing '80 10(6):78–81, 1980

Scott CS: Health and healing practices among five ethnic groups in Miami, Florida. Pub Health Rep 89(6)524–532, 1974

Smith WD, Burlew AK, Mosley MH, et al: Minority Issues in Mental Health. Reading, MA, Addison-Wesley, 1978

Snow LF: Folk medical beliefs and their implications for care of patients (a review based on studies among black Americans). Ann Intern Med 81(1):82–96, 1974

Stanhope M, Lancaster J: Community Health Nursing, 2nd ed. St. Louis, CV Mosby, 1988

Staples R: Introduction to Black Sociology. New York, McGraw-Hill, 1976

U.S. Department of Commerce: Statistical Abstract of the United States: National Data Book and Guide to Sources, 103rd ed. Washington, DC, US Department of Commerce, 1982–1983

Walker J: Prevention of premature death and disability due to injury. In Last JM (ed): Public Health and Preventive Medicine, 12th ed, pp 1543–1576. Norwalk, CT, Appleton-Century-Crofts, 1986

Watts W: social class, ethnic background, and patient care. Nurs Forum 6(2):155–162, 1967

Werner EE: Cross-Cultural Child Development: A View from the Planet Earth. Monterey, CA, Brooks/Cole, 1979

White EH: Giving health care to minority patients. Nurs Clin North Am 12(1):27–40, 1977

Wolff HG: Stress and Disease. Springfield, IL, Charles C Thomas, 1953

6 | HEALTH: ADAPTATION TO THE STRESS OF LIFE

KEY WORDS	After completing this chapter, students will be able to:
Adaptation	Develop a nursing perspective of health and adaptation.
Anxiety	Describe reciprocal interactions between persons and the
Behavior	environment as systems.
Coping	
Coping behavior	Recognize various models of health.
Crisis	Discuss the relationship between health and adaptation.
Distress	Describe the phenomena of change, stress, crisis, anxiety, and
Eustress	coping, and their effects on persons.
Health	
Health behavior	Identify theories of adaptation as they relate to persons and
Homeodynamics	their environment.
Illness behavior	Identify ways the professional nurse promotes health and
Maladaptation	adaptation.
Self-care	
Stress	Describe the concept of self-care.
Stressor	

As a nurse, you will be in a unique position to learn how to help yourself at the same time you learn how to help others. You will be privileged to assist persons in dealing with some of their most difficult and intimate life experiences. As a health professional, you will make life and death decisions in collaboration with clients, their families, and other health professionals. Nurses need to know a great deal about life and persons and health.

The goal of nursing, as stated earlier, is to help persons maintain optimum biological, psychological, and social functioning by adapting to a changing environment and functional alterations or deviations from health. To accomplish this goal, nurses need to understand the interaction between persons and their environment.

Currently, we are learning more and more about human health and survival, stress, crisis, coping, prevention, biofeedback, fitness, and wellness. Research findings support the belief that many illnesses and health problems are stress-related and preventable. Many psychophysiological disorders—often labeled *psychosomatic illnesses*—are now recognized as stress-related, occurring when persons do not cope effectively with change. Certain disorders—such as asthma, ulcers, hypertension, some cancers, depression, phobias, alcoholism, drug abuse, periodic attacks of epileptic seizures, and migraine headaches — are also considered by some authorities to be linked to stress.

With so many health problems apparently associated with ineffective coping, every individual is presented with the opportunity and the challenge to learn how to stay well. This chapter explores the concept of health and the relationship of health, environment, and adaptation. Several models of health and adaptation are discussed as well as concepts of crisis, coping, anxiety, and stress. The relationship of health and adaptation to self-care and applications to nursing practice is also explored.

PERSONS, ENVIRONMENT, AND THEIR INTERACTION

Environment

The *person* was described in Chapter 4 as an open system composed of biological, psychological, and social variables. The environment, discussed in Chapter 5, also can be considered an open system composed of subsystems and their variables, whether they be social, natural, or manufactured. The social environment consists of other human beings with whom persons interact in the family, in the community, and in society. The natural environment includes those aspects of the environment that exist independently of humans, such as climate or topography. The human-made environment includes human achievements in service to others, as well as undesired consequences of human creativity. All are essential to the study of persons.

Examples of environmental variables are presented in Table 6–1. These examples point out how complex each subsystem is. Consequently, the survival and health of each of us is dependent on our own strengths and resourcefulness in dealing with forces to which we are subject.

Both persons and environments are living, dynamic systems with porous boundaries capable of exchanging matter, energy, and information. The person, for example, receives internal information from the body indicating hunger, and the response is to take food from the environment. The same food becomes a source of energy for the person's body.

Picture the interaction between living systems that occur with a man lost on a rainy day in a noisy, crowded city in a foreign country whose language he does not speak. Figure 6–1 shows the reciprocal interaction between these two systems: person and environment. Note the multiple complex systems and subsystems within the environment that each person with his or her multiple subsystems is likely to encounter. Considering the amount of matter, energy, and information that is exchanged between these systems, it is remarkable that we complex persons are able to maintain disequilibrium in an equally complex environment.

Person — Environment System

When living systems operate in an effective or healthy state, they interact to produce a balance within each system and a balance among the various systems. When change occurs in either the person or the environment, disequilibrium or disorganization may result. This disequilibrium requires an adjustment. For example, a person responds to a change in the weather by altering the amount of clothing worn for protection. Such a response maintains health against the threat of heat or cold.

TABLE 6-1
EXAMPLES OF ENVIRONMENTAL VARIABLES

Social Variables	Natural Variables	Human-Made Variables
Human relationships	Water	Tools and machines
Interpersonal communications	Air	Buildings
Community groups	Land	Towns and cities
Family groups	Plants	Business and industry
Interest groups	Animals	Transportation
Culture	Microorganisms	Technology
Societal norms	Minerals	Pollution
Lifestyle	Space	Chemical
Philosophy	Solar systems	Noise
Social roles	Natural laws of physics	Accidents
Societal institutions	Energy	Overcrowding
Education	Weather	Privacy
Marriage	Heat	Urban decay
Government	Cold	Drugs
Economy	Light	Violence
Religion	Sound	Conservation
		Art
		Music
		Architecture
		Books

If the person and his or her environment do not interact in an effective way, a threat to health occurs. For example, a woman who smokes heavily may eventually develop respiratory disease. If she also lives in an area with high concentrations of air pollutants, this likelihood becomes even greater. Health, then, is linked to the effective interaction of persons with their environments. As stated in *Healthy People: The Surgeon General's Report on Health Promotion and Disease Prevention:*

> For decision makers in the public and private sector, a recognition of the relationship between health and the physical environment can lead to actions that can greatly reduce the morbidity and mortality caused by accidents, air, water, and food contamination, radiation exposure, excessive noise, occupational hazards, dangerous consumer products and unsafe highway design. (Department of Health, Education, and Welfare, 1979, pp 1–12, 13)

As informed decision makers, nurses ought to influence health-promoting action both in their private lives as citizens and in their professional lives as nurses concerned with person-centered care. For example, with a knowledge of both the community environment and local health practices, the community health nurse may alert citizens to hazards they have not recognized. The mechanism by which persons adjust to their environment is the process of adaptation.

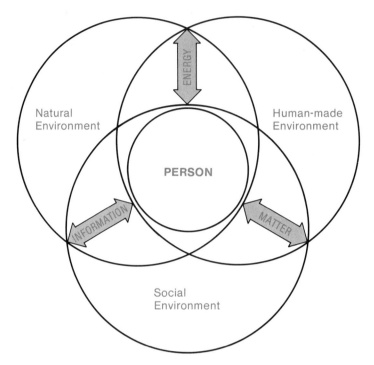

Figure 6-1   A reciprocal interaction exists between person and environment.

| WHAT IS HEALTH?

Nurses promote health by helping the person to preserve and strengthen adaptation and to develop new strategies for coping. Therefore, it is essential that we understand the concept of health and the process of adaptation.

Health means different things to different persons; nevertheless, the term is a familiar one. It is easy to relate the concept of health to ourselves by recalling past experiences of illness as well as those activities performed to keep well. Some consider health the opposite of illness. Others view health as something one has or does not have, as shown in these statements: "When you have your health, you have everything." "My health is good." "I lost my health when. . . ." "I have a health problem." "How's your health?"

Control over one's health may be implied when persons refer to various activities or substances: "It is healthy to exercise and eat well." "Smoking may be hazardous to your health."

These examples illustrate a variety of perspectives about the concept of health. Definitions developed over the past several years demonstrate the effort being made by the scientific community to define health more precisely.

Definitions and Models of Health and Illness

The World Health Organization was hailed for recognizing the whole person when, in 1947, it stated a new, broad definition of health in its constitution. This definition was unique because it introduced a more humanistic perspective than previously accepted. The definition of **health** was as follows: . . . a state of complete physical, mental, and social well-being, not merely the absence of disease or infirmity (p 29).

Smith (1983) described four models of health based on her reviews of literature on fundamental concepts of the nature of health: (1) the clinical model, (2) the role-performance model, (3) the adaptive model, and (4) the eudaimonistic model.

Clinical Model

The clinical model represents the medical model of health. Health is defined as the absence of disease. Illness is viewed according to directly observable aberrations such as the presence of microorganisms, toxic bacteria or viruses, or trauma. The focus of care in this model is "primarily the elimination of morbid physical or mental conditions and relief from concomitant pain" (Smith, 1981, p 46). Optimal function of mind and body is not considered. The health-care provider's role ends when symptoms of disease are no longer present and relief is obtained.

Role-Performance Model

The role-performance model represents health as the ability of a person to perform effectively his or her roles. It is based on the work of medical sociologists and the writings of Parsons (1972). Roles can include wage earning and parenting, among many others. Illness is viewed as incapacity to perform social roles and tasks based on feelings of not being well. Illness may be difficult to define in this model because persons may perform some roles yet fail in others.

Adaptive Model

The adaptive model of health is based on the work of Rene Dubos, a 20th-century biologist and philosopher. He wrote, "Health or disease is the expression of success or failure by persons in their efforts to respond adaptively to environmental challenges" (1965, p xvii).

Many nursing writers adhere to this model. Among them, Murray and Zentner defined health as

> a state of well-being in which the person is able to use purposeful, adaptive responses and processes physically, mentally, emotionally, spiritually, and socially, in response to internal and external stimuli (stressors) in order to maintain relative stability and comfort and to strive for personal objectives and cultural goals. (1985, pp 4–5).

Within this model, health is a reaction of the whole organism, the consequence of factors including internal and external stimuli and predisposition of the individual. Health care focuses on restoring the ability to cope with environmental changes.

Eudaimonistic Model

Eudaemonia, from which this model's name is derived, refers to a state of "happiness as the result of an active life governed by reason" (*The American College Dictionary*, 1962, p 414). This model is represented by the work of humanistic psychologists, particularly Abraham Maslow. These psychologists based their work on a belief in the uniqueness and wholeness of persons and recognized qualities such as potential for growth, individuality, autonomy, self-realization, and productivity. As a result of the humanistic movement, perspectives of health began to broaden; perceptions of human potential expanded. Health was defined as actualization or realization of one's potential. Illness is a condition that prevents self-actualization.

H.L. Dunn, a physician with the U.S. Public Health Service for many years, reflected the views of the humanistic psychologists when he wrote

> Good health can exist as a relatively passive state of freedom from illness in which the individual is at peace with his environment—a condition of relative homeostasis. Wellness is conceptualized as dynamic—a condition of change in which the individual moves forward, climbing toward a higher potential of functioning. (1959, p 447)

He defined high-level wellness as "an integrated method of functioning which is oriented toward maximizing the potential of which the individual is capable within the environment where he is functioning" (1959, p 447). High-level wellness involves the following:

- A continuing improvement in the way we function
- Continuing progress in our ability to respond to life's challenges
- Increasing oneness of our whole being—mind, body, and spirit—in the way we function

Within the eudaimonistic model, the "patient" emerges as a liberated, rational, creative, free-thinking person capable of self-realization and autonomy. "Patients" become "clients" who take responsibility for their own health care. The role of nurses and other health professionals within this model is to assist clients to achieve self-actualization.

Other Models of Health

These concepts of health, although not identified in Smith's work, also can be found in literature reviews on health.

Primitive Model.   In the primitive model, health and illness are controlled by forces external to humans. Ancient humans viewed natural phenomena, including illness, as the work of gods or spirits and religious and health practices were often closely interwoven. Medicine men or priests were employed to dispel evil spirits from the unfortunate sick. Even today, nurses may encounter many persons who view their illness as a punishment for wrongdoings or as an autonomous, amorphous force that attacked without provocation. "Why me?" is a common question among these individuals.

Ecological Model.   The ecological model is based on person-environment relationships. The three components of this model include a host or susceptible individual, an injury- or disease-producing agent, and the environment, which if poor or unhealthy may predispose persons to disease. Illness is a directly observable aberration caused by interaction of these three factors.

Health-Illness Continuum.   The health-illness continuum model perpetuates the medical model by equating health with absence of illness. This model pictures a horizontal scale with health at one pole and illness at the other. Health is viewed as the opposite of illness. Many find the health-illness continuum model unsatisfactory because most persons are neither totally healthy nor totally ill. It is difficult to accept a model that places persons at one particular point of the continuum. Jahoda rejected the health-illness continuum in reference to mental health, and wrote, "As with every other typological classification, pure types do not exist. Every human being has simultaneously healthy and sick aspects, with one or the other predominating" (1958, p 75).

Analysis of Models

The models just presented pose questions about health. If we believed that persons were defenseless victims of disease as described in the primitive model, we could do little to prevent or treat those who are affected. Of course, we recognize the fallacy of this belief because we have seen persons recover from many serious afflictions. Yet, some depressed persons who are grieving and guilt-ridden over their past behaviors (which they may view as sins) may be operating according to this model.

On close examination, other models also exhibit shortcomings. Using the clinical model, how do we explain the variety of responses we see among persons exposed to the same organisms or traumas? Not everyone becomes ill when exposed to the same environment. The ecological model describes the susceptibility of individuals to illness. Yet, how do we evaluate who is susceptible and who is not when all other factors are present, as in the ecological and clinical models? The adaptive model includes concepts from the four previous ones and focuses on the organism as a whole.

The role-performance model has long been in existence among many societies and cultures. Persons who give complaints of illness are excused from their social roles and responsibilities. However, subjective feelings alone are not always considered sufficient determinants of illness. For many, such illnesses are seen as avoidance behavior. Consider how many years women were excused from physical exertion and other activities during menstruation. For many others, such as the combat soldier or migrant farmer, the excuse of "not feeling well" would be scorned.

These models suggest a number of perspectives about health. Today, nurses encounter a variety of views about health held by persons from different cultures in the United States and other parts of the world. Actually, wellness and illness are determined culturally: what is healthy, normal behavior is one culture may be considered unhealthy, abnormal behavior in another. Therefore, the nurse is challenged to understand the biological, psychological, sociocultural, and environmental facets of persons who may be patients or clients.

Health Behavior and Illness Behavior

Efforts by others to define health have been directed toward objective criteria, namely, behavior. The term **behavior** refers to an emitted response (action or reaction); it is overt, observable, and measurable. Consequently, scientists in the health-care fields have begun research to define and clarify behavior as outcomes of health that can be measured and evaluated.

The concept of **health behavior** is quite complex and extensive, as evidenced by the literature on the subject. However, Wu's definition is one of the most succinct and provides direction for both nurses and consumers. Wu wrote that health behavior is "any activity undertaken by an individual who believes himself to be well to avoid an encounter with illness," (1973, p 112). Behaviors such as regular hygienic practices and participation in "well-balanced programs of rest, exercise, diet, and elimination" may be considered health behaviors (1973, p 112). Health-wellness, Wu writes, is a behavioral manifestation characterized by "a feeling of well-being, a capacity to perform to the best of one's ability; it is evidenced by an ability to adjust to and adapt actively to varying situations, to perceive correctly, free from need distortions, complemented with a wholesome outlook on life" (1973, p 86).

Illness behavior, on the other hand, is defined as follows:

> behavior that is triggered by such cues as pain, discomfort, signs of malfunction, and/or by confirmation by word of mouth that the individual is experiencing illness. (It) is the initial response of the person to aberrations of the body and psyche which he perceives as incapacitating and therefore as a sign of illness. (Wu, 1973, pp 136–137)

In the growing field of health behavior, health-care professionals join with behavioral and social scientists to study the effectiveness and the results of health care.

| WHAT IS ADAPTATION?

Adaptation includes the concepts of persons as biopsychosocial beings, the interaction or process of exchange with the environment, change or transformation, and health (the goal of adaptation). A working definition reads as follows: Adaptation is the process of changing throughout life by persons faced with new, different, or threatening experiences without loss of health, a sense of wholeness, or integrity of self.

The essence of adaptation is change; it is a process of dynamic equilibrium that is vital for survival. In broad terms, adaptation consists of biological, psychological, social, and spiritual facets. The concept of health, discussed previously in this chapter, is closely related to adaptation. Adaptation moves a person toward health and growth; **maladaptation**, on the other hand, occurs when a person uses inadequate ways of dealing with stress in an attempt to maintain equilibrium.

When change occurs in the environment, the person must adapt. This process requires energy, and rapid change may require more energy than the person has available. When the rate or amount of change exceeds our capacity to adapt, illness may occur, however, successful adaptation may strengthen integrity of self or lead to an even higher level of functioning.

Adaptation Theories

Historical Development

The concept of adaptation, as developed over the past century, is outlined in Table 6–2 and summarized below.

Bernard (Steady State).   Claude Bernard, a physiologist, was one of the pioneers in the study of the body's attempts to achieve a steady state while dealing with change. He pointed out that the internal environment of all organisms remains fairly constant even though the external environment changes. For example, the body maintains a stable core temperature despite changes in the weather.

Cannon (Homeostasis).   In the early part of this century, Walter B. Cannon, another physiologist, introduced the concept of "homeostasis" (1939). Homeostasis means the maintenance of equilibrium or a steady state of the body. For instance, the oxygen concentration within arteries remains fairly constant, even though carbon dioxide is continually given off by cells and oxygen is taken in by the lungs. Cannon recognized that this steady state was not completely fixed; rather, it varied within certain limits.

The term *homeostasis* has been criticized by some theorists because it implies inability of a system to develop or evolve. Martha Rogers (1970) supported the use of the

TABLE 6-2
PERSPECTIVES ON ADAPTATION

Scientist and Profession	Theory
Claude Bernard, physiologist	The internal environment of all organisms remains fairly constant even though the external environment changes.
Walter B. Cannon, physiologist	Homeostasis is the ability of living organisms to maintain their own equilibrium.
Hans Selye, endocrinologist	General adaptation syndrome: The body's response to stress of any kind occurs as a unified defense mechanism with specific structural and chemical changes. The reaction elicits resistance by the body to stressful agents and protects against disease. When the reaction is too long or faulty, disease or death may occur.
Rene Dubos, biologist	Health or disease is the expression of the success or failure by persons in their efforts to respond adaptively to environmental challenges.
Alvin Toffler, experimental psychologist and author of *Future Shock*	The faster the rate of change in a given time span, the more difficult it becomes for persons to adapt.
T.H. Holmes and R.H. Rahe, psychiatrists	Use of the Social Readjustment Rating Scale demonstrates a correlation between stressful life events and illness and may be a predictor of illness.

term **homeodynamics**, which implies a state of balance leading toward growth and evolution.

Consider the expected changes that occur to cells and organs from conception through aging. We know that certain changes are likely to occur at specific times in our lives. The growth and developmental processes are relatively constant; at the same time, they are self-regulated. "The wonder increases," Cannon wrote, "when we realize that the system is open, engaging in free exchange with the outer world, and that the structure itself is not permanent but is continuously being broken down by the wear and tear of action, and is continuously built up again by processes of repair" (1939, p 20).

Selye (Stress).   More recently, the work of Hans Selye has stimulated great interest in the concepts of stress and adaptation (1956). Selye, an endocrinologist, defined **stress** as the normal wear and tear of daily living and defined a **stressor** as anything that induces stress. He described the body's response to stress as a unified defense mechanism with specific structural and chemical changes and called this the "general adaptation syndrome" (GAS). The GAS response elicits resistance by the body to stressful agents, enhancing its ability to ward off these stressors. However, if this reaction is faulty or prolonged, disease or death may result.

The GAS has three phases: alarm reaction, resistance, and exhaustion. The responses in each stage are as follows:

Alarm. Defenses mobilize to respond to stressor.
Resistance. Body tries to adapt to stressor.

Exhaustion. If stressor persists or is severe, or if the person has limited adaptive capacity, the body loses ability to adapt; exhaustion and death follow.

Selye's early work concentrated on the physiological response to stress, although he subsequently recognized the role of psychological stress in the adaptation syndrome. However, the relationship between psychological stress and physiological response is still under study.

Dubos. Another perspective is that of biologist Rene Dubos, previously described in the discussion of the adaptive model of health.

Toffler (Culture Shock). Alvin Toffler, an experimental psychologist, described adaptation in his famous work *Future Shock* (1970), in which he discussed what happens to persons who encounter change of any kind. Toffler pointed out that the faster the rate of change in a given time span, the more difficult it becomes for persons to adapt. The term *culture shock* has become a byword to convey "profound disorientation suffered by the traveler who has plunged without adequate preparation into an alien culture" (1970, p 308). Today we recognize that the ability of persons to adapt in our rapidly changing world is being tested as never before.

Holmes and Rahe. Research on the relationship of adaptation to wellness has increased in recent years. Holmes and Rahe stimulated well-known research in this area (1967). They developed the Social Readjustment Rating Scale to demonstrate the correlation between stressful life events and serious illness. The ranking of life events was the result of perceived changes in life style following the events. The life events identified were not necessarily undesirable; rather, they included any experience that required some degree of adaptation (Table 6–3).

Studies showed that the number of life changes and subsequent alterations in the life styles of persons did have an effect on physiological adaptation; that is, persons who experienced a number of stressful events within 1 year were more likely to develop illness. Later studies by Holmes, Rahe, and others supported this belief. Therefore, it is reasonable to expect that persons experiencing too many life changes (multiple stressors) in a short span of time may be suitable candidates for intervention to prevent serious illness.

Development of the Concepts of
Adaptation and Health in Nursing

The concept of adaptation has been the focus of studies by professional nurses in education, research, and practice. Because adaptation is essential to maintain health, these concepts are important to nursing as a profession. Florence Nightingale, Myra Levine, Imogene King, Martha Rogers, and Sister Callista Roy are among those nurses who have contributed to the development of a nursing perspective on adaptation and health.

Nightingale. Often called the founder of modern nursing, Florence Nightingale was the first to consider the nature of health (1859). Nightingale believed that the condition of the environment affected a person's ability to adapt. Although she did not specifically use the term *adaptation*, her writings about the importance of the environment have affected all of the nursing theorists who followed her. A poor environment requires that a sick person use much of his or her energy to deal with these conditions rather than to recover from illness. Nightingale thought that a nurse's function was to provide a favorable

TABLE 6–3
SOCIAL READJUSTMENT RATING SCALE

Rank	Life Event	Mean Value*	Rank	Life Event	Mean Value*
1	Death of spouse	100	23	Son or daughter leaving home	29
2	Divorce	73			
3	Marital separation	65	24	Trouble with in-laws	29
4	Jail term	63	25	Outstanding personal achievement	28
5	Death of close family member	63			
			26	Wife begins or stops work	26
6	Personal injury or illness	53	27	Begin or end school	26
7	Marriage	50	28	Change in living conditions	25
8	Fired from work	47	29	Revision of personal habits	24
9	Marital reconciliation	45	30	Trouble with boss	23
10	Retirement	45	31	Change in work hours or conditions	20
11	Change in health of family member	44			
			32	Change in residence	20
12	Pregnancy	40	33	Change in schools	20
13	Sexual difficulties	39	34	Change in recreation	19
14	Gain of new family member	39	35	Change in church activities	19
15	Business adjustment	39	36	Change in social activities	18
16	Change in financial state	38	37	Mortgage or loan less than $10,000	17
17	Death of close friend	37			
18	Change to different line of work	36	38	Change in sleeping habits	16
			39	Change in number of family get-togethers	15
19	Change in number of arguments with spouse	35			
			40	Change in eating habits	15
20	Mortgage over $10,000	31	41	Vacation	13
21	Foreclosure of mortgage or loan	30	42	Christmas	12
			43	Minor violations of the law	11
22	Change in responsibilities at work	29			

*Values were assigned to life events according to the degree of change in life style they require.
(Holmes TH, Rahe RH: J Psychosom Res 2:214, 1967)

environment (adequate ventilation, water, cleanliness, and warmth) so that the person would be in the best possible position for the natural healing processes to occur.

Although many of the housekeeping activities that once were performed by nurses have been delegated to nonnursing personnel today, nurses still are concerned with environmental factors that affect health. For instance, a nurse in the hospital tries to provide adequate stimulus in the environment to prevent boredom or withdrawal. In the community, a nurse might recognize that an overcrowded apartment potentially affects a family's health and might assist them to find a more suitable living space.

Levine.   Like Nightingale, Myra Levine believed that nursing is based on the person's response to the environment. She wrote, "The nurse participates actively in every patient's environment and much of what she does supports his adaptations as he struggles in the predicament of illness" (1973, p 13). Levine defined adaptation as a process of change to meet the realities of the environment, enabling the person to retain integrity or wholeness of self. She defined health as a pattern of adaptation characterized by enhancement of the person's wholeness and well-being. Nursing involves recognizing the person's needs and adaptive responses and assisting persons to maintain and conserve integrity.

Levine defines two types of nursing actions: *supportive* (those actions that help the person adapt to an altered level of health, such as with dying persons) and *therapeutic* (those that promote healing and restoration of health). Note that both Nightingale and Levine considered only the nurse's role with ill persons; today we recognize the nurses assist persons in any state of health.

King.   Imogene King also considered the environment and its relationship to adaptation and to health (1981). She believed that persons are constantly in the process of using energy to change so that they can meet the requirements of the environment. King defined health as dynamic life experiences of persons, which implies continuous adjustment to stressors through optimum use of resources to achieve maximum potential for daily living (1981). The goal of nursing, according to King, is to help persons cope with health problems or adjust to interference in their health state. In other words, nurses help persons to cope with health and illness.

Rogers.   Martha Rogers (1970) believed in interaction of man and environment, which results in change and growth (homeodynamics). This belief is in opposition to the traditional notion of adaptation leading to a steady state (homeostasis). Change is an ongoing, irreversible process that prevents a person from going back to what he was before. Rogers used systems theory (discussed in Chapter 4) to describe the relationship between persons and the environment. She believed that a person and his or her environment need to be considered as a single system, because both are energy fields with no real boundaries between them. Each is continually affecting and being affected by the other; thus, health is described as "characteristics and behaviors emerging from interactions between man and environment." *Health* is a relative term because various cultures perceive health differently. Rogers viewed the nurse as a part of the person's environment; the nurse's goal is to promote a harmonious interaction between persons and environment.

Roy.   Sister Callista Roy defined adaptation as a positive response to the demands made on a person by the changing environment (1984). Adaptation is a function of the stimulus to which a person is exposed and is his or her adaptation level, while health is a state and a process of being and becoming an integrated and whole person. Persons use biological, psychological, and social mechanisms to cope with their world. The goal of nursing is to promote adaptation in four modes:

- Physiological needs (e.g., elimination, nutrition)
- Self-concept (sense of who we are)
- Role function (socially expected behaviors)
- Interdependence (balance between independence and dependence in our relationships with others)

A person needs nursing care when his or her adaptive responses are inadequate.

Orem.   Orem (1985) did not use the concept of adaptation in her model but rather focused on the person's capacity for self-care; her model of self-care is presented later in this chapter. Health is a state of a person that is characterized by soundness or wholeness of developed human structures and of bodily and mental functioning. Nursing is concerned with the person's "need for self-care action and the provision and management of it on a continuous basis in order to sustain life and health, recover from disease or injury, and cope with their effects" (1980, p 6). Nurses deal with health-related self-care deficits. As a person's health state becomes more favorable, his or her nursing care needs are modified and eventually eliminated.

Common Themes

Several common themes can be found among these authors' views about health and adaptation:

1   Persons continually interact with their environment.
2   Adaptation is the person's response to a change in the environment.
3   Environmental changes occur constantly, so adaptation is a continuous process.
4   The goal of nursing is to promote adaptation.
5   As we help persons to adapt, we are helping them to maintain or achieve health.

The importance of adaptation as a nursing concept should be apparent from this summary. Health depends on using our powers to respond effectively to the environment. It is true that all nurses do not practice using adaptation theory as a base. Yet each of us, whether we realize it or not, is actively helping our clients to adapt.

Rogers, Erickson, and Maslow, whose theories have been represented earlier, also used the concept of adaptation even though they were not nurses. They referred to adaptation indirectly when they stated that persons have the power within themselves to achieve their potential. In other words, because each of us has the power to adapt, adaptation is a key concept for any professional who assists persons with their health.

Process of Adaptation

To understand the process of adaptation, nurses must be familiar with several of its subconcepts:

- Stress and stressor
- Anxiety
- Adaptive and maladaptive coping behavior
- Crisis

None of the subconcepts is a synonym for the others; yet, each is related to the others as indicated in the following statement (subconcepts are italicized):

> Wear and tear of a *stress*ful event may produce disequilibrium, especially if persons are unprepared or unskilled to deal (*cope*) with the event. The failure to regain equilibrium will lead to *anxiety*, and excessive anxiety that remains unrelieved may lead to a *crisis*.

Stress

Stress has been defined as both a state and a response by various authors. Selye defines stress as "the nonspecific response of the body to any demand made upon it" (1975, p 14). Selye emphasized that stress is a normal part of life. Freedom from stress occurs only with death (Selye, 1956). Any stressful event produces disequilibrium; however, each person's perceptions of an event are unique.

The term *stressor* is often used in lieu of stress. The stressor (stimulus) places demands on persons to prepare for a change, for instance, pain, cold, a test. Stressors such as those identified in the Social Readjustment Rating Scale by Holmes and Rahe may or may not be happy events. **Eustress** is a state induced by a pleasant stimuli, whereas **distress** is a state induced by unpleasant stimuli. Persons themselves define whether stimuli are pleasant or unpleasant, because perceptions of such events are an individual matter. For this reason, how persons respond to stressful events is critical to health.

Nurses need to obtain information about their clients' strengths, risk-taking behaviors, past successes, and present abilities to change and adapt.

Anxiety

Any threatening situation can produce anxiety. **Anxiety** is a diffuse, unpleasant, vague feeling of apprehension, nervousness, or dread expressed both somatically and psychically. Like fear, it is a reaction to a threat; however, unlike fear (which is a response to a known, definite, external and immediate danger), anxiety is felt as a threat from something unknown, vague, internal, and in the future (Henderson and Nite, 1978, p 1617).

Anxiety is a normal response to a stressful event; everyone experiences it. Caplan describes anxiety in a crisis situation: "When the individual's usual problem solving methods fail, and the problem persists, he or she experiences a rise in inner tension, unpleasant emotional feelings, and disorganized functioning" (1964, pp 38–39).

Because the discomfort (anxiety) of a stressful situation needs to be relieved, the individual will utilize coping behavior to protect against disorganization or an unstable state of physical and emotional health. Therefore, some kind of adaptation or reorganization takes place; the result may be either growth or regression.

Nurses need to understand the phenomenon of anxiety when working with persons in crisis. Individuals who are experiencing a high level of anxiety often have limited ability to solve problems and, therefore, to adapt. These persons need assistance to lower their anxiety to a functional level. A mild degree of anxiety may be beneficial because it motivates persons to make needed changes in their behavior. Determining the level of anxiety is essential for choosing successful nursing actions.

Coping

The term **coping** refers to the way we deal with our life experiences. It means "to fulfill our needs, to find safety and love and self-respect, freedom from worry, opportunities for growth, and ultimately, a satisfying meaning for our existence" (Allport, 1965, p 262). As defined by Allport (p. 243), coping is characteristically

- Purposive
- Determined by the needs of the moment and situation
- Formally elicited rather than spontaneously emitted
- More readily controlled
- Aiming to change the environment

Coping implies action in response to our environment; effective coping leads to health. **Coping behaviors** consist of use of the cognitive functions (perception, memory, speech, judgment, reality testing), motor activity, affect, and psychological defenses (Mattsson, 1979, p 257).

Coping behavior may involve muscle activity, such as withdrawing one's hand from a hot stove, or it may require the use of knowledge, skills, recall from past experiences, and judgment. Sometimes effective coping behavior may be to ignore certain stimuli in favor of other stimuli that have meaning in one's life. For instance, most students can remember studying for an examination despite fatigue or a headache. The importance of getting a passing grade exceeded the need for sleep or comfort and was reflected by the choice of coping behaviors. Whatever form they take, successful coping behaviors result in adaptation.

Adaptive Versus Maladaptive Coping. Coping behaviors may be either adaptive or maladaptive. Adaptive behaviors lead persons toward effective biopsychosocial functioning within their environment; maladaptive behaviors deter achievement of or move persons away from health and growth. Maladaptive behavior does achieve some goal for the persons at the time it is used, however. Roy wrote, "An adaptive response in general is behavior that maintains the integrity of the individual. A maladaptive response is one that does not maintain integrity and is disruptive of the person" (1976, p 13). Therefore, adaptation is successful when the person responds to stressful events in a way that maintains or enhances integrity.

Maladaptation occurs when inadequate or ineffective methods of coping are used to maintain equilibrium. Illness may be considered the result of maladaptive coping. It should be noted, though, that maladaptive coping is not to be considered a fault, because a person is never prepared for all the contingencies of change. On occasion individuals find themselves in new situations for which previous coping methods may not be effective, and their attempts to survive in the situation may fail. Under such circumstances they may need to seek help and learn coping methods. Unfortunately, many times persons who cope maladaptively with changes in their environment may not be aware that they need help. Some persons may find it extremely difficult to seek help even when they recognize their problems. For instance, a woman who discovers a breast lump may delay seeking help because she cannot cope with the possibility of having cancer. If persons reach the state of exhaustion, as in a serious illness, help may be imposed on them. However, the need for action will be perceived differently by each person. For example, many of us can recall delaying health care because other needs took priority.

When circumstances warrant help, nurses, as well as other professionals, become resources in the environment — nurses assist persons to cope adaptively. It should be remembered that behaviors considered maladaptive in one culture may be adaptive in another. Consequently, nurses need to understand a person's sociocultural beliefs before making plans to intervene.

Crisis

The phenomenon of **crisis** is universal; no one escapes crisis because no one escapes change. The term *crisis*, like the term *stress*, has been used frequently to imply that which is positive and desirable as well as that which is negative or undesirable. Also, *stress* and *crisis* have been used interchangeably by some. Sheehy wrote, "Our culture's interpretation of the Greek word 'Krisis' is pejorative, implying personal failure, weakness, and inability to bear up against stressful outside events" (1974, p 16). Erikson, however, used the term *crisis* to describe a turning point, a crucial period of increased vulnerability and heightened potential (1963); both interpretations have merit.

The period of crisis is temporary and usually lasts no longer than 4 to 6 weeks. Because a person's usual coping mechanisms do not work, this period may be both a time of danger and an opportunity for learning new coping patterns. Whereas crisis may be overwhelming to some — for example, a woman who considers suicide after the death of her husband — others may use this time as a period of growth. Whether a crisis has a positive or negative outcome depends on its nature and the person's adaptive abilities and resources.

Situational Versus Developmental Crises.   Crises may occur as the result of a sudden and significant change in a person's life. During crisis, a person may be helpless and less able to find a solution; his or her functioning becomes disorganized.

Crises are of two types: situational or accidental; and maturational, normative, or developmental. A situational or accidental crisis occurs when the sense of biological, psychological, and social integrity is threatened due to unexpected events such as death, illness, divorce, loss of job, moving, unwanted pregnancy, or natural disaster. "Potential crisis areas occur during the periods of great social, physical, and psychological change experienced by all human beings in the normal growth process" (Aguilera and Messick, 1978, p 132).

A maturational, normative, or developmental crisis occurs when the person is unable to make appropriate changes to new life situations, such as in marriage, beginning school, adolescence, or parenthood. During periods of maturational crisis, the person learns to develop coping strategies for these new life situations.

Coping with Crises.   Figure 6-2 describes the balancing factors that determine health. The paradigm illustrates how health, well-being, and integrity of self are dependent on the person's ability to cope with crisis, adapt to life stresses, and maintain a stable state. Likewise, the person unable to cope with crisis and adapt to stress suffers disequilibrium and potential illness.

Figure 6-3 is a paradigm of the development of crisis, originated by Aguilera and Messick (1986). Figure 6-4 is an illustration of the paradigm using two students' responses

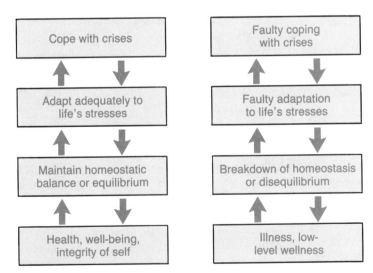

Figure 6-2. Balancing factors for health. (Harms MB. Adapted in Lindberg JB, Hunter ML, Kruszewski AZ: Person-Centered Nursing, p 86, Philadelphia, JB Lippincott, 1983)

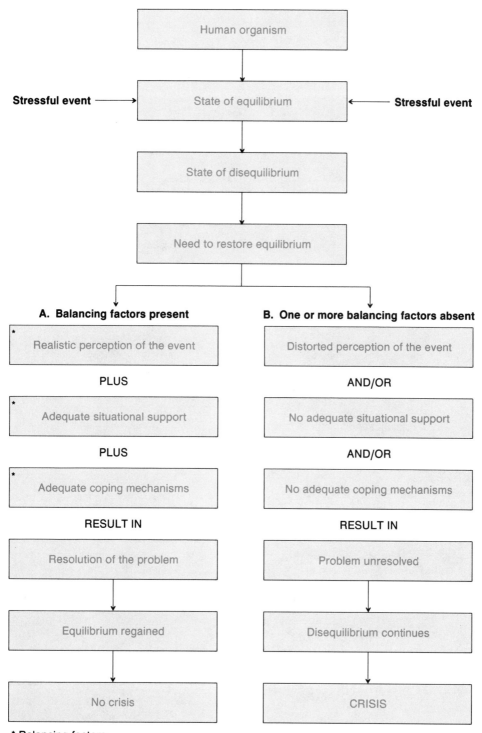

Figure 6-3 Effect of balancing factors in a stressful event. (Aguilera DC, Messick JM: Crisis Intervention: Theory and Methodology, 5th ed, p 69. St. Louis, CV Mosby, 1986)

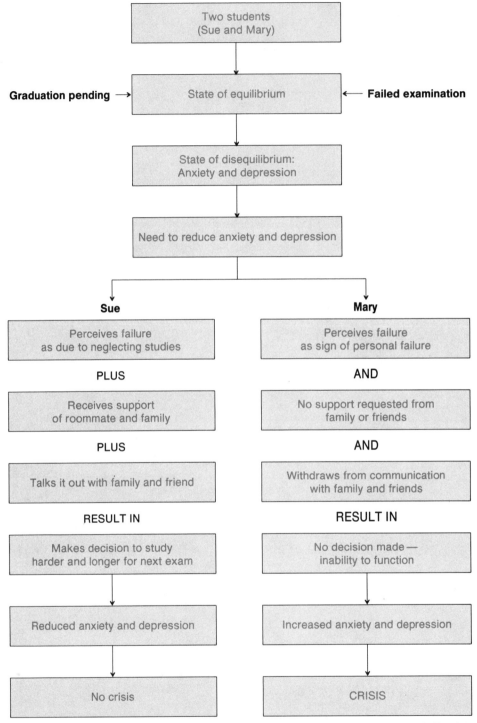

Figure 6–4. Illustration of effect of reducing factors in a stressful event. (Aguilera DC, Messick JM: Crisis Intervention: Theory and Methodology, 5th ed, p 71. St. Louis, CV Mosby, 1986)

to the same event: failing an examination. This example shows how a stressful event experienced by two individuals can lead to different outcomes, depending on which coping mechanisms the person uses. Note that maladaptive coping hinders problem solving, whereas adaptive coping enhances it. The coping behaviors used may make the difference in whether a stressful situation becomes a crisis.

The positive outcome of crisis is that persons may function at a higher level than before. Therefore, the nurse focuses on the person's strengths and abilities to change and adapt and provides positive reinforcement by pointing out the person's past successes. Nurses often provide support during crisis periods. In a situational crisis such as acute illness, they identify persons' strengths and provide emotional or physical support (e.g., being a sounding board or giving physical care). During developmental crises, nurses provide guidance to give persons the necessary skills for helping themselves.

| SELF-CARE

Self-care is related to concepts of health and adaptation. **Self-care** has been defined as activities that individuals perform that are directed to themselves or their environments to regulate their own functioning and development to maintain or enhance life, health, and well-being (Orem, 1985, p 31). The term connotes self-reliance, independence, and autonomy and, indeed, many health-care consumers are assuming increasing responsibility

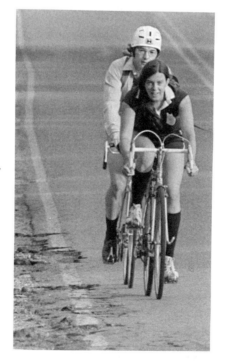

Exercise promotes health.

for their health. One author estimated that 75% of all health care in the United States consists of informed self-care (Levin, 1976). The tremendous growth in the number of self-help groups in the last two decades gives evidence of clients' increased role in maintaining or recovering their health. Alcoholics Anonymous and Weight Watchers are two of the best-known self-help groups.

Many definitions of nursing imply that the nurse assists others with health-care practices and activities of daily living when they are unable to care for themselves. Thus, nurses have long been supportive of clients' health-related self-care activities. Let us examine the concept of self-care from a nursing perspective.

Orem

Dorothea Orem's definition of self-care was presented earlier in this section. Her ideas about self-care include the following:

- *Self-care agency*: the acquired ability of individuals to meet requirements for care that regulates life processes and promotes health, development, and well-being.
- *Therapeutic self-care demand*: the measure of care required for persons to meet their self-care requisites to maintain or promote health and well-being or promote development.
- *Self-care deficits*: occurs when self-care agency is not adequate to meet therapeutic self-care demand. Persons who have self-care deficits have legitimate need for nursing care (1985, p 31).

Practitioners who use Orem's concept to organize and govern their nursing actions have elaborated on its application in various situations of nursing, especially in acute-care units of hospitals. Because Orem placed emphasis on biophysical aspects of care of acutely and chronically ill persons, her concept stresses problem solving in nursing situations and places a heavy emphasis on patient or client education. We note that this concept is often used in actual practice to individualize an essentially standard form of care prescribed, recommended, and often imposed on a person by members of the health team.

Kinlein

M. Lucille Kinlein, a former student and colleague of Orem, practiced according to her own self-care concept, a modification of that of Orem, whom she credited as her original inspiration (1977). Kinlein's concept applies particularly well to nursing persons who are essentially healthy but want to maintain or enhance their present state. Kinlein's many years in a private practice of nursing showed that persons want verification and expansion of their own knowledge and self-care practices. She expected her clients to express their particular need or desire for her care through their verbalization as she gave them her undivided attention. Nurses violate Kinlein's self-care concept when they introduce, either by consciousness raising or by direct statement, a problem or potential problem that was not first suggested by the client.

Erickson

Helen Erickson's concept of self-care incorporates ideas common to many nurse experts, including Orem and Kinlein, into her own special perspectives. Erickson's concept of self-care, when applied from her comprehensive conceptual framework or model for nursing, is equally useful with persons who are ill or well, young or old, in whatever place they may be receiving or needing nursing care.

At the heart of Erickson's concept of self-care is the notion of client-identified needs and goals. Individuals know the kind of help they need to mobilize their own strengths and resources. Erickson has said that those who are ill know what has made them ill and what will make them well. According to Erickson, if a person does not know this at a conscious level, he or she knows it subconsciously and may need expert nursing to identify the particular help the person wants and needs.

Caring (well) for oneself, taking (good) care of oneself, and that which some call "self-care for health" involve learning to know and exercise one's power to choose as well as creating conditions within one's relationships with persons and one's environment wherein personal growth and development toward an ever-healthier state occur.

The nurturance or "nursing" of these self-care powers is the ultimate goal of nursing judgments and action. Some would call this the nurturance of autonomy — a state of knowing and freely exercising persons' actual, reality-based choices. The choices are either to do alone what persons are perfectly capable of doing for themselves or to ask their associates or support systems openly, directly, and kindly for what they want or need from them. They do this to attain, maintain, or increase a state of health.

The notion of helping persons reach their own goals is vitally linked to Erickson's central self-care assumption. A capacity for healing and movement toward health and wholeness exist at both conscious and unconscious levels of individuals whom she described as multisystem persons. Quality nursing is not doing activities for, to, or at a person; rather, it provides care a person values at important levels of his being. It is given through an interactive process, in which the person perceives himself or herself to be deeply respected as a participant executor to the fullest possible extent in the decisions that affect his or her care.

| IMPLICATIONS FOR NURSING

The following is an example of a client who has experienced a situational crisis. The elements of health, adaptation, and self-care are evident in this situation. The client has experienced a crisis and has begun to cope with it.

Jan is a 42-year-old female client who underwent a hysterectomy 1 month ago. After leaving the hospital, she noticed that her surgical wound had reddened, was swollen, and had begun to drain pus. She was readmitted with a wound abscess. Jan also has been diabetic for 12 years and takes daily insulin injections. She is very knowledgeable about her disease and has developed a strict schedule for herself to control it.

Jan has a difficult family life. She states that her mother has a history of emotional problems and relies on her to make even the simplest decisions, and her father is experiencing memory loss due to aging and often forgets where he is. Jan expresses concern about caring for her parents. Jan is very close to her sister and a niece and has many friends in her church group. She also has a dog whom she describes as "almost human . . . we really understand each other." Jan is unmarried.

Jan weighs 242 pounds. She states she often feels lonely, depressed, or anxious and overeats to "feel better." She is trying to change by recognizing her habits and developing new eating behaviors.

In the hospital, Jan's infected wound is cleaned and bandaged three times daily. Jan will need to do this for herself after discharge. She experienced blurred vision soon after this hospital admission, for which no physical cause could be found. She states, "I realized that I was probably feeling overwhelmed at having to take care of my parents and their problems after I went home, on top of doing all those dressing changes and watching my diabetes. I guess my vision problem was a way to get out of all of the demands on me. As soon as I recognized this, my blurred vision went away."

Jan has established a strict routine in the hospital. When this routine is followed, she feels comfortable in the hospital environment. However, if the nurses do not include her in planning her care, such as determining times for dressing changes, she becomes visibly anxious and angry.

Jan is open and expresses her feelings readily. She can identify her own weaknesses and strengths and is usually able to solve problems. She assumes responsibility for as much of her hospital care as possible, yet asks for assistance when she needs it.*

*Data contributed by Charlotte Myers.

Several elements of the adaptation process that are affecting Jan's health can be identified in this situation. Jan is currently experiencing several stressors, including her parents' increasing dependence on her, her own health problems, and hospitalization. She is undergoing a situational crisis because her usual coping methods are not effective in helping her deal with those stressors. Notice that when Jan felt totally unable to cope with stress, she developed a physical symptom (blurred vision). This point illustrates the relationship between health and adaptation. Jan had inadequate energy to cope with psychological stress; she drew energy from her biological subsystem, causing it to become less healthy also. Jan has an absence of balancing factors as described in Figure 6–2. She has little situational support from her family and few effective coping mechanisms to deal with this situation. Her usual coping mechanisms include overeating, controlling situations through strict schedules or routines, and problem solving. Note that when the nurses interfere with one of her most important coping mechanisms (control), Jan has no way to deal with anxiety, as evidenced by her reaction of anger.

Nursing care is focused on assisting Jan to resolve her crisis. Jan's nurse will use elements of the self-care concept to help her become independent. This aid requires knowledge of Jan's strengths, her current level of anxiety, her past methods of coping, and the current stressors in her life. Because Jan is in a moderate state of anxiety, her nurse can help to think of new ways of dealing with her situation. The nurse and Jan set goals together for crisis resolution. Because control is the coping mechanism that Jan is currently using, her nurse develops ways of returning a sense of control. These methods involve teaching her to care for her infected wound, following her schedule as closely as possible, and encouraging her to make her own decisions about her hospital care. In this way, Jan's nurse supports her in her self-care activities, which leads to development of healthy adaptive mechanisms and wellness. The nurse might also talk with Jan about how she can use her social supports to help her deal with her parents' health needs. Other resources, such as a community health nurse or social worker might be called to give additional support after her discharge from the hospital.

| CONCLUSION

The concept of health has been discussed from the perspective of changing perceptions of humankind. Health has been described from different points of view without reaching a conclusive definition; nevertheless, ideas about health may be summarized in the following statements:

- Health is a dynamic process.
- Health is determined subjectively and objectively.
- Health is a goal.
- Health is being able to take care of yourself.
- Health is optimal functioning in body, mind, and spirit.
- Health is integrity of self.
- Health is a sense of wholeness.
- Health is coping adaptively.
- Health is growing and becoming.
- Health is a broad concept.

This chapter also described the process by which persons adapt to changes in their environment. Adaptation is dynamic because movement or change from one condition to another is expected all of our lives. As stressors impinge on us, we respond accordingly. Although the number and type of stressors may vary, there is no escape from them. Therefore, each of us is involved continuously in the process of adaptation. Because adaptation is vital to the health and growth of persons, nursing's goal is to facilitate this process. Nurses have the knowledge and skills to deal with planned change of persons and their environment. In this way, we assist persons to achieve their potential.

The chapter concluded by examining the concept of self-care. Although ideas about self-care may vary among nurses and laypersons, the term is widely used. Caring for self may be a reaction to the confusion and complexity of health-care delivery. Clients' desires to practice self-care are also a statement of belief about controlling individual destiny and potential.

Nurses who seek to give person-centered care will recognize that their clients are the source of much valuable information about themselves and their own self-care. Nurses will use the person's knowledge, strengths, and goals to provide meaningful individualized care. The challenge of self-care is one of collaboration between nurse and client. The subject is a broad and engrossing one, and we encourage you to take advantage of the readings listed at the end of this chapter.

| STUDY QUESTIONS

1   Explain environment and its variables as they relate to health and adaptation.
2   Discuss the various perspectives on health. What are the strengths and weaknesses of each view?

3 What is your personal definition of health? Of illness?
4 Describe several theories of adaptation. How can nurses use these ideas in their practice?
5 Describe the difference between the concepts of crisis, anxiety, stress, and coping.
6 Give three examples of life events that may lead (a) to situational crisis and (b) to maturational crisis.
7 List some ways in which the nurse may facilitate adaptation of persons.
8 Define *self-care*. What are your own self-care practices?

| REFERENCES

Aguilera DC, Messick JM: Crisis Intervention: Theory and Methodology, 3rd ed. St. Louis, CV Mosby, 1978
Aguilera DC, Messick JM: Crisis Intervention: Theory and Methodology, 5th ed. St. Louis, CV Mosby, 1986
Allport GW: Pattern and Growth in Personality. New York, Holt, Rinehart & Winston, 1965
The American College Dictionary. New York, Random House, 1962
Cannon WB: The Wisdom of the Body. New York, WW Norton, 1939
Caplan G: Principles of Preventive Psychiatry. New York, Basic Books, 1964
Department of Health, Education and Welfare: Healthy People: The Surgeon General's Report on Health Promotion and Disease Prevention. Washington, DC, Office of the Assistant Secretary for Health, 1979
Dubos R: Man Adapting. New Haven, Yale University Press, 1965
Dunn HL: What high level wellness means. Can J Public Health 50:447–457, 1959
Erickson E: Childhood and Society, 2nd ed. New York, WW Norton, 1963
Henderson V, Nite G: Principles and Practice of Nursing, 6th ed. New York, Macmillan, 1978
Holmes TH, Rahe RH: The Social Readjustment Rating Scale. J Psychosom Res 11(2):213–218, 1967
Jahoda M: Current Concepts of Positive Mental Health. New York, Basic Books, 1958
King IM: A Theory for Nursing: Systems, Concepts, Process. New York, John Wiley & Sons, 1981
Kinlein ML: Independent Nursing Care with Clients. Philadelphia, JB Lippincott, 1977
Levin L: The layperson as the primary health-care practitioner. Public Health Rep 91:206–210, 1976
Levine ME: Introduction to Clinical Nursing. Philadelphia, FA Davis, 1973
Mattsson A: Long-term physical illness in childhood: A challenge to psychosocial adaptation. In Garfield CA (ed): Stress and Survival: The Emotional Realities of Life-Threatening Illness, pp 253–263. St. Louis, CV Mosby, 1979
Murray AB, Zentner JP: Nursing Concepts for Health Promotion, 3rd ed. Englewood Cliffs, NJ, Prentice-Hall, 1985
Nightingale F: Notes on Nursing: What It Is and What It Is Not. London, Harrison, 1859. Facsimile edition: Philadelphia, JB Lippincott, 1966
Orem DE: Nursing: Concepts of Practice, 3rd ed. New York, McGraw-Hill, 1985
Parsons T: Definitions of health and illness in the light of American values and social structure. In Jaco E (ed): Patients, Physicians and Illness, 2nd ed, pp 107–127. New York, Free Press, 1972
Rogers M: An Introduction to the Theoretical Basis of Nursing. Philadelphia, FA Davis, 1970
Roy SC: Introduction to Nursing: An Adaptation Model, 2nd ed. Englewood Cliffs, NJ, Prentice-Hall, 1984

Selye H: The Stress of Life. New York, McGraw-Hill, 1956

Selye H: Stress Without Distress. New York, Signet, 1975

Sheehy G: Passages: Predictable Crises of Adult Life. New York, EP Dutton, 1974

Smith JA: The idea of health: A philosophical inquiry. Adv Nursing Sci 3:43–50, 1981

Smith JA: The Idea of Health. New York, Teachers College Press, 1983

Toffler A: Future Shock. New York, Random House, 1970

World Health Organization Interim Commission: Constitution of the World Health Organization. Chron WHO 1:29, 1947

Wu R: Behavior and Illness. Englewood Cliffs, NJ, Prentice-Hall, 1973

Part Three

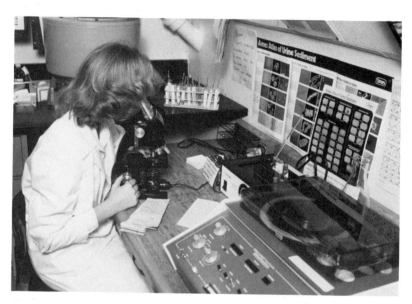

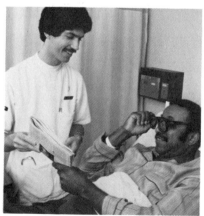

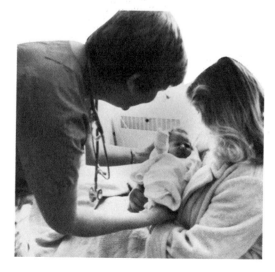

7 | HEALTH-CARE DELIVERY

KEY WORDS	After completing this chapter, students will be able to:
Client advocate Consumer Consumer movement Health maintenance organization National health insurance Preventive health care Primary nursing	Identify the major problems of health-care delivery. Discuss the contribution of nursing to health-care delivery. Discuss several ways in which government and the private sector have attempted to manage health-care delivery. Identify health problems of persons in the United States. Discuss the consumer movement in health care.

Health-care delivery in the United States is a huge and heavily stressed system. Health-care services are frequently inconsistent but miraculously life-saving and curing. The needs of the people of this large and diverse nation are often beyond the resources of this system; that is, the system deals fairly well with immediate crises, but has fewer capabilities when longer term, consistent care is needed. For example, in the past 20 years, major advances in life support systems, transplant programs, and chemotherapy have saved thousands of lives. However, we have encountered several new health-care challenges requiring long-term solutions. Among these are substance abuse, AIDS, Alzheimer's disease, longer but not always healthier life spans, and survival of persons with serious birth defects or major disabilities resulting from accidents. These are serious but more chronic problems that do not fare well with current programs. In addition, millions of homeless persons throughout our cities experience health problems largely ignored by the present focus of health-care delivery. As the costs of programs to solve these various problems escalate, we find our abilities to intervene severely limited. As a nation, however, we are learning to come to terms with the health-care crisis. The nursing profession has the opportunity to be a major force in the development and improvement of our delivery system.

All of us are consumers of health commodities and health services. Several problems are associated with buying commodities and services. Although consumers want to spend money wisely and to receive something of value in return, they frequently settle for less than the best because of the expense involved, a lack of awareness, or a lack of time to find out about other available products. In times of illness, it is even more difficult to make effective decisions concerning health care. Such are the variety of problems facing consumers of health-care delivery. Nurses who understand the characteristics of the consumer of health care and the variables that influence health behavior will be able to act as client advocates and also assist clients to participate in preventive health care.

HEALTH-CARE DELIVERY AS A SYSTEM

An exploration of health-care delivery as we know it may provide an understanding of its problems. Some of the literature on the methods and approach to health care in this country describe it as a "system." As indicated in Chapter 4, a *system* is an organized unit with a set of components that mutually react and function as a whole or total entity. Health-care delivery is composed of thousands of smaller systems. The question is whether or not these smaller systems are subsystems of a greater system. In small towns, for example, the doctors' offices, the pharmacies, the health department, and the community hospital may function as components of the town's larger system of health care. Other kinds of agencies such as Heart or Diabetic Associations, the Visiting Nurse Association, and the United Way may all work together with the other components of the system. When this is the case, health-care delivery in the area can be described as a system.

If, however, a person in that town is referred to a large medical center, he or she may find a totally unfamiliar environment that appears very "unsystematic" in comparison with previous experiences. Too often, persons entering large health-care facilities feel lost or overwhelmed by the system. They encounter various specialists from several professions, many clinics, painful diagnostic procedures, long waits, and difficulty in finding their way around. Moreover, conditions attached to the various payment plans are confusing and frequently result in unexpected expense that is both devastating financially and stressful personally. When describing his concerns about the cost of health care, Dougherty stated, "There are many, many Americans, especially among those already seriously disadvantaged in other ways, who are effectively denied the full benefits of modern health care . . . they represent a large and unconscionable pocket of health care poverty in the midst of America's health care affluence" (1988, p 190).

Procedures, policies, and payment plans vary among agencies and states. If one buys a car or house or enters an educational institution, these variations can be tolerated; however, where health is concerned, the added stress of trying to enter and cope with a health-care system may increase the person's susceptibility to disease. The frustration described by persons who have attempted to obtain health-care services indicates that physiological changes can actually occur as a result of the stress experienced. To cite one example, a person with asthma reported experiencing respiratory distress after a frustrating wait in a hospital clinic.

Consider the experiences that you, your family, and friends have encountered in the health-care system. Perhaps you have known someone who needed several services in the course of one illness. Perhaps this person had seen a family doctor and then been sent to a surgeon at a large hospital. There, he or she was referred to the social-service department for financial assistance, given physical therapy, and received nutritional counseling from a dietitian. After returning home, the person was visited by a public-health nurse and bought medicines and supplies from the nearest pharmacy. Consider this example and the following questions:

- Is there a common philosophy of health and health care among the agencies and care-givers?
- Are the person's basic needs considered when care is planned and does the person participate in this plan?
- Is there effective transfer of records and appropriate data about the person among agencies, care-givers, and the person seeking health care?
- Do nurses function as coordinators of care?

If you answered "no" to these questions, you have validated for yourself that the concept of "system" does not apply well to health-care delivery. We lack both a system for financing health care and a philosophy from which our programs emanate. Problem solving does not necessarily require a single controlling body such as the federal government, although government agencies are involved. Instead, any solution requires that health-care professionals collaborate and base health-care delivery on a common philosophical framework.

Problems in Health-Care Delivery

At present, the most appropriate word to describe health-care delivery is *industry*. Health care is a huge business that offers a multitude of products and services for sale that often emphasize illness rather than improved health. Some of the broad problems associated with our current structure of health care are listed below:

- Emphasis on crisis and illness rather than on preventive health care and promotion of health
- Inadequate enforcement of standards to ensure quality of care
- Minimal consumer participation
- Poor coordination of services
- Poor communication and collaboration among providers of services
- Extremely high costs

Health-Care Providers

Those who provide health care constitute a major component of the health-care delivery system. Table 7–1 lists the statistics for the approximate numbers of professional health-care workers in this country. These figures indicate that the nursing profession is twice the

TABLE 7–1
APPROXIMATE NUMBERS OF ACTIVE HEALTH-CARE PROFESSIONALS

	Actual for 1986	Projected for 1990	Per 100,000 Population	
			Actual	Projected
Nurses (RNs)	1,602,400	1,842,000	667.0	739.0
Physicians (MDs, DOs)	544,800	597,000	224.9	239.1
Pharmacists	161,500	171,900	67.1	68.9
Dentists	143,000	150,300	58.9	59.9

(Adapted from the Sixth Report to the President and Congress on the Status of Health Personnel in the United States. Pub. HRS-P-OD-81-1, 1988)

size of any other health profession. Clearly, nursing ought to have a great effect on the health of this nation. However, health and illness care provided by nurses is often difficult to quantify. Significantly, nursing is the only group to provide regular, consistent, around-the-clock care. For real changes to occur in the health-care delivery industry, nursing leadership in collaboration with other professionals must be as evident as the numbers indicate it should be.

Our health-care professionals and providers include nutritionists, dietitians, physical and occupational therapists, optometrists, and audiologists. Other professionals closely associated with the health-care industry assist with rehabilitation (e.g., social workers, psychologists, speech therapists, and vocational rehabilitation counselors).

Studies are frequently done by the health professions and the federal government to determine whether current personnel supplies are meeting society's needs. With the information obtained, plans may be made to raise or lower the numbers of professionals in a particular group. It is useful to note that changes in one group may have an impact on the functions of another. For example, if there are not enough physicians to meet medical care needs, nurses may discover that others consider them to be capable of performing tasks and procedures heretofore considered to be medical in nature. As the number of physicians increases, nurses may find that the same people no longer consider nurses to be competent for those duties.

The functions as well as the supply of health-care providers should also be considered. The team approach is often thought to be essential for effective care. Each professional has

Nurses are the most numerous health-care professionals.

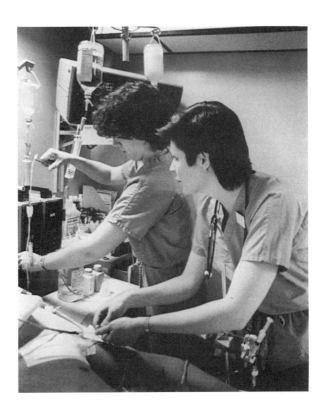

a set of skills that he or she believes is necessary to provide the kind of care the person is seeking. Unfortunately, we can overwhelm our clients when we ask them to relate to a team that may consist of nurse, doctor, pharmacist, dietitian, physical therapist, social worker, and chaplain. Clients' needs will vary, and they may indeed need direct care from these professionals. However, as nurses, we must consider the many skills we have. As the person who has the most direct contact with the client, you act as a *coordinator of care* and can help the client use other professional resources. The nurse relates to the team while the client relates to the nurse as care-giver. Nurses can assist the client in making more effective use of the physician. Nurses also find that persons will seek them as a care provider at least as often as they seek the doctor, especially in the community.

HISTORICAL INFLUENCES IN HEALTH-CARE DELIVERY

Table 7–2 identifies the changes that have occurred in the United States since World War II. The advances in science and technology, with the accompanying movement from the country to industrial areas, have resulted in changing needs for health care. However, some needs may have existed long before they were recognized. For example, a growth in the number of nonwhites was followed by an increased incidence in health problems for this segment of the population. Yet, this phenomenon may reflect the improvement in census activities rather than an increase in actual numbers.

Changes in family structure, civil rights demonstrations, and the emergence of the consumer movement have affected our current method of health-care delivery. Persons who grow older in our society stay productive and are able to maintain their own homes for a longer period of time than was previously true. They often continue working at their careers or engage in more meaningful recreational, social, and charitable activities. Many older adults are more independent than their forerunners and, as a result, do not often live with their adult children. When these persons become less active due to disabilities or diseases, they often need nursing home care. This need has added greatly to the costs of national health care.

Although substance abuse, eating disorders, and sexually transmitted disease have been with us for years, they have increased greatly in the last 5 to 10 years and have produced a heightened awareness of society regarding these problems. In particular, cocaine addiction and AIDS have presented us with a series of new challenges similar to those of infectious diseases and mental illness in the early part of the century.

As indicated in Chapter 3, changes in nursing have also influenced health-care delivery. In the process of pursuing its professional development, nursing has become more autonomous and independent. Nurses are recognizing their unique contribution and finding more creative ways to distribute their services to society; they are beginning to influence health-care legislation and the politics of health-care delivery. The discussion on nursing as a profession provided details of these and related issues.

Legislation represents another historical influence on health care. For example, legislation has provided monies for physical facilities—often hospitals—resulting in a prominence of tertiary care. *Tertiary care* can be defined as care that takes place in highly specialized institutions providing sophisticated diagnosis and treatment. Although persons

TABLE 7–2
HISTORICAL INFLUENCES IN HEALTH-CARE DELIVERY

Changes	Influences
Population dynamics since 1940	Increase in General population Nonwhite population Life expectancy and birth rates among nonwhite persons Proportion of foreign-born persons
Urbanization	Movement into suburbs
	Increase in Marriage and divorce rates Illegitimacy and teenage pregnancy Pregnant women who do not receive prenatal care Unemployment rate Adult crime and juvenile delinquency Numbers of persons living in substandard housing Numbers of persons living at the poverty level Older adult population Automobile accidents, homicides, and suicides Infant mortality rate and birth defects
Industrialization	Decrease in Farming Self-sufficiency once common among rural population
Literacy and education	Increases in Knowledge about health care Demand for more care of higher quality
Economic status	Wider range between high and low economic status
	Increase in government and private health-insurance programs
Advances in science and technology	Control of infectious diseases
	Development of drugs for control of many serious illnesses
	New and life-saving surgical techniques
	Life-maintenance techniques and equipment
	Hazardous industry
	Pollution resulting in increase in lung cancer and heart disease
Family structural changes	Breadwinner other than father
	New family structures, e.g., communal living
	Single-parent families
	Working mothers
	Grandparents in own homes, far from adult children
Civil rights movements	Equality in health care as a right
	Equality regardless of race, creed, sex
	Women's liberation movement
Consumerism	Change in consumer concept of health and illness
	Self-help groups
	Increase in litigation

(TABLE 7–2 continued)

Changes	Influences
Nursing profession	Increase in sense of accountability and responsibility
	Greater independence and autonomy
	More involvement in health policies and politics
Legislation	Hill–Burton Act (1946)
	Amendments to the Food, Drug and Cosmetic Act Durham–Humphrey (1952) Kefauver–Harris (1962)
	Department of Health, Education and Welfare (1953)
	Regional Medical Program (1965)
	Comprehensive Health Planning Program (1966)
	Social Security Amendments: Title XVIII Medicare (1966) Title XIX Medicaid (1966)
	Comprehensive Drug Abuse Prevention and Control Act (1970)
	Health Maintenance Organization Act (1973)
	Professional Standards Review Organization Act (1973)
	Child Abuse Prevention and Treatment Act (1974)
	National Health Planning and Resources Development Act (1974)
	Generic and Brand Names for Drugs Legislation (1977)
	The Tax Equity and Fiscal Responsibility Act of 1982 — TEFRA (Introduced DR6)
	Social Security Amendment of 1983: Medicare prospective payment, PL 98–21
	National Organ Procurement Act 1984
	Consolidated Omnibus Budget Reconciliation Act of 1985 — COBRA
	The Medicare Catastrophic Coverage Act of 1988
	Legislation prior to World War II
	United States Public Health Service (1798)
	Pure Food and Drug Act (1906)
	Social Security Act (1935)
	Federal Food, Drug and Cosmetic Act (1938)

may receive care in either the hospital or the ambulatory-care setting, tertiary care is generally considered to be long-term care.

Legislation has attempted to place controls on the accessibility, quality, and cost of health care. Specific legislation has been enacted to ensure the safety and efficacy of the drugs that are developed and distributed for general use in society. Several of these pieces of legislation will be discussed later in this chapter.

HEALTH PROBLEMS OF PERSONS
IN THE UNITED STATES

Despite the many problems discussed in this section, we should emphasize that Americans are a healthy people and have become progressively more so since 1900.

Consider the following facts from the book *Healthy People* (Department of Health, Education and Welfare, 1979, pp 1–4):

- Diseases such as tuberculosis, gastroenteritis, diphtheria, and poliomyelitis — major causes of disability and death in the early years of this country — are nearly nonexistent today.
- With the advent of antibiotics, many of the bacteria-related diseases, which used to carry a high mortality rate, have become readily treatable.
- In 1900 the death rate per year was about 17 per 1000 persons, compared to 9 per 1000 persons in the 1970s.
- Between 1950 and 1977 the mortality rate for children aged 1 through 14 years was cut in half.
- The life expectancy in 1900 was 47 years, whereas in 1977 it was 73 years.

Advances in our national health resulted from a variety of developments: improvement in sanitation, housing, and nutrition; the advent of antibiotics and immunization programs, as well as the development of numerous drugs to control diabetes, hypertension, and other diseases; a growing awareness of the impact of certain life styles and habits on our health; and the emergence of more self-help groups and techniques.

When the health statistics of the United States are compared to other industrial nations, it is frequently observed that certain other Western nations have better national health programs than the United States does. The facts and figures may verify this view and reflect our faulty methods of health-care delivery. However, the United States has a population far greater and more diversified than countries such as Sweden and Japan. In addition, because of its complexity our society produces many stressors that contribute heavily to health problems. Since World War II, the United States has been a refuge for persons fleeing political persecution and warlike conditions in Europe, Asia, and South America; that we may not provide proper care for these persons is only one issue in a very complex problem.

In truth, we have made numerous advances. Women with diseases such as diabetes and heart problems now are able to conceive and give birth. Many persons now survive serious illness and injury because of improved medical science, although they are often left with disabilities or compromised health. That we do have many preventable and treatable health problems must certainly be recognized, yet, in this regard, we should be aware that statistics do not tell the whole story.

HEALTH PROBLEMS ACROSS THE
LIFE SPAN

Several examples of health problems that may occur across the life span have been listed in Table 7–3. The list is long and varied. One interesting fact is that injury is the leading cause of premature death in the United States (National Center for Health Statistics, 1988, p 11). That many of these deaths are the result of homicide and suicide is noted by the Office of Disease Prevention and Health Promotion (1988 p. 40).

TABLE 7-3
HEALTH PROBLEMS ACROSS THE LIFE SPAN

Age	Health Problems	Rank as a Cause of Death
Infants	**Congenital anomalies**	1
	Sudden infant death syndrome	2
	Respiratory distress syndrome	3
	Low birth weight	
	Accidents	
	Influenza and pneumonia	
	Unfavorable resolution of trust versus mistrust	
Children, 1-14 years	**Accidents**	1
	Malignant neoplasms	2
	Congenital anomalies	3
	Abuse and neglect	
	Dental caries	
	Inadequate school functioning	
	Lead poisoning among inner-city children	
	Learning disorders	
	Problems begun in childhood as precursors for adult problems	
	Unfavorable resolution of	
	Autonomy versus shame and doubt	
	Industry versus inferiority	
	Initiative versus guilt	
Adolescents and young adults, 15-24 years	**Accidents**	1
	Homicide	2
	Suicide	3
	Alcohol and drug abuse	
	Injuries	
	Life-style and behavior pattern as precursors for chronic disease	
	Mental illness	
	Risk-taking behavior	
	Sexually transmissible disease	
	Smoking	
	Unfavorable resolution of	
	Identity versus role confusion	
	Intimacy versus isolation	
	Unwanted pregnancy	
Adults, 25-44 years	**Accidents**	1
	Malignant neoplasms	2
	Heart disease	3
	Alcohol abuse	
	Cirrhosis	
	Diabetes	
	Feelings of stagnation and self-absorption	
	Homicide	
	Hypertension	
	Mental illness	
	Obesity	
	Peridontal disease	
	Unfavorable resolution of generativity versus stagnation	

(Table 7-3 continues)

(TABLE 7-3 continued)

Age	Health Problems	Rank as a Cause of Death
Adults, 45–64 years	**Malignant neoplasms**	1
	Heart disease	2
	Cerebrovascular disease	3
	Other problems similar to those in the age group 26–44 years	
Older adults, 65 years and older	**Heart disease**	1
	Malignant neoplasm	2
	Cerebral vascular disease	3
	Arteriosclerosis	
	Decreased ability to care for self	
	Dependency	
	Depression	
	Diabetes	
	Fluid, electrolyte, and metabolic disturbances	
	Influenza and pneumonia	
	Injuries	
	Insufficient finances to meet basic needs	
	Neglect, loneliness	
	Nutritional deficiencies	
	Overmedication	
	Preventable and reversible mental deterioration and behavioral changes	
	Stress of loss and grief	
	Unfavorable resolution of Ego integrity versus despair Visual and hearing alterations	

(Monthly vital statistics report [final data from The National Center for Health Statistics]. 1988, 37(6): Adv Rep Final Mortal Statistics 1986)

Solutions

Many solutions for these problems have been proposed and, indeed, a variety of health promotion policies and activities are already in place. Table 7–4 suggests some of the current programs available.

The aim of health-related programs is to increase society's awareness of existing needs. It is an attempt to help persons realize their options and take better care of themselves, thereby retaining control over their lives.

MANAGEMENT OF HEALTH-CARE DELIVERY

Over the years, we have employed various strategies to manage the health-care delivery industry. These strategies have involved the government, the private sector, or a combination of both. The following discussion presents several key points in the history of health-care management. A review of these ideas may suggest new solutions for the future.

TABLE 7 – 4
POSSIBLE SOLUTIONS FOR HEALTH PROBLEMS

Solution	Examples
Community support systems	Abuse prevention
	Parent counseling
	Runaway centers
	Stress control
	Suicide prevention
Counseling programs	Family planning
	Genetic counseling
	Nutritional counseling
Educational programs	Cardiopulmonary resuscitation classes
	Health education throughout the school year
	Nutritional education
	Physical fitness activities and programs
	Information about signs of cancer
	Unemployment programs, teaching youth how to be employable
Health and safety protection	Automobiles designed for safety
	Changes in fabric (not inflammable)
	Childhood immunizations
	Control of firearms
	Control of disease (i.e., sexually transmissible disease, hypertension)
	Fluoridation of community water supply
	Lowering speed limits
	Occupational health and safety programs
	Poison control centers
	Proper reporting of disease, institution of regulations, and use of statistics
	Seat belts in moving vehicles
	Toxic-substance control
	Toy manufacturing safety regulations
Prevention programs	Dental hygiene
	Papanicolaou (Pap) smear
	Prenatal care and mental health
	Self breast examination
Screening programs	Screening and diagnosis for high-risk factors across age groups
	Screening programs for diseases such as diabetes and hypertension

Government Structures

The Department of Health, Education and Welfare (HEW) was established in 1953. Its purpose was to organize the various health and welfare agencies of the government under one administrative unit for more coordination and efficiency. There were four major branches at that time: the Public Health Service, Social and Rehabilitation Services, the Social Security Administration, and the Office of Education. The department is now called the Department of Health and Human Services and education has its own organization. In the future, the Department may be altered further to meet the needs of the time.

Of the four branches, the Public Health Service is of major concern to nursing. It was established by a congressional act in 1798 and is the oldest of the organizations making up the Department of HEW. It is intended as a vehicle for health professionals and scientists to discover and apply knowledge in order to cure disease and improve health.

The Public Health Science is composed of six major agencies, (Table 7–5), the combined purpose of which is to provide better health services for the American people. Activities of the service include the following:

- Review of the health care — quality and appropriateness of medical care provided to Medicare and Medicaid subscribers
- Provision of grants to study widespread health problems such as venereal disease and hypertension
- Assistance with plans to raise public awareness of serious health problems
- Operation of hospitals for national health concerns such as narcotics addiction, tuberculosis, and mental illness
- Research on health problems
- Provision of training grants to educational institutions in the health services
- Publication of vital statistics pertinent to public health programs

Particular emphases associated with different presidential administrations such as increased or decreased expenditures for health care will alter the philosophy and functions

TABLE 7–5
AGENCIES OF THE UNITED STATES PUBLIC HEALTH SERVICE

Agency	Mission
National Institutes of Health	Research
Food and Drug Administration	Regulation related to consumer protection
Health Services Administration	Establishment of responsibility related to the delivery of health care and quality of care
Centers for Disease Control	Responsibility for preventive medicine and public health
Health Resources Administration	Development of health-service resources and improvement of their use
Alcohol, Drug Abuse and Mental Health Administration	Development of strategies to deal with medical problems

of the Public Health Service. Note that the new Center for Nursing Research, established in April 1986, is housed in the National Institutes of Health. This research center provides the first visible national governmental center devoted to nursing research — research about the human responses to persons' actual or potential health problems and also the nursing interventions to promote, maintain, and restore health.

Financing Health-Care Delivery

Health-care costs have mounted alarmingly since 1900; accordingly, many agencies can no longer be supported by fee for service alone and must rely on voluntary contributions or tax dollars. Many persons cannot afford to pay for health care and find it necessary to join insurance programs or to receive help from the government.

Funding Health-Care Agencies

Agencies are funded from two basic sources: tax support and private support. Tax-supported agencies receive public aid through city, county, state, or federal agencies funds. Often, several levels of government combine to provide assistance. These agencies are not necessarily free to those whom they serve and usually charge a fee for service to offset operating costs.

Most tax-supported agencies are nonprofit. Those that make a profit return monies to the agency for expansion of services and the purchase of new equipment. Examples of tax-supported agencies include health departments from all levels of government; many hospitals; the Bethesda, Maryland, hospital complex; other army, navy, and veteran's hospitals; state mental hospitals; and neighborhood health clinics.

Non-tax-supported agencies include private profit-oriented agencies such as pharmacies, some hospitals, nursing homes, and private practices that are run on a fee-for-service basis.

Private, nonprofit agencies are supported by fees for service and voluntary contributions. Examples of this kind of agency include certain hospitals, the Visiting Nurses' Association, and programs such as Motor Meals. Most voluntary agencies are also private and nonprofit oriented. They usually concern themselves with a single problem. The American Cancer Society, The American Heart Association, and the National Foundation (The March of Dimes) are examples of voluntary agencies. Figure 7–1 indicates the funding structure of health-care agencies.

Financing Personal Health Care

Private Insurance.   Private insurance is one way of financing personal health care. Nonprofit, tax-exempt organizations such as Blue Cross – Blue Shield provide payment for the health-care needs of many Americans. Private, profit-oriented insurance companies also deal with the payment of health-care needs. To become insured, members must pay monthly premiums either by themselves or in combination with an employer. The best method of buying insurance is as a member of a contracting group through a union, an employer, or a club. This approach reduces the cost of insurance, because the pooled risks of all group members determine charges. These plans commonly pay about 80% of health-care costs; the client must pay the remainder.

Many other insurance plans are available that offer varying coverage. Many do not cover preventive health-care costs or screening procedures such as routine chest radio-

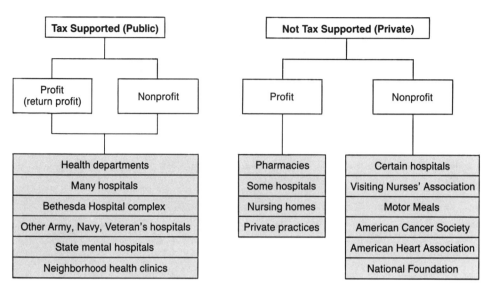

Figure 7-1   Funding of health-care agencies.

graphs. Some include benefits for psychiatric care and cancer follow-up care, but often coverage is limited for long-term disease. A certain amount of time must elapse between hospitalizations for a given disease before benefits resume. Although nurses will not know specifics of each insurance program, we assist our clients to learn about their coverage and plan their health care through the insurance agency resources. Although we do not usually question the need for emergency or intensive-care treatment, there may be a number of treatment plans to consider for less crisis-oriented concerns. As nurses, we can help clients to make sound decisions.

Medicare.   Medicare (Title XVIII of the Social Security Act), which has been in existence since 1966, is another prominent insurance program. It is administered by the federal government and is thereby uniform from state to state. Medicare serves persons age 65 or over regardless of financial resources. It also covers disabled persons under 65 years who have been entitled to social security benefits for 2 consecutive years and certain other persons with renal failure. These persons are insured through a monthly premium deducted from their social security benefits, with additional amounts being paid by the federal government. These monies are placed in trust funds that pay medical expenses for insured persons. Medical expenses covered include costs of physician services, home health care, and outpatient services such as rehabilitation therapy. Hospital insurance under Medicare is financed by workers' payroll deductions. Hospital expenses covered include semiprivate rooms, meals, the intensive-care unit, drugs, laboratory and x-ray tests, operating room use, dressing supplies, appliances such as wheelchairs, and rehabilitative services such as occupational and physical therapy. Psychiatric hospital care is covered for up to 190 days.

Services sometimes cover certain hospital and home health-care agencies, independent laboratories and x-ray services, some ambulance firms, chiropractors, and a variety of independent practitioners. Agencies and independent practitioners can make the decision not to accept persons insured by Medicare if they find the bookkeeping necessary for reimbursement too time consuming and expensive. In addition, Medicare often will not pay the fee charged by independent practitioners for a particular visit or procedure.

Services not covered by Medicare include personal services in hospitals (such as television and telephones), private rooms or private-duty nurses, routine foot care, eye and hearing examination, eyeglasses and hearing aids, and immunizations for infectious diseases. To be covered, care must be considered reasonable and necessary. Care that can be provided by unskilled care-givers such as home health aides is not covered. Drugs or meals delivered to the home are also not covered.

Nurses who provide care for persons receiving Medicare should be aware of the following facts.

- Persons should always carry their Medicare cards and present them whenever seeking services.
- The person's claim number should appear on any bills or correspondence sent to the claims offices.
- The agencies and services the person is seeking should be checked beforehand to determine that they are approved for reimbursement by Medicare and that they accept Medicare.
- The services covered within a given agency should be clarified before the agency is used.
- Persons disagreeing with the coverage by Medicare in a specific instance have the right to appeal.
- All persons insured by Medicare should have a copy of *Your Medicare Handbook*, distributed by the Department of HHS (1987).

Medicare does not address certain common needs of persons age 65 or older, and preventive and promotional health-care coverage is inadequate.

Medicaid.   Medicaid (Title XIX of the Social Security Act), a third way of financing personal health care, has also been in existence since 1966. It is administered by both federal and state governments in a partnership arrangement. The states develop their own programs within federal government guidelines, so benefits vary from state to state. The program provides benefits for certain eligible needy and low-income persons who are under 65 years of age. In addition, it pays for certain expenses for persons over 65 who are below a certain income level, including services that Medicare does not cover. Medicaid pays for medical expenses incurred by persons with complete visual loss and those classified as disabled, as well as by members of families with low income and dependent children. The program is funded by federal, state, and local taxes. Table 7–6 lists services covered by Medicaid.

. As with Medicare, nurses can assist clients who are eligible for Medicaid by providing them with information concerning the program, making sure that they understand the necessity of always carrying their Medicaid card, and checking agencies to determine whether they accept Medicaid clients and which services are covered. Nurses will want to

TABLE 7-6
SERVICES COVERED BY MEDICAID

Covered	Covered in Some States
Inpatient services	Dental care
Outpatient services	Prescribed drugs
Skilled nursing-home care	Eye glasses
Physician's services	Intermediate-care facilities' services
Laboratory services	Diagnostic
X-ray procedures	Screening
	Preventive
Diagnosis and treatment of children under 21	Rehabilitative
Home health-care services	
Family planning services	
Rural health-clinic services	

stay current with government reimbursement policies related to Medicare and Medicaid. For example, in 1988, the largest expansion of Medicare instituted assistance for catastrophic illness. Similarly, at that time Medicaid underwent significant change to prevent financial disaster of a spouse caused by nursing home care of a mate. As the administration of all levels of government changes, programs and their rules, regulations, and benefits change also.

Both programs expect high standards of care and they support the development of needed services. They encourage innovations in medical care delivery and require a review of the care provided. Both programs are also concerned about cost containment. An amendment to the Social Security Act, called the Professional Standards Review Organizations (PSRO), was enacted in 1972. This amendment mandated that physicians develop a mechanism for monitoring care and assuring quality care to beneficiaries of Medicare and Medicaid. Physicians were the first target group of this law. However, nursing is now included and nurses are involved in peer review and quality assurance programs.

National Health Insurance

A major proposed solution for the financing of health-care delivery in the United States is **national health insurance**, which would provide guaranteed coverage so that health care could be obtained by everyone. The Advisory Committee on National Health Insurance, charged by President Jimmy Carter (1977-1980), was instructed to develop a plan that would provide the following:

- Fair and equitable treatment
- Redistribution of health-care resources
- Meeting manpower needs
- Training of health-care professionals
- Quality assurance systems
- Illness prevention means
- Planning and control of resources
- Origin and delivery of services

- Administrative simplicity
- Eligibility standards (Mauksch, 1978, p 1323)

This list indicates that the Carter administration wished to examine other major problems in addition to financing. Other administrations will have their own view of the issues. The Reagan administration, for example, halted most discussions on this proposal.

Overall, the proponents of a national health insurance program seek to reflect the generally agreed on notion that everyone is entitled to health care that is financially equitable, accessible, available, comprehensive, and uniform in quality of care.

Two nursing leaders, however, caution us to be alert to the limitations of national health insurance. Mauksch stated, "The crucial issue here is that a national health insurance package that does not alter the manner in which care is administered or change the attitudes fostered by caregivers simply will not meet the needs of the people." She went on to explain, "The true success of national health insurance depends to a large extent upon the way providers and consumers deal with it. . . . [They] will need to mount a national effort toward the improvement of health and illness care attitudes, so that the new system [national health insurance] may serve society well" (1978, p 1327). In the same vein, McGee cautioned, "It should be kept in mind that national health insurance deals only with cost coverage, not the health care system itself" (1980, p 37).

It behooves us to be aware of these concerns. Federal legislators have asked nurses to testify during hearings on national health insurance. Proposed nursing solutions could make a difference in the overall effectiveness of health-care delivery. For example, Barbara Nichols, president of the ANA (1978–1982), testified before the Senator Edward Kennedy hearing in Denver on November 29, 1978 (Brewer, 1979).

Nichols pointed out that the United States provides a medical or acute-care system designed to treat persons after they become ill or injured, rather than to emphasize preventive services. She indicated that the acute-care focus relies heavily on physicians and institutions, thus adding significantly to national health-care costs. Nichols reported that Senator Kennedy's plan for national health insurance did not consider nursing services as a covered benefit. She indicated that a separate identification of nursing service costs would more accurately describe the financial situation, and she suggested a number of key ways in which nursing services could deal effectively with many of today's health problems. For example, health education programs and plans of care for chronically disabled and dying persons in the home could provide cost-effective care.

Just a year later, Sister Rosemary Donley (1979) indicated that the Kennedy proposal now delineated nursing service as a separate factor. She stated that the proposal opens the possibility of expanding the system of reimbursing nurse practitioners. This statement suggests that nursing can have an impact on the development of national health insurance policy.

Several plans for national health insurance have been proposed, each of which covers a variety of services. For example, some would provide payment for catastrophic illness only. Catastrophic illness is defined in terms of cost. Other proposals suggest additional coverage and improved benefits for the aged, pregnant women, and children. Some would require membership of our entire population while others consider voluntary participation. Some programs would be supported by tax dollars; others might involve private enterprise.

Although, as times change, specific persons such as Senator Kennedy may not be as vocal in health-care issues, others will take their place. Nurses must be active in shaping legislation that would delineate appropriate nursing services; in this way we may be able to protect our clients from exorbitant expense and to ensure that preventive health care becomes a priority.

Donley stated, "The ANA is on record in support of comprehensive national health insurance. ANA is on record in support of nursing service as a benefit and the professional nurse as a provider" (1979, p 4). She urges us to press this issue.

Nurses will want to consider the following questions concerning any form of national health insurance:

- How does the government plan to deal with overuse of the system?
- Can we expect a change from illness-oriented care to preventive health care and health promotion?
- Will national health insurance provide reimbursement of nursing services?
- Does the federal government understand the difference between medical insurance and health insurance?

What the Bush administration will do about national health insurance remains to be seen.

Diagnostic-Related Groupings

The diagnostic-related groupings (DRG) system represents a major thrust by the Federal Government to contain the cost of health care. The system was devised by a group of researchers at Yale University and is based on the International Classification of Diseases drawn up by the World Health Organization in the 1920s. The code letters *ICD-9-CM*, which stand for International Classification of Diseases, 9th revision, Clinical Modification, now appear on hospital records of Medicare clients to identify in which category of the DRG system they have been placed for payment. The system officially went into effect on April 20, 1983, when President Reagan signed Public Law 98-21 (the Social Security Amendments of 1983). Title VI of this law deals with Medicare payments for hospital inpatient services under the DRG system. Private insurance companies, while not specifically using the DRG system, have developed similar criteria for reimbursement.

Simply described, the DRG system works in the following way. A client enters a local hospital emergency room with severe lower abdominal pain. After appropriate studies, the diagnosis of appendicitis with a need for surgery is made. The client is assigned the DRG number covering this condition that indicates that clients undergoing an uncomplicated appendectomy may stay in the hospital for three days. If his or her postoperative course is smooth and he or she indeed leaves in 3 days, the hospital is reimbursed accordingly. If the client is able to leave in just 2 days, the hospital will receive the same reimbursement as if he had stayed for 3 days and consequently will make money. On the other hand, if the client remains more than 3 days and the hospital could not justify the necessity, such as a demonstrated complication from surgery, reimbursement would be paid for 3 days and the hospital would assume the rest of the cost. If the client develops a complication, such as a wound infection, the original DRG code number can be changed to ensure proper reimbursement to the hospital. The code number can also be changed for other reasons, such as if the client is diagnosed with an additional disease while in the hospital.

Under the DRG system, clients are admitted to the hospital later in an illness and discharged earlier in convalescence than ever before. For example, in the past, clients about to undergo planned surgery were usually admitted one or more days ahead of the scheduled date. This time was spent in diagnostic studies and general preparation for the surgery. This work is now done more often in ambulatory care clinics and clients enter the hospital on the day of surgery. Postoperatively, clients proceed through a planned program and are discharged as soon as possible, often leaving with a need for nursing care in the home.

The implications for nursing under the DRG system are many. The client acuity (severity of illness) in the hospital is greater than ever before because only the sickest or those who have had surgery are admitted. Joel stated, "Increased volume under DRG's equals more admissions. And new admissions demand significantly more nurse time and energy," (1987, p 794). Although administrators may note that they are employing more nurses than ever before, nursing states that the number of nurses is still inadequate to meet this increased need. This situation creates tension between nursing and administration because nurses are frequently required to justify their demands for more positions by proving their productivity.

In addition to the sicker client issue, implications exist for nursing regarding, in particular, the surgical client who arrives on a nursing unit only after surgery. Time-honored nursing research has clearly indicated that postoperative complications are reduced when clients are given preoperative education and coping skills regarding the surgical experience. During the preoperative period, the nurse can develop rapport with the client as well as assess the client for baseline data with which to compare his or her postoperative response. Although assessment and education are being handled in some ambulatory clinics, the programs are often not well developed and clients may not receive adequate preparation.

Nursing in the community has also been affected by the DRG system. While hospital acuity is higher, so is acuity in the community. Because clients stay home longer and return home sooner, a need exists for more acute nursing care in this setting as well — often involving sophisticated equipment. It is not unusual to find clients at home with oxygen, intravenous therapy, open wounds, or various drainage tubes. Even clients on ventilators (breathing machines) can sometimes be cared for at home.

Depending on the hospital, the DRG system can negatively affect nursing job security. Although tertiary care hospitals generally will not experience a decrease in client populations, some community hospitals already have, requiring the closure of sections, or even entire hospitals. In these instances, nurses may want to consider a new setting. While there may be more nurses than necessary in some places, there are shortages in others.

Health Maintenance Organizations: A Possible Solution

Health maintenance organizations (HMOs) are group health practices whose major distinguishing feature is prepayment and whose existence suggests one major solution to the problems of health-care costs. Members pay a fixed fee on a yearly basis and receive health care whenever they need it, either for a nominal additional charge or no charge, depending on the plan. The HMO provides comprehensive health-care services that include wellness care as well as illness care. The program is arranged so that a broad group of specialists participates in care and is available for referral. Most HMOs have participating hospitals as well.

The emphasis on preventive health services and wellness care encourages persons to seek care early in a disease process, thereby avoiding hospitalization: the healthier the clients, the more financially stable the HMO. The traditional approach to health care has been to pay doctors and hospitals to provide care to the sick, thus giving incentives for illness care. The HMO has sought to change that by providing incentives for health care.

One of the most successful HMOs is the Kaiser-Permanente prepaid care plan, which provides medical and hospital services to more than 3 million persons. Agencies and physicians over a large portion of the western United States as well as Ohio and Hawaii participate in this program. Kaiser-Permanente has developed six basic principles from which it operates:

- Group practice
- Integration of facilities (combining both hospital and outpatient facilities)
- Prepayment
- Preventive health care (emphasis on keeping the person well in addition to treating the sick)
- Voluntary enrollment
- Physician responsibility (for client care, financing, planning, and allocation of resources

Central to the operation of Kaiser-Permanente is the principle that the program must be self-sustaining. Equipment and facilities are paid for by client fees and long-term loans, and less than 1% of Kaiser-Permanente's costs has been supported by either private or government sources.

A summary of the characteristics of HMOs and traditional health-care delivery suggests the following differences:

- *Traditional care* — fee for service to physicians and cost reimbursement for hospitals provides incentives for delivering illness care; third-party insurance coverage relieves the person from much of the cost of his or her health care, thus providing the individual with little incentive for questioning that cost.
- *HMO care* — prepayment of fixed fees to hospitals and physicians provides a strong incentive to keep costs reasonable and to provide wellness care. When the cost barrier is removed, persons come in earlier for care and thus avoid long-term and expensive illness problems.

Using the Kaiser-Permanente plan as a model, the federal government enacted the Health Maintenance Organization Act in 1973. The act was developed to study various methods of health-care delivery in the hope of generating a model for comprehensive health care. It was intended to deal with such issues as the distribution and availability of quality health care, cost containment, and quality control. It provided for members of the Department of HEW (federal government) to collaborate with the PSROs (health care professionals) to ensure quality of care.

"Between 1976 and 1986, the number of health maintenance organizations [HMOs] increased from 174 to 623 and enrollment rose from 6 million to 26 million" (National Center for Health Statistics, 1988, p 4). Although during the past 10 years the number of HMOs has burgeoned, their future is uncertain. Much depends on what course the government takes with regard to national health insurance. A combination of the two concepts — HMOs and national health insurance — is a distinct possibility.

Nursing Solution for Cost Containment in Health-Care Delivery

Continuity of Care

Nurses have long known that continuity of care — that is, discharge planning — starts with admission to the hospital; however, this concept has become even more critical with the advent of the DRG system. Many hospitals have nurses, often called home-care coordinators or discharge planners, who assist the general staff nurse in continuity of care activities. In other systems the primary nurse or other staff nurses are responsible for this planning.

Planning for discharge as soon as the person is admitted requires nursing expertise in anticipating the usual needs of a particular client population as well as expertise in assessing individual clients and their families for special needs. It also requires knowledge of general issues such as the operations of other departments within the hospital that affect the client (e.g., physical therapy, social work), how to help with transportation, identifying pharmacies where medications and supplies can be obtained, and determining how much nursing care will be needed at home after discharge.

Fagin, in her article describing various ways in which nursing can be an alternative to the high cost of health care, referred to Georgopoulus and Mann when she stated, "Research data accumulated over the past twenty years indicate the importance of nursing and nursing care in affecting patient outcomes in and out of hospitals and show that nursing services can contribute immeasurably to the goals of a competitive delivery system" (1982, p 59). Fagin went on to suggest that specialization in nursing is one solution to burgeoning costs and mentions such specialties as nurse-midwifery, nurse practitioner (pediatric, psychiatric, cardiovascular, etc.) and nurse-rehabilitator.

An excellent example of how nurse specialists in rehabilitation and neurological conditions can foster preventive health care is evident with the Feet First Program. This national program is directed at preventing head and spinal cord injuries. Originally aimed at teaching young persons the importance of testing swimming areas first with their feet before diving in head first, it has developed into a more comprehensive program with education focused toward taking better care of themselves in all activities that could cause injuries. Nurses take this program to the schools and include, when possible, a peer counselor and a young injured person with quadraplegia (paralysis from the neck down) who describes his or her accident, injuries, and current life style. Although it is difficult to place a dollar value on prevention (we rarely know what we have prevented), it is nevertheless an important area that nursing can attend to well.

Primary Nursing

Marie Manthey is recognized as the first person to describe the concept of **primary nursing**. She indicated that this is a system of nursing care delivery that renders the nurse responsible and accountable, though not necessarily present or available, on a 24-hour basis. This accountability is possible through coordination, management, and communication of the care so that others can provide that care in the absence of the primary nurse.

Joel spoke harshly of those who would not see the value of professional nursing care: "faced with patients who are less functionally able and more acutely ill, the fool's answer to economic constraints is to dilute staffing: the foolish will sacrifice two professional positions to hire three ancillary workers. This reasoning proves disastrous" (1987, p 794).

Nursing has been accused by some of providing the "Cadillac model" of client care. Administrators and economists in health care believe that a less luxurious and more cost-effective model would serve as well. It is unfortunate for nursing and our clients that we do not more adequately describe our care. As it happens, this Cadillac is one we must afford. Anything less would markedly decrease the ability to meet our clients' basic needs, will increase acuity and complications and, in turn, hospital admissions and longer stays. Nursing care is a major reason why many clients can stay within the limits of the DRG system. Consider the following example:

> Paul, a 21-year-old man, had been through a rugged experience with kidney stones, pain, hemorrhage, and infection. Because he was otherwise healthy, everyone expected that following appropriate treatment he would get well and be discharged. Instead, he became weak and depressed. Finally, the primary nurse uncovered the problem. Paul said that he was exhausted but could not sleep because he was afraid of suddenly hemorrhaging during the night. He thought that if his sister could spend the night with him he would not be afraid. The primary nurse was criticized by some for encouraging dependence when she permitted his sister to stay. However, the nurse recognized that his unmet need for safety was contributing to the dependency. Criticism evaporated when Paul slept through the night for the first time in several weeks, showed considerable improvement the next day, and was discharged the day after. He told the nurse that "it was because you let my sister stay that I got well."

PERSON-CENTERED HEALTH-CARE DELIVERY

Students, in their learning years, can be observers of health-care delivery. For example, watching and listening while sitting in waiting rooms of health-care agencies provide opportunities for obtaining information about the system. Be aware of how often the person becomes a number and how often needs of the agency or the practitioner take priority. The following example comes from a nurse and mother of a 20-year-old man waiting to have an angiogram (x-ray film of the vascular system using a radioactive dye) for a possible subclavian artery aneurysm.

> Tony's angiogram was scheduled for 10 A.M. that morning. However, as we left the house, a severe thunderstorm began. Upon arriving at the hospital, we learned that only an emergency generator for essential electrical equipment was operating. Although many radiographs were cancelled, Tony was asked to wait until electrical power could be restored, which made him very anxious because he had expected to have the procedure over quickly. The receptionist was kind but could not offer much assistance. No nurse came to console the clients. Tony's doctor appeared briefly but did not stop to commiserate, which was unfortunate—I knew that just talking to him for a minute would have helped Tony feel better.
> Despite my personal concerns, I found myself viewing the situation as a professional

nurse and systems observer. I watched the frustration and anxiety persons demonstrated when their radiographs were cancelled. I noted that health professionals did not come to assist the receptionist or the clients. One doctor appeared and spoke to the waiting room in general, saying he was sorry and that clients would be rescheduled as soon as possible. Some clients were unreasonable and rude to the receptionist, who then became defensive and told them loudly that it was not *her* fault.

I kept thinking how much difference a nurse would have made. A nurse, using a Maslovian framework, understands the anxiety and insecurity that this kind of situation creates for clients. A nurse understands that frustrated persons irrationally heap abuse on whomever is available. Nurses can be objective and use therapeutic communication skills to help persons focus on reality and do problem solving. They can use their professional knowledge to establish logical priorities for rescheduling. Their presence would provide leadership for persons who do not have these skills.

CONSUMERISM AND PREVENTIVE HEALTH CARE

Consumers are persons who use a commodity or service. As consumers, we use a continuous array of products every day, even when we sleep. All of us are consumers of health commodities and services. Some of these services require the specialized knowledge and skills of health-care professionals while many of the commodities may be purchased by our own choice. Toothpaste, antidandruff shampoos, aspirin, and bandages are a few of the items we buy for health purposes.

The appeal of packaging as well as the media — that is, television, magazines — often figure in our decisions of what to buy. Television, articles, or pamphlets — such as the one distributed by the American Cancer Society providing a checklist of cancer symptoms — add to our knowledge about health.

As mentioned in the introduction to this chapter, there are problems associated with buying health commodities and services. For a variety of reasons, consumers may settle for less than optimum value, especially when illness may affect the ability to make rational choices.

Unfortunately, consumers may not shop for health-care services but instead accept those readily available. When buying products for personal use, we consider their value per dollar; when seeking a special service, we try to learn about the providers. However, when purchasing health services, we are deplorably reluctant to check on the type of health care available.

Characteristics of the Consumer of Health Care

Consumers of health care, like all persons, have certain characteristics that must be taken into account when health-care services are rendered. As such, these characteristics have important implications for nursing.

Interrelated Biophysical and Psychosocial Concerns

Consider the following examples. Mrs. Jones, the single mother of a teenage daughter, is hospitalized for surgery. The nurse is concerned with providing preoperative teaching, but

Mrs. Jones is worried about leaving her teenager with inadequate supervision and cannot focus on preoperative teaching. Clinical studies have indicated that preoperative teaching instruction shortens a hospital stay if barriers to the client's learning are removed.

Helping Mrs. Jones to plan for her daughter will ease her worries so that she can absorb important information. Ideally, a well-prepared client will have a smoother postoperative course and return home quickly, thus alleviating the family situation.

Next, consider the client who must convalesce for several weeks following a heart attack. He is discharged and told to rest and relax. This task may be difficult, because long illnesses usually compound pre-existing job, financial, or family concerns.

Such examples focus on physiological problems and suggest that psychosocial needs increase the harmful effects of physical illness. Viewing this example in another way, we note that pre-existing psychosocial needs may precipitate physical problems. The interrelationship of these factors reinforces the need for nurses to treat clients from a holistic perspective.

Ill-Matched Concerns

The consumer of health care has a set of concerns that may differ from those of the health-care providers. Persons often consider a long-term illness as normal for them rather than a health problem. One woman with diabetes, during an interview, was asked if she knew what had made her sick. She stated that she was not sick and that as a diabetic she was hospitalized only for sugar control. However, she pointed out to the nurse that her real problem was not being able to do her housework since a heart attack 4 years ago.

Martha Weinman Lear, in her book *Heartsounds* (1980), described the last 3 years of her husband's life as he tried to cope with progressive heart disease. Although concerned about his heart condition, he discovered, to his horror, that his mental abilities had declined following heart surgery. He had lost his memory and often could not grasp the meaning of monosyllabic words. Driving or shopping left him exhausted and confused. His cardiologists told him to be patient, that his mind would recover. They thought he should be more concerned about his heart disease, which was life-threatening.

Personal Priorities

Community nurses often consider immunizations a top priority. However, a mother with chronic fatigue and financial burdens may not have the time or energy required to take her children to even a free immunization clinic. Her other problems are more important to her: the possibility of her children contracting a disease such as polio seems remote.

Self-Care Abilities and Knowledge of Personal Needs

The philosophy of self-care purports that persons have knowledge and abilities regarding their health. However, because they sometimes cannot communicate their knowledge or mobilize their strengths, they become consumers of health care. As nurses, we provide health services because we are hired by consumers and not because we have the right to exert authority over their choices.

Variables that Influence Health Behavior

Health behaviors are learned and develop from customs particular to one's social system, culture, and family. A person adopts a health behavior if he or she perceives it to have value, meaning, and relevance to his or her particular needs. Although care-givers regard certain health behaviors as important, we may discover that the person disagrees, or, having agreed, does not practice those behaviors as expected. If we examine the variables that affect health behaviors, the cause of this variance between the ideal and reality becomes clear.

Biophysical Variables

The following physical symptoms are those that most commonly motivate a person to seek health care:

- Pain
- Respiratory distress
- Insomnia
- Visual and auditory alterations
- Dizziness
- Malfunction of a body part

Health care is sought more quickly if a symptom interferes with the person's functioning. For example, a person who reads a great deal will want glasses as soon as his or her vision becomes impaired; others may wait longer. Some persons neglect their dental health until pain occurs, or they cannot eat as before. Some persons seek health care as soon as they experience pain, while others, athletes, for example, may function well in their sport while suffering from pain related to old injuries.

Psychological Variables

Hesitancy to Consult a Physician or to Enter a Health-Care System. Consumers prefer to seek health care from professionals they know or have previously consulted; they want affordable health care without the confusion of a large system. When their experience does not meet these expectations, they may put off seeking the care they need. Some persons have grown up in families that used home or cultural remedies rather than traditional care, and these individuals may be suspicious of practices with which they are unfamiliar.

The Need to Know and the Fear of Knowing. Some persons who are fearful that they might have a serious illness seek medical care immediately, while others minimize symptoms hoping that they will go away. Those who put off obtaining health care usually seek help once they accept the idea of coping with serious illness. Sadly, sometimes the extra time taken shortens a person's life.

Knowledge Levels. Our knowledge of health and disease frequently affects the way in which we seek health care. Some persons can determine that symptoms are serious and can seek appropriate help. Knowledge of health services and health systems helps many of us to pursue health care with less difficulty than those who know little. Understanding where to go and how one is expected to function can decrease hesitancy to consult health-care professionals.

Self-esteem. Our sense of self-worth may affect when we seek health care and how we adhere to treatment plans. Feelings of self-esteem may not be conscious; persons may not recognize how these feelings affect behavior. For example, persons with decreased self-esteem may not believe that they will receive attention unless they are ill, which may motivate them to seek health care repeatedly for the secondary gain it provides.

Sociocultural Variables

Availability of Health-Care Services.   Persons generally desire health-care services that are near their homes. Healthy persons may prefer not to drive long distances for care, and ill persons may find long distances or public transportation especially difficult.

Financial Status.   For many years, persons with limited financial resources had difficulty obtaining care. They may have refused or been denied health services because they were unable to pay. Today, insurance programs cover a large percentage of health-care costs for those who can pay the program premiums, and government programs have been developed that assist needy persons to obtain health care. However, depending on the plan, certain necessary services may not be covered. For example, some insurance plans do not cover nurses visiting in the home. Families must find other means to obtain needed care.

Alternative Healing Systems and Specific Religious Philosophies.   Some individuals trust the medicine man or curandero and practices such as acupuncture or astrology more than the Western cultural practice of calling the doctor. Others from the Judeo-Christian tradition have been attracted by the laying on of hands and other faith-healing practices. Often, these alternative practices can be very effective — remember that persons have survived on this earth for centuries prior to the advent of modern health care.

Media.   Television and news publications have had a far-reaching effect on our lives, especially in the last 35 years. Through these sources, we receive health-related information that is not always accurate or useful. Nurses can assist clients to develop decision-making skills to judge the quality of information from the media.

In one instance, information from a television program about a hospital emergency unit helped a young girl save a young boy's life. When he accidentally electrocuted himself, his 11-year-old sister performed cardiopulmonary resuscitation that she had learned from watching the program.

The foregoing discussion suggests that all consumers of health care have their own definitions of health and illness. Decisions about whether and when to seek health care and to engage in health practices are based on many variables. Although our health practices reflect our cultural and family customs, our uniqueness has an even greater influence on how we perceive health. As nurses, we believe persons are holistic and we consider the interaction among all variables that influence perceptions of health.

Consumer Movement

Prior to World War II, there were few medicines or surgical techniques. Chemotherapy, dialysis, radiation or other technological advances to help persons manage disease were minimal. Sick persons were often kept at home and families used private duty nurses for help, if they could afford them. During this time, persons were fearful of contracting dreaded diseases such as tuberculosis, pneumonia, strep throat, or polio. The summer months were stressful for parents who feared a polio outbreak and, therefore, kept their children away from crowded areas. Going to a sanitarium for tuberculosis carried a social stigma; having a nervous breakdown often meant entering a state hospital from which no one ever returned.

Advances in medicine and science began to change this picture. In 1921, insulin was first used successfully in the treatment of diabetes mellitus. By the early to mid-1940s, antibiotics were introduced to combat bacterial infections. Miraculous drugs turned life-threatening diseases into treatable problems, while tranquilizers changed the whole concept of care for mentally ill persons. Steroids treated a range of inflammatory diseases such as arthritis and dermatology disorders. At the same time, surgical techniques and hemodialysis were developed and perfected, making a number of fatal diseases treatable or curable. In 1953, the polio vaccine arrived, solving one of our major national health problems.

Throughout the 20th century, many new drugs became available, including medicines for hypertension and cancer as well as drugs for infertility and birth control. We were a nation of drug users long before the term came to have legal or abusive connotations. We believed there was a pill for everything and became resentful when told there was no remedy for a particular problem, nor could we easily understand that antibiotics were effective against bacteria but not viruses. Too often, we demanded antibiotics inappropriately and the physician would agree.

Eventually prescriptions, rather than the person's individual needs or self-care abilities, became the focus of treatment. Although drugs were often appropriate (as when antihypertensive drugs were prescribed for persons with high blood pressure), they were relied on completely without giving much thought to other aspects of the person's life, such as are emphasized in the holistic view. It is conceivable that if persons had examined some of the factors precipitating hypertension, they might have learned other ways to control blood pressure. Professional nurses possessed skills to assist clients to do this, but the emphasis remained on the new miracle drugs and the easy solutions they provided for health problems.

As the age of science and technology progressed, consumers no longer remembered the effects of polio or strep throat. Doctors and nurses became more controlling with their advanced knowledge and often indicated that they knew what was best, without consideration for the client's ideas, while large hospitals and clinics provided less individualized care than settings in which the person was known. As persons wondered how they had come to have minimal say in their health care, they often voiced the following concerns:

- Drugs and surgical procedures that were expected to cure patients sometimes made them sicker.
- Return visits to doctors were expensive and often seemed unnecessary.
- The cost of health care was escalating beyond reasonable levels.
- Scandal was frequent: nursing-home administrators pocketed money provided for client care; physicians received percentages of prescriptions costs from pharmacists to whom they sent customers.
- Nurses were often perceived as uncaring and unavailable.

The **consumer movement** in health care originated from these concerns. It probably began with Ralph Nader's book, *Unsafe at Any Speed*, written in 1965. Nader berated car manufacturers for their failure to respond to the needs of the public and for their disregard for safety. Nader has continued his fight for consumer protection in a wide variety of products and services, and others have followed his lead, contributing to the growth of the movement.

As consumer pressure developed, consumer advocates were hired by hospitals and other health organizations. Hospital boards and committees were required to have consumer representation. Human subject protection committees developed in institutions where research was being done.

The consumer movement has produced many positive effects, especially in promoting protective and educational functions. Committees have been formed to set standards for many kinds of commodities and services, and organizations have created boards of review to ensure that these standards are followed. In the health-care industry the consumer movement has clearly established that persons have a right to receive information about their disease and treatment, to participate in decision making, and to understand the charges for treatment. These rights have been outlined in the Patient's Bill of Rights developed in 1972 by the American Hospital Association (Table 7–7). A variety of pamphlets and books have been written to increase health consumers' knowledge and decision-making abilities. These publications are available from government, private agencies, and individuals; the words "The Consumer's Guide" often appear in the title.

The consumer movement has helped create responsible consumerism. Consumers control and provide input into those things that affect them as individuals. Responsible consumerism is an obligation. If persons wish to receive value for their dollars, they have a responsibility to see that this happens.

A negative effect of the consumer movement is the proliferation of malpractice lawsuits. Consumers have recently discovered their rights and have taken to the courts. As a result, malpractice insurance premiums have become astronomical, particularly for physicians.

Some persons who merit payment due to physician error would prefer to settle quickly without litigation. One such situation involved a woman who was to have minor surgery for diagnosis of her infertility problem. Another woman was scheduled for a sterilization procedure on the same day. The physician confused the two women and tied the tubes of the one with the infertility problem. He stated,

> As soon as I realized my mistake, I called a surgeon in another city who was known for his ability to repair tubes, and made arrangements for him to see this woman the next week. Then I called my attorney and told him we would have to make a settlement for my error. Attorneys for both parties were able to negotiate a reasonable settlement that included payment for future medical expenses as well as reimbursement for the emotional distress and pain incurred by this lady.

Such reasonable settlement of problems might prevent malpractice insurance premiums from becoming prohibitive.

Still, many consumer complaints reach the courts. Some physicians may be reluctant to admit mistakes. Sometimes persons are looking for a reason to file suit in the hope of gaining special attention or a large sum of money, and some attorneys encourage this practice for their own financial gain. Whatever the reason for litigation, the result is increased malpractice insurance premiums, which are then passed on to the consumer through fees for professional service.

Although the increased incidence of malpractice suits is a real problem, it has had positive effects. The health-care professions have begun to review and evaluate their practices more carefully. Committees for standardizing diagnostic and therapeutic procedures are a part of most agencies that provide health care. Their purpose is to provide

TABLE 7–7
PATIENT'S BILL OF RIGHTS

The American Hospital Association presents a Patient's Bill of Rights with the expectation that observance of these rights will contribute to more effective patient care and greater satisfaction for the patient, his physician, and the hospital organization. Further, the Association presents these rights in the expectation that they will be supported by the hospital on behalf of its patients, as an integral part of the healing process. It is recognized that a personal relationship between the physician and the patient is essential for the provision of proper medical care. The traditional physician-patient relationship takes on a new dimension when care is rendered within an organizational structure. Legal precedent has established that the institution itself also has a responsibility to the patient. It is in recognition of these factors that these rights are affirmed.

1 The patient has the right to considerate and respectful care.
2 The patient has the right to obtain from his physician complete current information concerning his diagnosis, treatment, and prognosis in terms the patient can be reasonably expected to understand. When it is not medically advisable to give such information to the patient, the information should be made available to an appropriate person in his behalf. He has the right to know, by name, the physician responsible for coordinating his care.
3 The patient has the right to receive from his physician information necessary to give informed consent prior to the start of any procedure and/or treatment. Except in emergencies, such information for informed consent should include but not necessarily be limited to the specific procedure and/or treatment, the medically significant risks involved, and the probable duration of incapacitation. Where medically significant alternatives for care or treatment exist, or when the patient requests information concerning medical alternatives, the patient has the right to such information. The patient also has the right to know the name of the person responsible for the procedures and/or treatment.
4 The patient has the right to refuse treatment to the extent permitted by law and to be informed of the medical consequences of his action.
5 The patient has the right to every consideration of his privacy concerning his own medical care program. Case discussion, consultation, examination, and treatment are confidential and should be conducted discreetly. Those not directly involved in his care must have the permission of the patient to be present.
6 The patient has the right to expect that all communications and records pertaining to his care should be treated as confidential.
7 The patient has the right to expect that within its capacity a hospital must make reasonable response to the request of a patient for services. The hospital must provide evaluation, service, or referral as indicated by the urgency of the case. When medically permissible, a patient may be transferred to another facility only after he has received complete information and explanation concerning the needs for and alternatives to such a transfer. The institution to which the patient is to be transferred must first have accepted the patient for transfer.
8 The patient has the right to obtain information as to any relationship of his hospital to other health care and educational institutions insofar as his care is concerned. The patient has the right to obtain information as to the existence of any professional relationships among individuals, by name, who are treating him.
9 The patient has the right to be advised if the hospital proposes to engage in or perform human experimentation affecting his care or treatment. The patient has the right to refuse to participate in such research projects.
10 The patient has the right to expect reasonable continuity of care. He has the right to know in advance what appointment times and physicians are available and where. The patient has the right to expect that the hospital will provide a mechanism whereby he is informed by his physician or a delegate of the physician of the patient's continuing health care requirements following discharge.
11 The patient has the right to examine and receive an explanation of his bill regardless of source of payment.
12 The patient has the right to know what hospital rules and regulations apply to his conduct as a patient.

(Table 7–7 continues)

(*TABLE* 7–7 continued)

No catalog of rights can guarantee for the patient the kind of treatment he has a right to expect. A hospital has many functions to perform, including the prevention and treatment of disease, the education of both health professionals and patients, and the conduct of clinical research. All these activities must be conducted with an overriding concern for the patient, and, above all, the recognition of his dignity as a human being. Success in achieving this recognition assures success in the defense of the rights of the patient.

(Reprinted with the permission of the American Hospital Association, 840 North Lake Shore Drive, Chicago, Illinois 60611, copyright 1972)

quality and safety in the care of the individual, as well as to protect the agency from litigation. These committees, concerned with both medical and nursing procedures, have attempted to set standards for the most common medical diagnostic tests and procedures and for most technical nursing procedures.

Nurses as Client Advocates

An advocate is one who supports, upholds, defends, or intercedes on behalf of another. Nurses perform this function when they assist and support clients. The following list details ways nurses can function as client advocates.

1 Uphold the Patient's Bill of Rights.
2 Respond to the social and ethnic uniqueness of the person.
3 Provide scientifically current nursing care.
4 Establish continuity of care.
5 Provide for client participation and decision making in all aspects of health care.
6 Serve on a committee for standardizing agency procedures.
7 Become involved in health care at the community level.
8 Become involved in governmental programs that affect health care.
9 Intervene on behalf of a person with any other health-care provider involved in that person's care.
10 Coordinate all services used by the client in the attempt to restore, maintain, or promote health.

The following example describes a nurse who acted as a **client advocate** while she served on a standardizing committee at a large medical center.

The head nurse in a nursery intensive-care unit became concerned because of the large amount of blood that was being removed from the babies for the purpose of doing diagnostic tests. She pointed out that the amount of blood taken from the babies was often as much as that taken from adults for the same test. She stated that while 5 or 6 ml of blood was not a great deal for an adult to lose, it was too much for a baby, especially when more than one test was to be conducted on a given day. On occasions when this subject was before the committee, laboratory personnel were consulted. Often they indicated that the amount of blood specified was necessary. On each of these occasions the nurse persisted in the following way: she remained composed, she came to the committee with data about her tiny clients, she elicited support from other members of the committee (often before the meeting), and she was willing to compromise. She stated, "I know this is difficult for the labs, but we must try to reach a better solution because these little ones cannot tolerate the loss of so much blood." In this way she attained the respect of her colleagues and paved the way for protection of her clients.

Nurses can become involved in the community in a variety of ways. They can serve on the board of directors for agencies whose activities are designed to meet consumers' needs.

Because of their unique skills in understanding the biopsychosocial aspects of persons, nurses can identify consumers' needs and how these can be met. For example, one nurse sitting on a board of a community clinic — which served persons with special socioeconomic needs — was able to identify these needs for funding agencies. Using knowledge about perceptions of health and health behavior, the nurse could inform others more clearly of her clients' special needs.

Nurses can be advocates for individual consumers by assisting them to deal with the process of entering a health-care agency, by helping them to find information they need, and by encouraging them to solve problems and identify solutions for their health-care needs. Consumers often need someone who can consider their total needs; nurses, with their knowledge of biological, psychological, and sociocultural functioning, are well suited to this role. Since nurses spend more direct time with clients than other health-care providers, they are in an ideal position to listen to their problems, identify their needs, and assist them to find solutions. When the hospital nurse helps a client contact a dietitian for concerns about his or her low-sodium diet and when a community-health nurse helps a client identify an agency that provides needed financial assistance, both are acting as consumer advocates.

Journalist Fred Cook wrote about his wife's long battle against heart disease in *Julia's Story* (1977). The story is a tragic one, not so much because of the unhappy ending or even because of the constant stress Julia suffered at the hands of the various health-care delivery services she consulted. The real tragedy was that throughout their whole ordeal, she and her husband never really found anyone to whom they could turn. They needed someone who was willing to listen, to run interference for them, and to view them as whole persons. Nurses reading *Julia's Story* can hardly miss the need these persons had for nursing care. Yet there are few nurses of any significance described in this story; in fact, the most helpful nurse they met arrived too late to be of real assistance.

Our challenge is clearly marked: as professional nurses, we have the knowledge, skills, and numbers necessary to make a difference to the health of individuals and groups of persons. We can make ourselves seen and heard in a number of ways, for instance, we can insist on the consumer's right to have coordinated health care and, with other specialized professionals, we can help to provide it. We can assist consumers to use their self-care abilities so that they will remain in control of the health care they receive.

Table 7–8 presents a list of person-centered health-care goals. These goals reflect the philosophy of person-centered health care.

TABLE 7-8
PERSON-CENTERED HEALTH-CARE GOALS

1 To receive care that subscribes to the philosophy of the whole integrated person with spiritual, psychological, physiological, and sociological components.
2 To collaborate with health-care providers and direct the planning and implementation of one's own care
3 To receive information from health-care providers about the person's health concerns or disease to assist him or her in making appropriate decisions about his care.
4 To receive care that considers the person's unique needs when he or she has a diminished ability to participate.
5 To communicate the person's knowledge about his or her unique needs and expect that health-care providers will incorporate these into the care plan.
6 To have the person's strengths assessed by health-care providers and mobilized toward supporting, maintaining, or promoting health status.
7 To have the person's unique characteristics (biopsychosocial–spiritual) assessed and care provided that is safe and relevant given those characteristics.
8 To expect confidentiality concerning the person as a person and the care he or she is receiving.
9 To be provided with the most modern and scientifically sound medical and nursing care available.
10 To be advised of the rules, regulations, policies, and procedures of the agency or persons from whom he or she is seeking care.
11 To receive continuity of care.
12 To receive a full explanation of the expected costs of the health care for which the person is contracting and the actual costs of it after completion.

| PREVENTIVE HEALTH CARE

The consumer movement that has produced increased participation in health care has also generated interest in maintaining personal health. Persons have begun to lose weight, to stop smoking, and to participate in sports in order to stay healthy. **Preventive health care** is a term used to describe activities that promote health by reducing factors that contribute to illness and by reinforcing the person's strengths. As consumers have become interested in preventive health care, the concept has received increasing attention from health-care providers. This section describes the concept of preventive health care and the nurse's role in health promotion.

Development of Preventive Health Care

Prevention is not a new concept in nursing. Consider the words of Florence Nightingale to the nurses of 1859: "There are five essential points in securing the health of the house: (1) Pure Air, (2) Pure Water, (3) Efficient Drainage, (4) Cleanliness, (5) Light. Without these no house can be healthy. And it will be unhealthy just in proportion as they are deficit" (pp 14–15).

Nightingale's principles demonstrate an awareness of preventive health care in an era in which communicable diseases presented the most serious threat to health. A person who lived in the 1860s was fortunate to survive beyond the age of 40 and to escape the dread diseases of tuberculosis, cholera, and rheumatic fever.

Today, the factors that affect a person's health are often related to life style, environment, and psychosocial response to stressors. The leading causes of death have shifted from communicable diseases to conditions stemming from a complex interaction of heredity, environment, and personal health behavior. Death occurs for many persons who might have lived longer had they altered those behavior patterns that compromised their health. In addition, many persons are living restricted lives that are due to preventable conditions. The person with debilitating emphysema who continues to smoke, the child who develops polio because of a failure to be immunized, and the mother who delivers a low–birth weight infant because of poor nutrition during pregnancy are examples of persons whose quality of life has been impaired by failure to engage in preventive health care.

Society pays a price when preventive health care is not practiced. Increased technology, inappropriate utilization of hospitals, and the increasing complexity of health-care systems contribute to spiraling health-care costs. As the price of illness care climbs, interest in preventive health care increases. Nurses, physicians, and other health professionals are being challenged to collaborate with consumers to develop health promotion plans that focus on maximizing persons' strengths and modifying stressors before irreversible illness occurs.

Levels of Preventive Health Care

The concept of preventive health care can be applied at three levels: primary, secondary, and tertiary.

In primary preventive health care, the nurse intervenes with persons who have no symptoms at the time of the intervention but who are at risk for developing behaviors that could decrease their health. Exploring the implications of smoking with an adolescent who does not yet smoke, teaching the components of good nutrition to a 10-year-old child, and advocating the use of seat belts are examples of primary preventive health care.

In secondary preventive health care, the nurse identifies those risk factors in a person's life style that affect physical or mental health. The nurse explores the significance of these factors with the person and assists the individual to minimize these risks through education, counseling, and treatment. Assisting a new mother to adapt her life style to the birth of her daughter, weighing and measuring a premature infant, and examining and protecting the bony prominences of a person confined to bed to avoid skin breakdown are examples of secondary preventive health care. In these instances, the conditions are ripe for the activation of stressors, but the nurse and client attempt to identify and eliminate those factors that contribute to the potential for physical or mental illness.

Tertiary preventive health care focuses on persons who have encountered significant stressors that have already compromised their health. Here the nurse's role is to facilitate an adaptive response to this stressor. Tertiary preventive health care emphasizes use of the person's coping mechanisms. This process is closely linked to rehabilitation. A nurse who facilitates the grieving process in a severely depressed widow or teaches range of motion exercises to the person who has experienced a stroke is providing tertiary preventive health care.

Consider the following example, which exemplifies how nurses can integrate all three types of health care into their practice.

Sharon Richards is a staff nurse in a hypertensive clinic at a rural community hospital. She is often asked to speak to community groups about the causes and risk factors that contribute to hypertension. As she provides this service, she is practicing primary preventive health care. She is interacting with a population that is assumed to be healthy and that hopes to maintain good health.

One day a month, the clinic offers a hypertension screening program. During the screening clinic, Sharon Richards takes blood pressures, evaluates risk factors, counsels persons about their life styles, and refers persons with high blood pressure to the hypertension treatment clinic. At this time, she is practicing secondary preventive health care.

In the hypertension treatment clinic, Sharon works with clients who have active disease. She teaches them about diet, medications, and exercise. She counsels and assists them in adapting their life styles to reduce factors that contribute to the progression of hypertension. Disease may have caused irreversible damage in these clients; however, Sharon supports them in developing health behaviors that will minimize the effects of disease and reverse or impede the illness process. In this way, she is practicing tertiary preventive health care.

As a nurse, your role may focus on one of the levels of preventive health care, but in all likelihood, you will be involved in every level. You might work with a single client at all three levels — for example, you might teach a young woman how to do self breast examinations (primary) and help her to develop coping mechanisms to deal with the stress of impending motherhood (secondary). This client might also have a history of urinary tract infections for which you have developed a plan of care together (tertiary).

Preventive Health Care Throughout the Life Span

The preceding discussion illustrates that consumers are entitled to an evaluation of their risk factors and preventive health-care practices. Recall Table 7–3, which shows that there are specific health problems for specific age groups. Nurses can assist persons of all ages to identify the common stressors of their age group by using knowledge of growth and development. Many stressors are present throughout the entire life span because they affect basic needs such as good nutrition or a safe environment. Although a checklist approach to identifying stressors may be inadequate, knowledge of the individual's phase of development can assist nurses in planning preventive health care appropriately.

Nursing Implications for Preventive Health Behavior

The variables that affect a person's ability and willingness to adopt preventive health behaviors were described earlier in this chapter. One important way that nurses can advocate preventive health care is to help their clients explore their own health behavior. As clients become aware of their behavior, they can be guided to modify those factors they identify as stressors.

Various ways exist to assist clients to develop preventive health behaviors. Exploring the client's health values and beliefs can help develop positive attitudes toward health, while health counseling enables clients to identify the existence of any risk factors for certain health problems and to develop strategies for maintaining health. Some individuals become so anxious and immobilized by fear of disease that they delay preventive health care action. By exploring such fears, nurses can help these persons reduce their anxiety to a level that will enable them to seek health care.

When persons believe that the positive value of seeking health care outweighs the barriers, they will be more likely to take action. Finally, teaching is an important nursing action that assists clients in developing programs for wellness. Health education that actively involves the client has been shown to have a positive effect on willingness and ability to practice preventive health care. It often provides an impetus for health action. For instance, telling a person to relax and avoid stress will have little meaning if his or her self-esteem is built around achievement at work. Specific information on how to incorporate techniques of relaxation into such an individual's life style will be more useful in helping him or her to decrease stress. The processes of teaching and learning are described further in Chapter 10.

To develop strategies for preventive health care, nurses must synthesize knowledge and concepts from all areas of their education and experience. Interviewing and physical examination skills increase nurses' abilities to help clients examine their own risk factors. Knowledge of the principles of adaptation provides an insight for supporting clients to make changes in behavior that interferes with good health. The focus of preventive health behavior is assisting persons to identify and maximize their strengths. Building on strengths and facilitating preventive health behavior at primary, secondary, and tertiary levels are central to establishing a plan for health maintenance for consumers.

CONCLUSION

The current approach to health-care delivery is complex, unsystematic, and often described as being in a state of crisis. Historical influences shaped the system, making it illness-oriented, industrial in nature, and extremely costly. Financing health care involves funding both the agencies and the private and government insurance plans to pay for the health-care services persons need. Americans are basically healthy people, and the leading health problems in various groups are well known. Americans recognize, however, that health-care delivery in the future may require both a different focus and different management strategies to maintain and increase the nation's health. These changes seem likely because of both cost factors and consumer complaints about a health-care delivery system that dehumanizes the individual person.

Nurses work with many persons who have difficulty taking preventive health-care action. Nurses need to determine which factors that are known to delay action may be relevant for particular clients, while clients, as consumers of health care, with the help of their nurses, can learn to make appropriate decisions on how to take care of themselves.

STUDY QUESTIONS

1 Consider a health-care agency with which you are familiar (i.e., hospital unit, pharmacy, doctor's office crisis center).
    a Identify the professionals and nonprofessionals in the agency. Consider how geographically accessible it is to a broad spectrum of people.
    b Identify the philosophy and standards of care in the agency.
    c Identify the larger system of which it is a subsystem.

2   Considering the problems of health and health-care delivery, suggest some ways nursing could advance health in the United States.

3   Examine the ideas behind national health insurance and health maintenance organizations. Describe how these two concepts might work together toward a health-care delivery system for all Americans.

4   Assess and describe the biological, psychological, and sociocultural variables that influence your personal health behavior.

| REFERENCES

American Hospital Association: Patient's Bill of Rights. Chicago, American Hospital Association, 1972

Brewer K: Inclusion of nursing services vital to any national health insurance programs, p 31. Am Nurs Jan 20, 1979

Cook FJ: Julia's Story. New York, Kangaroo Book Publishers, 1977

Department of Health, Education and Welfare (DHEW): Healthy People: The Surgeon General's Report on Health Promotion and Disease Prevention. Washington, DC, Office of the Assistant Secretary for Health, 1979

Department of Health and Human Services: Your Medicare Handbook, p 4. Baltimore, Health Care Financing Administration. Pub. No. HCFA-10050, 1987

Donley R: Will we allow candidates to dodge the NHI issues? Am Nurse 11(4): 1979

Dougherty CJ: American Health Care: Realities, Rights, and Reforms. New York, Oxford University Press, 1988

Fagin C: Nursing as an alternative to high-cost care. Am J Nurs 82:56–60, 1982

Georgopoulus BS, Mann FC: The Community General Hospital. New York, Macmillan, 1962.

Joel LA: Reshaping Nursing Practice. Am J Nurs 87:793–795, 1987

Lear MW: Heartsounds. New York, Simon & Schuster, 1980

Mauksch IG: On national health insurance. Am J Nurs 78(8):1323–1327, 1978

McGee E: The national health insurance maze. Imprint 27(36):37–107, 1980

Nader R: Unsafe at Any Speed. New York, Grossman Publishers, 1965

National Center for Health Statistics: Health, United States, 1987. Hyattsville, MD, Department of Health and Human Services. Pub. No. (Public Health Service) 88-1232, 1988

Nightingale F: Notes on Nursing: What It Is and What It Is Not, 1st ed. London, Harrison, 1859. Facsimile edition: Philadelphia, JB Lippincott, 1966.

Office of Disease Prevention and Health Promotion: Disease prevention/health promotion: The facts. United States Public Health Service, United States Department of Health and Human Services. Palo Alto, CA, Bull Publishing Co., 1988

United States Department of Health and Human Services, Public Health Service, Health Resources Administration, Bureau of Health Professions: Sixth Report to the President and Congress on the Status of Health Personnel in the United States. Pub. HRS-0D-81-1. Rockville, MD, 1988

8 | THE NURSING PROCESS

KEY WORDS	After completing this chapter, students will be able to:
Aggregation **Analyzing** **Assessing** **Diagnosing** **Evaluation** **Goals** **Implementing** **Nursing diagnosis** **Nursing process** **Planning** **Problem** **Standard** **Strength**	**State the purpose of the nursing process.** **Describe how the nursing process has developed over time as the problem-solving process of nursing science.** **Describe how the nurse collects data about the person to individualize care.** **Describe how the nurse plans and implements individualized nursing care.** **Discuss how evaluation and revision enhance the nursing process and improve nursing care.**

The nursing process provides a way to identify the health, strengths, and needs of clients. This problem-solving process emphasizes the responses of persons to various situations and experiences, thus offering a means to plan effective and individualized nursing care. After years of development and testing, the nursing process has become the framework of professional nursing practice. Its importance is reflected in the Standards of Nursing Practice — developed by the ANA — which incorporate the phases of the nursing process. The nursing behaviors that are tested on the licensing examination for registered nurses are grouped under the five parts or phases of the nursing process.

BEFORE THE NURSING PROCESS

Historically, nursing focused more on health problems or specific disease conditions than on persons receiving care. Often, nursing care was based on the intuition of individual nurses or on orders written by physicians. Such care suggested that nurses were extensions of physicians rather than health professionals providing a different service called nursing. As the knowledge base of nursing expanded, it became clear that this approach to planning care did not view persons as holistic beings with unique strengths and needs. Schedules of activities or procedures, so common to this traditional method of planning care, omitted the purpose of nursing: caring. As nursing developed into both a science and an art, the problem-solving method of science — that is, the scientific method — was adopted as a systematic approach to nursing practice.

The Nursing Process Defined

The **nursing process** is a series of scientific steps that assist the nurse in using theoretical knowledge to diagnose strengths and nursing care needs of persons and to implement therapeutic actions for the purpose of attaining, maintaining, and promoting optimal biopsychosocial functioning.

The nursing process proceeds logically through this series of scientific steps or phases from data collection to evaluation of care. Most nurse scholars suggest that five distinct phases — assessing, diagnosing, planning, implementing, and evaluating — compose the nursing process. Additionally, diagnosing and the actual nursing diagnosis component of this phase are discussed extensively because of current national focus on these areas. Figure 8–1 depicts the sequence of phases in the nursing process.

Phases

The first phase in the nursing process, **assessing**, consists of collecting information, data, or facts about the person so that the nurse may better understand the individual's feelings, ideas, values, and biophysical responses. With this information, the nurse and the client work together to identify the client's strengths and needs and to develop an effective nursing care plan.

The second phase in the nursing process is **diagnosing**. **Nursing diagnoses** generated during this phase represent conclusions drawn by the nurse and the person from data collected and analyzed. Thus, analyzing follows assessing and precedes the actual care planning. And, nursing diagnoses, the outcome of analysis, summarize the client's strengths and needs within those specific functional areas for which nurses are qualified and licensed to provide support and care.

The third phase in the nursing process is **planning**. Here, the nurse and client plan achievable outcomes and actions that both will take. The client participates in this step as he or she is able and is assisted by the nurse as needed.

The fourth phase in the nursing process, **implementing**, is the activation of the care plan. The nurse and the client work to achieve mutually planned objectives using actual nursing interventions.

The fifth phase in the nursing process, **evaluating**, is the act of determining the client's progress toward outcomes planned in the third step. As before, the nurse and the client evaluate and revise the plan as needed to make continued progress toward the goals or to maintain identified strengths.

Aggregation: A Basis for Theory Development

The scientific steps as summarized above form the accepted standard for basic professional care by aspiring nurses and mature professionals. Guides for particular components of the process (e.g., assessment guides and standard diagnoses) evolved as nurses collectively gained experience in its use. As individual nurses progress from novice to expert status, the additional potential of such a scientific approach becomes apparent. For example, as nurses

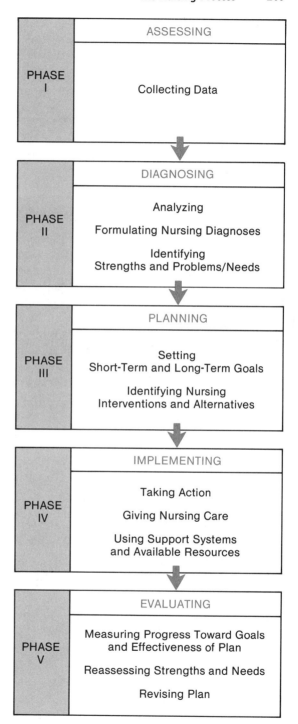

Figure 8–1 Five phases of nursing process.

mature from novice to expert status, they accumulate a wealth of experience while caring for many persons with similar needs, problems, and concerns (Benner, 1984). An extension of the nursing process which provides such an added potential is an activity called "aggregation." To aggregate is "to compile or gather together individual pieces of information" (Erickson and coworkers, 1983, p 252).

Although not usually identified as a phase in the nursing process, **aggregation** is defined as the process of collecting and summarizing many nursing interventions and their outcomes. Steps in aggregation follow:

1   Collect and summarize clinical interventions
2   Establish relationships
3   Synthesize nursing principles
4   Conduct nursing research
5   Develop nursing theory

From such summaries, nurses determine relationships among the outcomes to predict the most effective interventions for a given age, sex, culture, health concern, life style, and so forth. The idea of aggregation was first suggested by Swain (1973) and has since evolved as one method for developing a theory base for nursing practice.

Aggregation is a natural result of the many observations nurses make during the course of their practice, and it demonstrates how persons are unique yet similar. Based on this information, nurses can develop interventions that are useful for certain common needs, such as altered mobility, pain control, unmet basic needs, experiences of loss, or feelings of hopelessness. Interventions developed through aggregation can be researched in actual clinical practice. Informal hunches can be tried and formal hypotheses tested. It was from just such informal hunches that Dumas and Leonard's (1963) pioneering research arose concerning preoperative interventions to stem postoperative nausea and vomiting. Thus, aggregation — the process of synthesizing data collected from many persons — contributes to nursing principles, nursing theories, and general nursing knowledge. Ultimately, aggregation can expand the knowledge base of nursing and stimulate theory-based practice.

THE NURSING PROCESS AS A PROBLEM-SOLVING PROCESS

The nursing process can be compared to the problem-solving approach and the scientific method as shown in Table 8–1. All these processes follow a logical sequence of steps, beginning with the gathering of information and concluding with an evaluation of the outcome. Use of the scientific method is common to all professions but each profession alters the method to suit its particular focus. For example, two characteristics of the problem-solving method — interaction and a goal direction — are particularly well suited to the nursing process.

Interaction and Goal Direction

The interaction between client and nurse is the nursing profession's unique use of the scientific problem-solving process. The nursing process both guides nursing practice and is essential for effective, safe, quality care. Interaction is emphasized in the nursing process:

TABLE 8–1
COMPARISON OF NURSING PROCESS TO SCIENTIFIC METHOD AND PROBLEM-SOLVING METHOD

Scientific Method	Problem-Solving Method	Nursing Process
Define the problem.	Gather information in a situation.	Assess the situation, collect data.
Collect data from observation and experimentation.	Analyze information and identify the problem.	Make a nursing diagnosis after analyzing data
Devise and execute a solution.	Plan a course of action.	Plan care, set goals or expected outcomes, establish nursing interventions.
Evaluate the solution.	Carry out the plan.	
	Evaluate the plan and its outcomes.	Implement interventions.
		Evaluate and revise the process.

the nurse interacts while working *with* the client to set goals and devise a plan directed at the strengths and needs of the client. The patient is both the recipient of the nursing care and a participant in it. The goal direction is a process and an outcome of the interaction. Thus, the professional work of nursing is approached in a scientific manner, as suggested in the discussion of the criteria of a profession in Chapter 2.

The interactive component of the nursing process—listening, observing, and responding for a purpose—results in meaningful nursing care. Clients have described interacting with the nurse as helpful in identifying their health needs. Professional nurses have developed the knowledge and skill necessary for this helping role. Purposeful use of that knowledge and skill will help persons understand their needs, and identify and attain their goals. Gaining independence and self-awareness helps persons assume more control over their own care. Those who are more dependent and have complex needs may require more active involvement from the nurse. Achieving a balance between taking and returning control can be difficult for the nurse. However, it is the aim of nursing to promote self-care abilities through appropriate use of the nursing process. Nurse-client interaction is basic to the achievement of this end.

Now that the nursing process is the accepted professional practice method, nurses are becoming more sophisticated in its use. For example, initially, as the nursing process method came into vogue, most of the attention was focused on assessing—the data gathering phase. The pioneering McCain article (1965) reflects the era when general assessment skills predominated. Taking a history and performing a physical examination, much as a physician would do, received major emphasis. Gradually, however, assessment skills deepened and broadened to include psychosocial issues and data that would enhance nurses' diagnostic skills in specialty areas of nursing practice.

The creation of nursing diagnoses also signals increased sophistication in the use of the nursing process. The current emphasis on nursing diagnosis, including attempts to evolve standard nursing diagnoses, can be compared to nursing's earlier emphasis on assessment. The next developmental wave, the designation of interventions to be used with particular standard diagnoses, is beginning. Moreover, it is happening as nurses acknowledge the increasingly important aim of nursing research: to scientifically test nursing interventions in actual practice. Nursing's scientific development provides a legitimate scientific rationale for the care nurses give. This scientific development is also a necessary step toward aggregation, the important theory development phase that will expand the science of nursing.

The Nursing Process and Promotion of Self-Care

The nursing process as depicted here represents the client participating fully with the nurse in planning care. However, many variations exist in nurse-client approaches and responses. Ours, though perhaps an ideal, envisions persons as active participants and nurses as facilitators in the achievement of health promotion goals. In principle, this ideal is appropriate to all settings where professional nursing care is given and can be practiced even when nurses modify the process to meet certain reality situations. (Refer back to the discussion of self-care in Chapter 6.)

| STANDARDS OF NURSING PRACTICE

A **standard** is a specification set up and established by authority as a rule for the measure of quantity, weight, extent, value, or quality. A standard may be considered as a criterion on which individuals or actions are compared and judged. The practice of nursing involves various settings, specialty areas, and levels of care. Nursing practice also reflects varying individual perspectives (both nurse and client) regarding the process of effective care. Therefore, the use of standards for practice has become necessary for professional functioning. Standards provide a common base or unifying force in this diverse profession. In other words, although nurses may function in different ways, they still provide services from a shared understanding of the essence of nursing.

The ANA sets professional standards for the purpose of maintaining a high level of quality in the practice of nursing. Because there is a close relationship among the defining characteristics of nursing practice — that is, the development and application of theory through nursing action, the nursing process, and the standards of nursing practice — the standards are identified in this section. Students will note that the standards are stated with consideration for the phases of the nursing process as defined earlier in this section (Fig. 8 – 2).

| ASSESSING: COLLECTING DATA — PHASE I

The assessing phase of the nursing process consists of collecting data about the client. *Data* are information, facts, or findings that the nurse gathers to understand the person's feelings, ideas, values, and biophysical responses; these data are also used to identify the person's strengths and needs.

Purposes of Collecting Data

The nurse collects data during the assessing phase to obtain relevant information about the client's strengths and needs. The nurse uses these data to plan effective care collaboratively with clients, families, and other professionals. The collected data provide a basis for

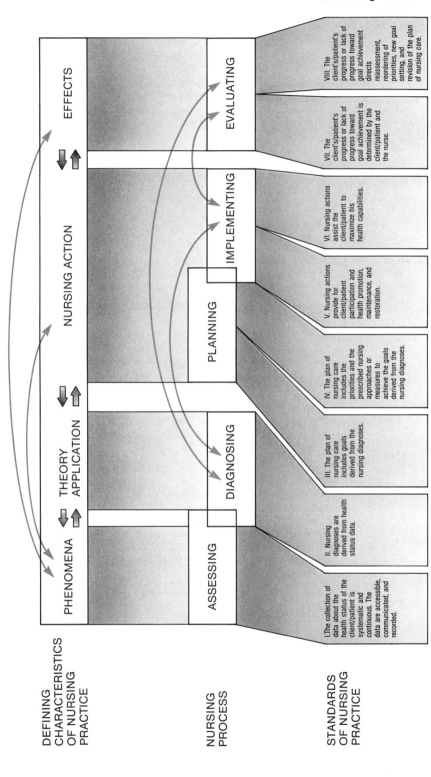

Figure 8–2 Defining characteristics of nursing practice: relationship to the nursing process and the standards of nursing practice.

expected outcomes and for planning interventions to maintain strengths or to cope with particular problems. Table 8–2 describes purposes for collecting data as discussed by nurse scholars. Additional important priorities of data collection include the following:

- The nurse communicates with the client rather than secondary or tertiary sources to gather a major portion of the data.
- Data collection includes information about both strengths and needs.
- Data collection includes the client's responses to current alterations, and to past biopsychosocial stressors that may have precipitated the current alteration.

TABLE 8–2
PURPOSES OF COLLECTING DATA

Nurse-Scholar	Quotation
Yura and Walsh	"The purpose of this phase [assessment] is to identify and obtain data about the client that will enable the nurse and/or client or his family to designate problems relating to wellness and illness" (1978a, p 95).
LaMonica	"Data collection is the continuous process of obtaining information needed in providing care" (1979, p 2).
Jones	"Assessment is defined as an interactive process through which the nurse gathers information about the client and the client's responses and interprets the information to derive an understanding of the level of wellness and the pattern and level of coping" (1980, p 196 of the Proceedings).
Marriner	"To deal with a problem one must first determine what the problem is. Therefore assessment is the first phase of the problem-solving process. It begins with the collection of patient data that have implications for nursing actions and ends with the nursing diagnosis, a statement of the patient's problems" (1983, p 27).
Carpenito	"The purpose of collecting data is to identify the client's: —Present and past health status —Present and past coping patterns (strengths and limitations) —Response to present alterations —Response to therapy (nursing and medical) —Risk for potential alteration developments. Nurses collect data to determine nurse activities and to assist other professionals (pharmacists, nutritionists, social workers, physicians) in determining their activities" (1987, p 5).
Erickson, Tomlin, and Swain	"—To develop an overview of the client's perspective —To develop an understanding of the client's personal orientation in terms of the client's expectations for the present and future —To determine the nature of the external support system —To determine the client's strengths and virtues —To determine the client's currently available internal resources —To determine the current developmental status in order to understand the client's model (view of the world) and to utilize maximum communication skills. The purpose for data collection within each of these major categories is to be able to interpret the data and specify nursing diagnoses" (1983, p 118).

Classifying Data

Data can be classified as subjective or objective. The literature describes these two types of data as follows:

- *Subjective data* (symptoms) represent the person's description of his or her strengths, needs, perceptions, feelings, and experiences, that is, data that cannot be seen or felt by the observer. Examples include the client's statements, "I feel warm," or "I am very tired."
- *Objective data* (signs) consist of information obtained from clinical observation, examination, and diagnostic studies. Examples include skin lesions, blood pressure readings, and swelling associated with a bone fracture.

Both types of data are essential for accurate data analysis. Although these definitions of subjective and objective data are generally accepted, some would suggest that they ought to be reversed in keeping with the emphasis on person. That is, the client's own observations may be more objective than those of the nurse (Finch DA: Personal communication, September, 1984). In research terminology, this would be using a phenomenological approach. The term suggests that it is the client's perceptions of or the meanings he attaches to his or her experience that provide the most objective data about the phenomenon.

Sources of Data

Data about a person can be obtained from primary, secondary, or tertiary sources:

- The *primary* source is the person himself.
- *Secondary* sources include the nurse's own observations, and data from family and friends.
- *Tertiary* sources are the person's record and other health-care providers such as other nurses, physicians, and dietitians.

When evaluating data sources, the nurse considers the person or client as the first point of observation, hence the word *primary*. When collecting data from one whose communication abilities are limited (e.g., from an infant, or a comatose or confused person), the primary source is obviously limited. Therefore, the nurse uses data from secondary and tertiary sources as well to develop a more complete understanding of the client.

Tools for Collecting Data

Several tools can be used for collecting data. These tools are helpful for the examination or testing of a phenomenon against established norms to make comparisons. Table 8–3 describes the most common tools. Figure 8–3 illustrates physical assessment tools.

The Environment for Collecting Data

Selecting a Time and Place

Data collection occurs whenever a person is under the care of an agency such as a hospital, clinic, or nursing organization. Peace, quiet, and privacy are essential elements of the environment in which nurses and their clients talk. Difficulty in finding this environment is a common frustration. In the home, family members, phone calls, and the television provide distraction. In health-care settings, interruptions occur frequently. In hospital ward settings,

TABLE 8–3
TOOLS FOR COLLECTING DATA

Assessment	Definition	Tools Needed	Examples
Observation	The art of seeing or sensing	Senses: sight, hearing, smell, touch, taste	Severe pallor Respiratory wheezing Cold, clammy skin Verbal and nonverbal behavior
Interview	A conference held in a face-to-face situation for the purpose of discussing and exploring a particular point	Conducive environment: comfortable, private Communication skills	Informal or unstructured —that is, when bathing client Formal or structured —that is, planned conference for initial assessment data
Listening	The act of purposefully attending in order to hear another person express his or her feelings, beliefs, strengths, and needs	All senses Conducive environment: comfortable, private Communication skills	Recognition of a person's underlying grief statement, "I don't really care."
Consultation	The use of additional resources to supplement data	Expert knowledge Literature Agency records Family, friends and others who know client Client	Read literature or speak with expert regarding a subject or technique Discuss with client, family how to arrange house for disabled person
Inspection	A close and purposeful observation involving the visual and auditory examination of a client to obtain qualitative and quantitative data	Vision, hearing Tools such as scale, otoscope, stethoscope, thermometer, etc. Standard charts for comparison	More focused than observation Color and integrity of skin Height and weight Blood pressure Body temperature, etc.
Palpation	The use of the hands or fingers to examine the external surface of the body to determine surface or underlying characteristics	Hands Senses: touch, vision	Location of pain, tenderness, hardness Degree of edema Location, rate, quality, and strength of peripheral pulses
Percussion	Light but sharp tapping on an area of the body to produce vibration, resonance, and pitch of sound or resistance	Hands Senses: touch, hearing Reflex hammer tool	Determine position, size, and density of the underlying structure Presence of fluid in a cavity —for example, normal: urine in bladder —for example, abnormal: fluid in the lungs Reflexes of the extremities

(Table 8–3 continued)

Assessment	Definition	Tools Needed	Examples
Auscultation	The act of listening with a stethoscope or other similar instrument for sounds in organs or body cavities	Stethoscope Doppler, ultrasonic probe Sphygmomanometer Fetoscope	Heart, lung, and bowel sounds: duration, frequency, relative intensity, quality of pitch as well as adventitious sounds, that is, rubbing, rumbling, gurgling Apical and brachial pulses Fetal heart tones

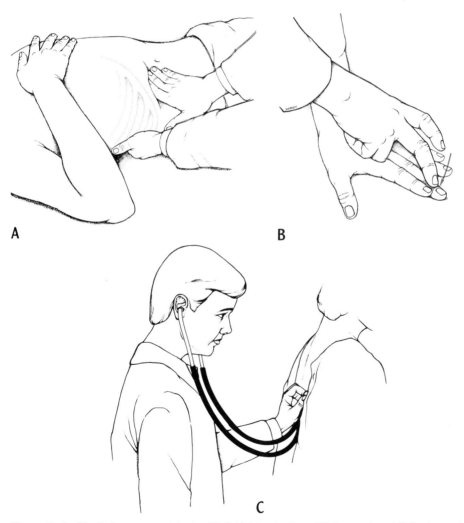

Figure 8–3. Physical assessment tools. (*A*) A Light palpation. (*B*) Percussion. (*C*) Stethoscopic examination.

others may hear the client's responses. Despite these difficulties, nurses usually create a comfortable atmosphere so that persons can share private thoughts and information.

Establishing Trust

In addition to having a peaceful, private environment, clients need a sense of trust in the interviewer. Trust is developed as people work together. The nurse can begin to build trust by establishing a harmonious atmosphere of honest acceptance and empathy. Table 8–4 outlines interventions that encourage the development of trust.

TABLE 8–4
INTERVENTIONS TO DEVELOP TRUST

Develop rapport:
- Demonstrate
  - Concern
  - Belief in the intrinsic value of the person
  - Unconditional acceptance of the person with his or her strengths and limitations
  - Empathy
  - Compassion

Develop trust:
- Demonstrate
  - Consistency in behaviors exhibited toward the person
  - Willingness to clarify communications
  - Genuine interest
  - Truthfulness
- Remember that trust is not spontaneous but must be earned:
  - Spend time with the person.
  - Use a relaxed and unhurried manner.
  - Visit when there is nothing specific to do.
  - Address the person by name.
  - Do not invade privacy; hesitate at the door; ask the person if he or she feels like talking; ask if you may sit down.
  - Do not interrupt.
- Do not issue direct commands, such as "you should."
- Ask for clarification of statements you do not understand.
- Let the person know you remember what he or she has told you on another occasion. For example, ask how the situation is now; say, "I remember when you told me. . . ."
- Communicate that you wish to understand what the client is experiencing.
- Offer touch; assess the person's comfort level with touch, and start slowly and gently.
- Move your body toward the person as he or she speaks.
- Allow the person to tell his or her complete story, even when it is uncomfortable for you, or explain your discomfort honestly and find someone else to listen.
- Inform the person early of your time limitations.
- Be reliable. It is all right to forget or change your plans, but be honest about what you did and why.
- Be consistent in behavior.
- Facilitate the person to regain control over his or her care and life.
- Help the person plan and carry out goals.

(Kennison B: Personal communication, January, 1980)

Issues of Confidentiality

During interactions with the nurse, clients often share personal information. The nurse must decide which data to report. The key is to protect the client from exposure and yet to provide enough data so that others may give consistent care. Nurses must decide whether information has been revealed to them in confidence or can be generally known. How one conveys data is often more important than the actual information given. Consider the following clinical example illustrating this point.

> One nursing instructor relates, "The students and I were listening to morning report. The night nurse, addressing the entire day staff, reported on a patient who had not slept. She then disclosed, in great detail, a disturbing incident about the woman's alcoholic son. Later I asked the students for their response to the nurse's report. They believed that the client had been exposed and the report had seemed like gossip. When I asked how data should be passed on so that relevant care could be given, the students came to the following conclusion: the nurse could have recorded some general statements and then talked privately to the day nurse. She might have explained the situation in some, but not total, detail. They reasoned that if the day nurse were aware of the problem, she could make herself available should the woman choose to talk. Furthermore, if this nurse approached the client with care, the woman would not feel that everyone knew her troubles. Many nurses find the confidential nature of client-nurse interactions to be both challenging and satisfying.

Approaches to Collecting Data

Frameworks

Several specific frameworks or guides have been created to help nurses collect and organize data. Tables 8–5 through 8–9 provide details of the following nurse scholars' frameworks:

- Faye Abdellah (1960), 21 nursing problems
- Faye McCain (1965), functional abilities or statuses
- Virginia Henderson (1966), activities of daily living
- Marjory Gordon, (1982), 11 functional health patterns
- Helen Yura and Mary Walsh (1978, 1982, 1983), human needs (Maslow adaptation)

Although these references are comparatively old, they are generally acknowledged as classics. Furthermore, they have withstood the test of time and present several enriching perspectives that contribute to a basic understanding of collecting data.

Although Abdellah referred to her framework as problems, and the others use more health-oriented titles, all of these frameworks emanate from a health perspective. Abdellah has developed her framework around nursing goals to be accomplished with each client. Henderson and McCain have both used a person-focused approach, that is, the areas for collecting data are suggested from the person or client's perspective. The word *status* — as used by McCain — means the person's condition, state, or situation and is used with a modifier, e.g., respiratory, circulatory, This notion suggests collecting data on the client's general state rather than on needs or strengths. Thus, the nurse uses an approach for collecting data that views the client as a holistic person with a variety of strengths and needs. Other writers use terminology similar to McCain's. Carnevali (1983) suggested "health status," which consists of three major components: normal biological development, the

TABLE 8–5
HENDERSON'S ACTIVITIES OF DAILY LIVING

1 Breathe normally

2 Eat and drink adequately

3 Eliminate by all avenues of elimination

4 Move and maintain a desirable posture (walking, sitting, lying, and changing from one position to another)

5 Sleep and rest

6 Select suitable clothing, dress and undress

7 Maintain body temperature within normal range by adjusting clothing and modifying the environment

8 Keep the body clean and well-groomed and protect the integument

9 Avoid dangers in the environment and avoid injuring others

10 Communicate with others in expressing emotional needs, fears, etc.

11 Worship according to faith

12 Work at something that provides a sense of accomplishment

13 Play or participate in various forms of recreation

14 Learn, discover, or satisfy the curiosity that leads to "normal" development and health

(Henderson V: The Nature of Nursing, pp 16–17. New York, Macmillan, 1966)

normal developmental tasks, and the pathology present. "Further, these components are viewed in terms of their interactive implications for Activities of Daily Living . . . (rather than as separate entities)" (Carnevali, 1983, p 16). Gordon's (1982) typology of functional health patterns provides groupings for the development of the nursing diagnoses currently accepted by the North American Nursing Diagnosis Association (NANDA).

Theoretical Perspectives

In addition to the frameworks mentioned above, nursing scholars have suggested theory bases from which nursing care may be practiced. Martha Rogers, Sister Callista Roy, Dorothea Orem, and Helen Erickson and colleagues provided varying theoretical perspectives for collecting/assessing data. These nursing theories have several concepts in common, namely, *nursing, person, environment,* and *health.* The various theoretical perspectives for collecting data differ, however, in their interpretation and application in clinical practice. These perspectives are mentioned here briefly; students are encouraged to consult the writings of these scholars for a more detailed discussion of their work.

Rogers.   Martha Rogers' science of unitary man suggested that nurses elicit data about factors affecting a person's ability to achieve maximum health potential. Rogers focused on the nature and direction of a person's development and continuous interaction with the environment. A nursing assessment from her perspective would emphasize data collection in the following areas (Rogers, 1970):

TABLE 8–6
ABDELLAH'S 21 PROBLEMS

1 To maintain good hygiene and physical comfort

2 To promote optimal activity; exercise, rest, and sleep

3 To promote safety through the prevention of accident, injury, or other trauma and through the prevention of the spread of infection

4 To maintain good body mechanics and prevent and correct deformities

5 To facilitate the maintenance of a supply of oxygen to all body cells

6 To facilitate the maintenance of nutrition of all body cells

7 To facilitate the maintenance of elimination

8 To facilitate the maintenance of fluid and electrolyte balance

9 To recognize the physiological responses of the body to disease conditions—pathological, physiological, and compensatory

10 To facilitate the maintenance of regulatory mechanisms and functions

11 To facilitate the maintenance of sensory function

12 To identify and accept positive and negative expressions, feelings, and reactions

13 To identify and accept the interrelatedness of emotions and organic illness

14 To facilitate the maintenance of effective verbal and nonverbal communication

15 To promote the development of productive interpersonal relationships

16 To facilitate progress toward achievement of personal spiritual goals

17 To create and/or maintain a therapeutic environment

18 To facilitate awareness of self as an individual with varying physical, emotional, and developmental needs

19 To accept the optimum possible goals in the light of physical and emotional limitations

20 To use community resources as an aid in resolving problems arising from illness

21 To understand the role of social problems as influencing factors in the cause of illness

(Abdellah FG, et al: Patient Centered Approaches to Nursing, pp 16–17. New York, Macmillan, 1960)

- Growth and development
- Life style
- Personal history
- Environment
(Rogers, 1970)

Roy. Sister Callista Roy viewed persons as biopsychosocial beings along a continuum of health-illness and uses an adaptation model to determine whether behavior is adaptive or maladaptive. Roy suggested that collecting data occurs in four adaptive modes which she defined as ways in which the person adapts:

- Physiologic needs—air, water, nutrition, rest, etc.
- Self-concept—how persons view themselves
- Role function—roles persons fulfill at home, at work, and in society
- Interdependence relations—support systems
(Roy, 1984, p 22)

TABLE 8–7
PERSON ASSESSMENT STATUS AND HUMAN NEEDS*

1 General appearance of client or family member

2 Sociocultural spiritual status

3 Life style status

4 Environmental status

5 Developmental task status

6 Psychological status—esteem needs

7 Rest and comfort status—needs for sleep and avoidance of pain

8 Mobility status—exercise and activity needs

9 Special senses status—stimulation and protection needs

10 Nutritional status and needs

11 Sexuality status and needs

12 Integumentary status—protection and hygiene needs

13 Fluid and electrolyte status—need for water and electrolyte balance

14 Circulatory status and needs

15 Temperature status and needs

16 Respiratory status—oxygen needs

17 Elimination status and needs

*Based on McCain's work.

TABLE 8–8
YURA AND WALSH: HUMAN NEEDS

Acceptance	Safety
Activity	Self-determination, self-control, and
Air	responsibility
Autonomous choice	Self-esteem
Effective perception	Sensory integrity
Fluids and electrolytes	Sexual integrity
Freedom from pain	Sleep
Interchange of gases	Spiritual integrity
Love	Stress management and adaptation
Nutrition	Tenderness
Rationality, conceptualization, and problem	Territoriality
solving	Wholesome body image

(Modified from Yura H, Walsh MB: Human Needs and the Nursing Process. New York, Appleton-Century-Crofts; 1978; Yura H, Walsh MB: Human Needs 2 and the Nursing Process. Norwalk, CT, Appleton-Century-Crofts, 1982; Yura H, Walsh MB: Human Needs 3 and the Nursing Process. Norwalk, CT, Appleton-Century-Crofts, 1983)

TABLE 8-9
GORDON'S TYPOLOGY OF 11 FUNCTIONAL HEALTH PATTERNS

1 *Health perception–health management pattern.* Describes client's perceived pattern of health and well-being and how health is managed

2 *Nutritional-metabolic pattern.* Describes pattern of food and fluid consumption relative to metabolic need and pattern indicators of local nutrient supply

3 *Elimination pattern.* Describes patterns of excretory function (bowel, bladder, and skin)

4 *Activity-exercise pattern.* Describes pattern of exercise, activity, leisure, and recreation

5 *Cognitive-perceptual pattern.* Describes sensory-perceptual and cognitive pattern

6 *Sleep-rest pattern.* Describes patterns of sleep, rest, and relaxation

7 *Self-perception–self-concept pattern.* Describes self-concept pattern and perceptions of self (e.g., body comfort, body image, feeling state)

8 *Role-relationship pattern.* Describes pattern of role-engagements and relationships

9 *Sexuality-reproductive pattern.* Describes client's patterns of satisfaction and dissatisfaction with sexuality pattern; describes reproductive patterns

10 *Coping–stress-tolerance pattern.* Describes general coping pattern and effectiveness of the pattern in terms of stress tolerance

11 *Value-belief pattern.* Describes patterns of values, beliefs (including spiritual), or goals that guide choices or decisions

(Gordon M: Nursing Diagnosis: Process and Application, p. 81. New York, McGraw-Hill, 1982)

Once data are collected in these modes, the nurse identifies various stimuli influencing the person's behavior:

- Focal—stimuli or stressors that are most immediate to the person and that precipitate the behavior
- Contextual—all other stimuli or stressors present that contribute to the behavior caused by the focal stimuli
- Residual—other relevant factors including beliefs, attitudes, traits, etc., that may be affecting behavior but whose effects are not validated (Roy, 1987, p 42)

The interrelationships among the three categories of stimuli result in the level of adaptation achieved by the person.

Orem. Dorothea Orem emphasized the person's *self-care ability* (or *self-care agency*), which she defined as the activities initiated and performed on one's own behalf in maintaining life, health, and well-being. In this self-care model, collecting data involves assessing six components of universal self-care:

- Maintenance of sufficient intake of air, water, and food.
- Provision of care associated with elimination processes and excrements.
- Maintenance of a balance between activity and rest.
- Maintenance of a balance between solitude and social interaction
- Prevention of hazards to life, functioning, and well-being
- Promotion of human functioning and development within social groups in accord with potential known limitations, and the desire to be normal (Orem, 1980, p 42)

In the process of collecting data, according to Orem, the nurse identifies whether the client is totally able, partially able, or totally unable to perform self-care actions in the above areas.

Erickson, Tomlin, and Swain.   Helen Erickson, Evelyn Tomlin, and Mary Ann Swain's theoretical perspective "Modeling and Role-Modeling" proposed that each person has a model of the world that is unique to him. This model grows out of all of his or her life experiences and is formed by his perceptions of life, events, people, and situations. Erickson and colleagues, believed that collecting data in the following categories will help nurses to understand more fully their clients' unique models of the world and thus to plan effective care:

- Description of the situation from the client's perspective including causes and how the nurse can help
- Expectations
- Resource potential
- Goals and life tasks
  (Erickson and colleagues, 1983, p 119).

Campbell and associates (1985) provided an assessment tool that suggests questions and observations useful for eliciting data in the categories developed by Erickson, Tomlin, and Swain. For example: How do you see your situation? What do you think caused your situation? What do you think will improve the situation?

The use of a theoretical perspective for assessing and planning care, as well as for theory-based practice in general, provides the following essential elements for nursing:

- A common language
- A purpose and rationale for care planned
- An approach for communication with other professionals
- A base for the development of research
- An increase in the body of knowledge
- Continued growth toward meeting the criteria for a profession
  (Chinn and Jacobs, 1987)

A General Approach

A person-centered approach is essential to this text's format for collecting data. Learning about the client's life experiences and understanding the client's particular view (model) of his or her life will provide a base for effective nursing care (Erickson and colleagues, 1983).

Choosing some general-purpose tool that facilitates the comprehensive, orderly collection of data is most important at this point. Regardless of the particular theoretical perspective used, common areas exist across which data may be collected. The data obtained can be analyzed to yield diagnoses that conform to the evolving diagnoses of NANDA. The work of this organization will be discussed in the diagnosis section of this chapter. The essential point is that collecting data, that is, assessing, is an ongoing process that takes place wherever and whenever it is needed. Consider the box for an example of data collection.

DATA COLLECTION FOR MRS. CARROLL

Physical Signs and Symptoms

72-year-old woman admitted in wheelchair for a mitral valve repair
Height, 5'11"; weight, 160 lb
Very pale complexion
Lungs clear on auscultation
Respirations regular and unlabored but audible
Dyspnea on exertion beyond dressing self and ambulating a few steps
Heart rate strong and regular
Skin clear and intact
Shoulders hunched
Sad affect
Speech slow and barely audible
States: "I can change my clothes, but it will take me a long time."
Sighs frequently

Mental and Emotional Concerns

NURSE: You do look very tired to me. Have you been unable to rest or sleep well lately?"
CLIENT: "I've stayed up all night crying this past week. I'm so afraid of this surgery."
NURSE: "Can you tell me more about your fears?"
CLIENT: "I'm afraid because I know they are going to put that tube down my throat during surgery. Then when they take it out they will rip my trachea and I'll die. That's what happened to my sister-in-law, right here in this hospital. My father died here, too, from cancer."
NURSE: "Have you discussed some of these worries with your family?"
CLIENT: "It has been 8 years since my husband died but I still miss him. My daughter and her family try to help, but I still feel as if there is no one to turn to."

| DIAGNOSING — PHASE II

Analyzing Data

Diagnosing is the second phase of the nursing process. This phase includes analyzing data, an important mental activity that follows collecting data. **Analyzing** is the cognitive (thinking) process where nurse and client form conclusions on which to base nursing care. Analyzing occurs whenever there are data, whether from a full assessment or a brief interaction. The focal points of the analysis are both the client's strengths and needs.

A classic and still helpful statement by Durand and Prince describes data analysis as the thought process leading to the recognition of a pattern that precedes the nursing diagnosis. They indicated that this thought process is influenced by scientific knowledge applicable to nursing, by a definition of nursing, and by past experiences that lead to the recognition of a pattern and thus the nursing diagnosis (Durand and Prince, 1966, p 55). LaMonica (1979) presented the data processing, or data analysis, segment of the nursing process as the bridge connecting rote nursing responsibilities with individualized client considerations (Fig. 8–4).

Carnevali suggested a strategy for analyzing data and thus developing nursing diag-

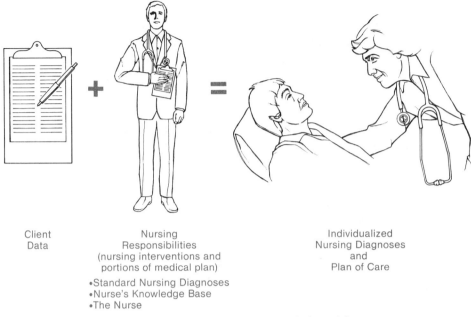

| Client Data | Nursing Responsibilities (nursing interventions and portions of medical plan) | Individualized Nursing Diagnoses and Plan of Care |

•Standard Nursing Diagnoses
•Nurse's Knowledge Base
•The Nurse

Figure 8–4   Lamonica's data analysis model.

noses. She stated: "the actual organization, storage, and creation of accessing pathways must be done by the individual clinician" (1983, p 38). Three basic activities are involved.

- Accumulating knowledge from reading, listening, observing, and analyzing experience
- Storing facts, cues, variations, contexts, and experiences in a purposeful and systematic way in one's long-term memory
- Engaging in ongoing critiqued clinical practice of using "accessing routes" to the stored knowledge . . . and testing the effectiveness of recognition features and treatment options
  (Carnevali, 1983, pp 38–39)

Thus, when analyzing data, the nurse compares facts gathered from the person with a number of accepted norms: anatomical, physiological, psychological, and developmental. At the same time, the nurse draws on accepted nursing knowledge and personal nursing experiences to recognize patterns in or relationships among the data. The conclusions drawn by the nurse are then discussed or checked with the client to determine their validity or soundness.

Analyzing data occurs in an ongoing way when working with a client. The nurse constantly considers, sifts, and sorts the facts presented. Often, conclusions are drawn quickly with little chance for discussion with the client or others. However, many interactions with a client may be required before the nurse has data suitable for planning comprehensive care. Frequently, during interactions between nurse and client, both form perceptions and begin analysis. In one research study, clients described the nurse's questions as helpful because in answering them, the client was able to do his own sorting, which assisted him in attaching more meaning to his experiences (Kennison, 1983). See Table 8–13, for details of the thinking process followed by the nurse in analyzing data and formulating nursing diagnoses for a specific client, Mrs. Carroll.

Nursing Diagnosis

Establishing a **nursing diagnosis** is the outcome of analyzing in the diagnosing phase. Diagnosing has long been considered the prerogative of the medical profession. Indeed, dictionaries frequently list the first definition of the term as the art or act of identifying a disease from its signs and symptoms. Nursing diagnoses, however, summarize the client's strengths and problems within those specific functional areas for which nurses are qualified and licensed to provide support or care. In differentiating the nursing diagnosis from other clinical problems—that is, medical problems—Carpenito suggested the following questions:

- Can the nurse identify the problem legally and educationally?
- Can the nurse legally order the necessary interventions to treat or prevent the problem?
- Can the nurse legally treat the problem?
  (1987, p 17)

Nursing diagnosis emphasizes the unique contribution nurses can make to the health of individuals and the community.

Definition of Nursing Diagnosis

Nursing diagnosis represents a nursing judgment drawn from data concerning client strengths and needs that guides decisions for care. The following are essential elements of the nursing diagnosis:

1 Represents a statement, judgment, or conclusion
2 Focuses on the person's responses (either strengths or problems)
3 Comes from and follows collecting data
4 Labels conclusions
5 Suggests interventions

Just as there are many tools for collecting data, there are numerous definitions of nursing diagnosis. See Table 8–10 for other definitions of nursing diagnosis.

Strengths.   The following definition of strengths describes this component of nursing diagnosis.

Strengths, also called *internal resources*, are biological, psychological, social, or spiritual qualities that contribute to a person's character, integrity, and uniqueness and that can be mobilized to cope with a problem or to attain a goal. Strengths are an inherent part of each individual, but may not be maintained or mobilized in an adaptive manner without nursing interventions.

Strengths represent inner health that promotes greater wellness. Strengths are important considerations when planning nursing care. See Table 8–11 for examples of strengths. Popkess-Vawter stated:

Without a strengths list, nursing care is planned in isolation; there is no recycling of patient energy back into his system to revitalize his recovery process. Without assessing

TABLE 8–10
DEFINITIONS OF NURSING DIAGNOSIS

Author	Definition
Mundinger and Jauron	"The statement of a patient's response which is actually or potentially unhealthful and which nursing intervention can help to change in the direction of health. It should also identify essential factors related to the unhealthful response" (1975, p 97).
Gordon	"Actual or potential health problems which nurses, by virtue of their education and experience, are capable and licensed to treat" (1976, p 1299).
Kim and Moritz	"The judgment or conclusion that occurs as a result of nursing assessment" (1982, p 107).
Marriner	"A statement of the patient's problems, including his strengths, limitations, and methods of adapting to that problem" (1979, p 2).
Thomas and Coombs	"A statement of a conclusion resulting from a recognition of a pattern derived from a nursing investigation of the patient" (1979, p 66).

TABLE 8–11
EXAMPLES OF STRENGTHS

Has resolved developmental tasks favorably:
    Trust versus mistrust
    Autonomy versus shame and doubt
    Initiative versus guilt, etc.
Meets own basic needs:
    Physiological
    Safety and security
    Love and belonging
    Esteem
    Growth
Values independence
Relates warmly with spouse, children, and others
Expresses spirituality and faith
Expresses a comfortable philosophy of life
Verbalizes knowledge about health problems
Displays a sense of humor
Uses pain control methods effectively
Displays unique talents and interests (music, art, languages, cooking, woodworking, needlework, gardening, extensive reading, athletic endeavors, etc.)
Demonstrates effective problem solving
Accepts help from the nurse and others
Gives and receives warmth, affection, friendship
Expresses readiness to learn about health concerns
Expresses readiness to start coping with health concerns
Has insight into personal situations and responses
Has progressed through stages of grief and loss appropriately
Sleeps well
Absorbs and digests food effectively
Maintains a stable blood pressure
Maintains effective breathing patterns
Moves about with ease
Maintains skin integrity

the patient's strengths, the nurse is second-guessing what would be a therapeutic approach to care for the patient's problems. (1984, p 435).

The client's *external resources* also assist the nurse when planning care and can be included in the individual client's diagnosis list because they provide important sources of support in coping with health problems. Consider the following categories:

- Support systems—family, friends, health-care professionals
- Financial resources—income, insurance
- Environmental resources—health care, recreation, shopping, transportation, education
- Education—level, training, and experience for an occupation

Problems and Needs.   Another element of nursing diagnosis is the problem and need category. **Problems** can be classified into three basic areas: actual problems, potential problems, and possible problems.

Actual problems or needs are those that can be identified from the current data. Some examples include the following:

- Decreased endurance
- Respiratory distress with minimal exertion
- Anxiety related to forthcoming surgery
- Chronic nausea

Potential problems or needs are those which the person is at high risk to develop, given his particular situation. Some examples include the following:

- Skin breakdown related to decreased mobility
- Increased respiratory secretions related to postoperative state,
- Diminished self-esteem related to alteration in usual functioning

Possible problems or needs are those for which the nurse has obtained enough data to suggest a hunch, but not enough to identify an actual problem. An example might be possible financial problems. The client may indicate that he is not worried about finances, yet the nurse notes that he wrings his hands when questions of finances arise.

Purposes of Nursing Diagnoses

In 1973, a group of nurses from the United States and Canada met to identify nursing functions and to establish a classification system of nursing diagnoses. These nurses represented all specialties and roles within the nursing profession. Foreseeing future needs, they envisioned a classification system suitable for the age of computerization. These and other nurses interested in nursing diagnoses have continued to meet at intervals to develop and establish the classification system further. The current list of accepted nursing diagnoses can be found in Table 8–12.

This international group, NANDA, has identified several purposes for the establishment of a classification system for nursing diagnoses:

- Identifying nursing's independent practice domain
- Providing a common reference system to assist in the growth in clinical knowledge through research
- Assisting computerization of the nursing process

TABLE 8-12
APPROVED NURSING DIAGNOSES
Nursing Diagnoses Accepted at the Fourth National Conference (1982)

Airway clearance, ineffective
Bowel elimination, alteration in: constipation
Bowel elimination, alteration in: diarrhea
Bowel elimination, alteration in: incontinence
Breathing pattern, ineffective
Cardiac output, alteration in: decreased
Comfort, alteration in: pain
Communication, impaired verbal
Coping, ineffective individual
Coping, ineffective family: compromised
Coping, ineffective family: disabling
Coping, family: potential for growth
Diversional activity, deficit
Fear
Fluid volume deficit, actual*
Fluid volume deficit, potential
Gas exchange, impaired
Grieving, anticipatory
Grieving, dysfunctional
Home maintenance management, impaired
Injury, potential for; poisoning, potential for; suffocation, potential for; trauma, potential for
Knowledge deficit (specify)
Mobility, impaired physical
Noncompliance (specify)
Nutrition, alteration in: less than body requirements
Nutrition, alteration in: more than body requirements
Nutrition, alteration in: potential for more than body requirements
Parenting, alteration in: actual
Parenting, alteration in: potential
Rape-trauma syndrome: rape trauma, compound reaction, silent reaction
Self-care deficit (specify level): feeding, bathing/hygiene, dressing/grooming, toileting
Self-concept, disturbance in: body image, self-esteem, role performance, personal identity
Sensory-perceptual alteration: visual, auditory, kinesthetic, gustatory, tactile, olfactory
Sexual dysfunction
Skin integrity, impairment of: actual
Skin integrity, impairment of: potential
Sleep pattern disturbance
Spiritual distress (distress of the human spirit)
Thought processes, alteration in
Tissue perfusion, alteration in: cerebral, cardiopulmonary, renal, gastrointestinal, peripheral
Urinary elimination, alteration in patterns
Violence, potential for

(Table 8-12 continued)

Nursing Diagnoses Accepted at the Fifth National Conference (1984)

Activity intolerance
Activity intolerance, potential
Anxiety
Family processes, alteration in
Fluid volume, alteration in: excess
Health maintenance alteration
Oral mucous membrane, alteration in
Powerlessness
Social isolation

---

*Two sets of defining characteristics with two etiologies for the same nursing diagnosis.
(Hurley ME [ed]: Classification of Nursing Diagnoses—Proceedings of the Sixth Conference, pp 513–514. St. Louis, CV Mosby 1986)

Other nurse-scholars concur and have given additional purposes such as the following:

- Meeting record keeping requirements
- Evaluating quality care
- Assessing charges for reimbursement

Given the number of definitions and purposes listed for nursing diagnosis, it is well to note the observation by Carnevali and associates: "Although several individuals and groups are in the process of developing classification systems of nursing diagnoses or problems, there is not yet widespread acceptance of a single approach, or an overall conceptual framework" (1984, p 101).

Let's consider writing nursing diagnoses or diagnostic statements in the form suggested by Gordon and Carpenito. As an illustration, consider the actual problems listed previously in an informal format:

- Decreased endurance
- Respiratory distress with minimal exertion
- Anxiety related to forthcoming surgery
- Chronic nausea

Now, using the more formal three-part wording, they are transformed to a format of

---

PROBLEM—related to—*ETIOLOGY*—manifested by—*SYMPTOM*

- **ACTIVITY INTOLERANCE related to ALTERATION IN OXYGEN TRANSPORT SYSTEM as manifested by DECREASED ENDURANCE and RESPIRATORY DISTRESS WITH MINIMAL EXERTION**

- **ANXIETY related to FORTHCOMING SURGERY as manifested by FEELINGS OF LOSING CONTROL**

- **COMFORT, ALTERED: NAUSEA related to STRESS as manifested by CLIENT COMPLAINS OF FEELING "SICK TO MY STOMACH"**

No one correct way exists to write such diagnoses. In part, the decision about how to write is based on the emphasis desired. For example, is nausea primarily a comfort problem or a long-standing manifestation of a nutrition problem? If the latter, the nursing diagnosis might have been written:

ALTERATION IN NUTRITION: LESS THAN BODY REQUIREMENTS
related to ANOREXIA as manifested by COMPLAINTS OF NAUSEA

Or, if the client can verbalize her concerns about surgery, the problem might be written:

FEAR related to FORTHCOMING SURGERY as manifested by patient statement,
"I KNOW I WON'T COME THROUGH THIS OPERATION."

When a standard diagnosis does not cover the specific situation, the nurse describes or creates a diagnosis as necessary to plan care and validates the statement with professional nurse colleagues.

Analyzing and Diagnosing: An Illustration

Analyzing and diagnosing have now been presented from several specific viewpoints. Using the analysis of data for the scenario with Mrs. Carroll (Table 8–13), nursing diagnoses can now be formulated for this client from a general person-centered approach. This approach incorporates the various theoretical frameworks introduced in the conceptual discussion of person in Chapter 4; however, the data presented are incomplete in the sense of a total person assessment. The facts, however, are considered accurate since the client's actual statements and the nurse's objective observations are provided. In addition, the nurse has validated some of her observations with the client through the questions she asked. In analyzing these data, the nurse notes that the client can communicate her fears and express at least some of her feelings. Mrs. Carroll can also perform certain activities of daily living, for example, changing her clothes. Using knowledge from physiology and pathophysiology, the nurse understands that the faulty mitral valve has compromised cardiac output and thus circulation throughout the body, which in turn contributes to the extreme fatigue. The nurse also recognizes from nursing theory and past experiences that fear and unresolved issues of loss and grief may contribute to fatigue. The Maslow, Erikson, and Piaget frameworks are helpful in understanding Mrs. Carroll's statements and her personal model of the world. The following list may be considered the nursing diagnoses or conclusions drawn from this data base. The first list uses the NANDA standardized diagnoses, and the second list individualizes or expands on these standard diagnoses, using the client's data base (Table 8–14).

Nursing diagnoses according to the NANDA list of standard nursing diagnoses are as follows:

- Activity intolerance
- Sleep pattern disturbance
- Dysfunctional grieving
- Anxiety, severe
- Thought processes, alteration in

Nursing diagnoses expanded according to individualized data set are as follows:

Strengths

- Able to express feelings
- Can establish rapport with a helpful person (nurse)

TABLE 8–13
ANALYZING DATA FOR SCENARIO WITH MRS. CARROLL

Summary of Nurse's Observation	Rationale
Communicates readily with the nurse and talks about feelings and experiences Can take care of self and activities of daily living Lungs clear on auscultation Breathing unlabored with limited exertion Heart rate strong Skin clear and intact	Strengths identified using both psychosocial and physical data (nurse's observations, past experiences, anatomy and physiology sources)
Demonstrates feelings of extreme fatigue, fear, grief, and abandonment.	Affect; slow, quiet speech; statement that she has no one to turn to (Engel's theory of grief and loss, Piaget's theory on object permanence.)

Demonstrates unmet needs in following areas:
  Physiological
  Safety and security
  Love and belonging
  Esteem
	Rest, sleep, cardiac output, circulation
	  Statements about what will happen to her
	  Statements that she misses husband and has no one to turn to
	  Statements suggest that she does not feel in control but that others will cause things to happen (Maslow's basic needs theory)

Distrustful of care-givers	Statements about what will happen to her during and after surgery (Erikson's psychosocial development theory)
Perceives little control over destiny	Statements regarding what others will do to her (Maslow and Erikson)
Unsure of boundaries between self and sister-in-law, self and father	Comments suggest that it happened to them so it will happen to me (Piaget's cognitive development theory—preoperational thinking)

TABLE 8–14
EXAMPLES OF STRENGTHS DERIVED FROM NORTH AMERICAN NURSING DIAGNOSIS
ASSOCIATION (NANDA) LIST

Accepted Diagnoses	Strengths
Breathing pattern, ineffective	Breathing pattern, effective
Communication, impaired verbal	Communication, effective
Contractures, potential joint	Joint motion, full range
Fluid volume deficit	Hydration, adequate
Grieving, dysfunctional	Grieving, appropriate
Powerlessness	Control, ability to maintain
Skin integrity, impaired	Skin integrity, maintained
Sleep pattern disturbance	Sleep pattern, restful

- Self-care asset: can dress self
  Problems
- Activity intolerance related to
  - decreased cardiac output and decreased circulation
  - feelings of fear, abandonment, grief
- Sleep pattern disturbance, insomnia related to fear of surgery
- Grieving, unresolved issues related to death of husband, father, sister-in-law
- Deficit in ability to meet basic needs
  - physiological
  - safety and security
  - love and belonging
  - esteem
  - growth (Maslow)
- Unresolved issues of
  - trust versus mistrust
  - autonomy versus shame and doubt
    (Erikson)
- Preoperational thinking mode related to death of father, sister-in-law (Piaget)

Note that the nurse has identified both strengths and problems derived from the available data. In this way, he or she can use the strengths to assist with problem solving. For example, Mrs. Carroll can express her fears and concerns. Therefore, the nurse knows that listening carefully and providing time for verbalization will help the client begin to work through her feelings. Mrs. Carroll's exhaustion does not prevent her from being somewhat independent. This fact indicates that the nurse can support Mrs. Carroll's independence and help the client maintain the abilities she still has. Further data collection will help the nurse determine how to promote the client's independence optimally.

If this process seems confusing, remember that nursing students have many opportunities for clinical practice under the guiding assistance of a clinical instructor.

Establishing Priorities
Among Nursing Diagnoses

After determining the nursing diagnoses, the nurse will rank them in a particular order to plan the most effective approach for the delivery of nursing care. When establishing priorities, the nurse considers the following questions:

- What strengths does the person have and how can they best be used?
- Are there acute or life-threatening problems?
- What is the client's stated most pressing concern?
- Which problems, not acute or pressing, does the client prefer to work on first?
- Which problems can the client work on by himself, and with which ones will he need nursing assistance?
- Which strengths can the client mobilize at the present time to facilitate his problem solving?
- Are there several problems that are acute or pressing, and if so, how can the approach to care accommodate the client's needs in several areas?

The nurse will often note that a client has many pressing needs that cannot be met at once. When this occurs, it is best to consider urgent safety issues and then comfort. Returning to the client and determining with him or her how to order nursing care uses both the client's model of the world and his or her strengths. Usually when life-threatening problems are involved, several persons are available to assist. In this way, emergency needs can be attended to by some personnel while others consider safety, security, and comfort needs. Maslow's hierarchy of basic needs may be helpful if used with the client to explore his or her needs. If the client is not conscious or is otherwise unable to make his or her needs known, the nurse reviews the physiological needs using a head-to-toe assessment process. At the same time, the nurse attends to psychological needs by talking to the person and providing comfort. During this time, it is useful and comforting to remind the client of strengths as the nurse has identified them, for example, strong heart rate, regular breathing, responses to care. Additionally, secondary and tertiary data sources are consulted as necessary. The nurse attempts to determine this particular person's perspective, as well as interventions that have been helpful in the past.

When writing a list of the person's nursing diagnoses, strengths are often listed first so that the nurse and the client are clearly aware of them. Strengths, as an integral part of the person's holism, are used to assist him generally. Strengths may be correlated with specific problems, however, if suitable.

Guidelines for Using Standardized Lists of Nursing Diagnoses

The standardization of nursing diagnosis has provided a way for the nursing profession to define and articulate practice. As this development continues, several nurse-scholars caution us to use this standardization format with care (see below).

It will become more holistic when clinicians from a wide variety of settings contribute diagnostic categories that include health behaviors, health assessments, and outcome criteria for self-care and optimum health. (Donnelly and Sutterley, 1984, p vi)

These general headings have their uses in each discipline, but that use may not be one that serves as a basis for individualized treatment. . . . General labels for categories of diagnoses have their place in nursing. They should not, however, be misused by substituting them for more specific working diagnoses that individualize care. (Carnevali 1983, p 165)

The current nursing diagnosis labels are the working papers of the profession. . . . From a professional perspective, the efforts being made not to limit the labels or systems prematurely are to be commended. (Westfall, 1984, p 87)

It is therefore inappropriate to be constrained by a predigested set of labels into which one must force bits of information. Rather, it is incumbent upon us to describe carefully and thoughtfully and fully the phenomena we see." (Shamansky and Yanni, 1983, p 48)

First, what are the dangers of packaged categories, that is, diagnoses that may simplify and even obliterate the client's experience? Second, what are the implications of prefabricated lists of labels for power relations between clients and professionals involved in health services? . . . . believe them [labels] to be prone to stereotyping. They are, after all, mere labels to be imposed on any situation or person. (Hagey and McDonough, 1984, p 151)

Donnelly and Sutterley (1984) shared their concern for the nature of present diagnoses' focus on disease and pathology. Additionally, we make the following suggestions:

1 Develop nursing diagnoses from a theoretical foundation rather than disease or pathology.
2 Develop a format for describing the phenomenon observed in the individual client's data base including both strengths and problems (e.g., maintains a stable blood pressure, unresolved trust versus mistrust).
3 Avoid using the standardized nursing diagnoses as labels or value judgments and develop a procedure for describing the individual client's perspective and experiences.

Nurses are encouraged to expand on or enlarge the standard diagnoses to describe the individual person's response and to develop new diagnoses as a situation warrants. Although a standard diagnosis assists the nurse by providing a general category, it should be made specific enough to give others an understanding of the problem. For example, "noncompliance" is a standard diagnosis used in instances where the client does not follow his medical or nursing care plan. This diagnosis provides us with the concern. However, the nurse also explores — with the client — why the plans are not relevant or useful to him or her. Nursing care can then be developed to deal with the client's perceived needs, changing the diagnosis and the nursing care as persons and their responses change.

Currently, nurse scholars are working to further classify standard diagnoses by developing a list of defining characteristics for each diagnosis. For example, the NANDA diagnosis of "Comfort, alteration in: pain," according to Gordon, includes the following defining characteristics:

- "Communication (verbal or coded) of pain description
- Narrowed focus (altered time perception, withdrawal from social contact, impaired thought process)
- Distraction behavior (moaning, crying, pacing, seeking out other people/or activities, restless)
- Facial mask of pain (eyes lack luster, "beaten look," fixed or scattered movement, grimace)
- Alteration in muscle tone (may span from listless to rigid)
- Physiological responses (excessive perspiration, blood pressure and pulse rate change, pupillary dilatation, increased or decreased respiratory rate)" (1985, p 150)

Panels of nurses with defined expert knowledge are polled to determine if, in their judgment, certain defining characteristics are generally present with a given diagnosis. This process will further clarify the actual diagnosis and, when used with an individual client's experience and perspective, can provide a basis for planning nursing care.

Legal Implications of Nursing Diagnoses

When nurses collect and analyze data and develop nursing diagnoses, they have a professional obligation to communicate and record these items; moreover, it is expected that the professional nurse will develop and implement a care plan relative to the diagnoses. Accurate record keeping that reflects the plan for nursing care and the person's response to the plan is essential. Documentation on the legal record, that is, the client's agency chart, is required for several reasons that will be discussed later in Chapter 11. However, one important reason for documentation is to have available, in the event of legal questions or litigation, an account of the person's care while associated with a particular agency.

Bernzweig's definition of nursing diagnosis leads the nurse to consider legal issues as well as holistic care: "A nursing diagnosis is one which involves the evaluation of all physical, mental, sociological, and economic factors which have an influence on the patient's recovery" (1981, p 121). This definition suggests that nursing must consider all aspects of the person to provide safe care.

Client Participation in Establishing a Nursing Diagnosis

A major challenge for nurses is determining how best to facilitate the client who disagrees with the nurse regarding a nursing diagnosis. Consider the following situation.

> On the basis of physiological principles and nursing knowledge, the nurse knows that ambulation (walking) following surgery facilitates the return to former functioning. Moreover, the nurse can identify problems that may occur if a regular ambulation regimen is not followed. However, because of postoperative fatigue and pain, the client may prefer to rest rather than ambulate.

Standards of care developed through research indicate that nurses would be negligent if they did not intervene at this point. The client's participation can usually be gained if the nurse first addresses his concerns and finds mechanisms to help him cope. For example, establishing a pain management plan and regular rest periods may help relieve pain and fatigue. This relief facilitates ambulation, a necessary part of postoperative care. The person who is still unable to become involved in his or her own care may be expressing a deeper unmet need, about which more data must be collected.

Respecting a person's right to ignore or deny an obvious health problem is difficult, particularly if doing so has serious implications. If nurses assess the meaning behind the avoidance behavior and consider the person's perception of his real need, they are more likely to intervene effectively. For another example, imagine a man who has high blood pressure and may not take his medications as prescribed. The nurse might identify the problem as noncompliance with the health-care regimen. The person, however, may feel that the pills cause unpleasant side effects, or that he cannot remember to take them. The nurse who respects the person's right to make decisions about his or her health care will spend time talking with the client and concentrating on the individual's perception of the situation. For instance, the client may tell the nurse that his or her family is struggling with complex problems. Working to solve some of these problems may seem more relevant to the person than trying to cope with the nurse's main concern. If the person is assisted to improve his or her family relationships, the person may decide to take the medication as scheduled. Moreover, if the person is happier in his or her family life, the client's high blood pressure may return to a more normal level.

Nursing Diagnosis Versus Collaborative Problems

The discussion of nursing as a science and a profession described nursing as having independent, interdependent, and dependent functions. The discussion of nursing diagnosis has focused primarily on those problems that are within the domain of nursing's independent function. In other words, these are problems for which nurses can legally determine the actions to avert, solve, or relieve the problems.

Nursing as a science and profession also is primarily concerned with persons' health generally and clients' specific responses to their particular health problems. However, many of nursing's clients also have diagnosed medical problems (disease); in addition, these same clients have a likelihood of developing difficulties or potential complications related to their disease or medical or surgical interventions used to treat the disease. Other clients are at risk for developing medical complications from diagnostic tests, whether they have actual disease or not. These actual or potential problems which are outside the realm of nursing's independent function are designated *collaborative problems*. Carpenito (1987) defines collaborative problems as, "The physiological complications that have resulted or may result from patho-physiological and treatment-related situations. Nurses monitor to detect their onset/status and collaborate with medicine for definitive treatment" (p 24).

Collaborative problems require nurses to collaborate with other health professionals for their resolution. This collaboration usually involves physicians but may involve health professionals other than physicians. For example, nutritionists, physical therapists, and dentists may be some of the professionals with whom nurses collaborate. This collaboration often involves nurses' interdependent and dependent functions. However, just as the greater part of professional nursing's functioning should be independent, the greater share of professional nurses' activities should be focused on resolving problems for which nursing has prime responsibility.

For example, Mr. Jones, age 75, is at high risk for increased respiratory secretions related to his recent surgery done under general anesthesia. The nurse may initiate teaching and positioning as well as coughing and deep breathing to assist the client's return to health. If, however, Mr. Jones develops pneumonia, a medical postoperative complication of

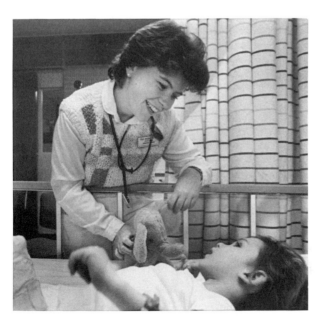

The recipient of the nursing process is the person, whatever his or her age or health status.

surgery, the nurse, and the physician will work together to solve the resulting collaborative problem of respiratory insufficiency. The physician may prescribe antibiotics and oxygen as specific medical treatments. The usual supportive care of the nurse, that is, positioning, coughing, and deep breathing may be supplemented by additional nursing measures to conserve energy and maintain comfort. The nurse will also continue to perform the monitoring interventions that are within nursing's independent functioning and will administer the prescribed medication, a dependent nursing function.

As a postscript to our discussion of nursing diagnoses versus collaborative problems, another point should be clarified. In its most general meaning, the word *collaborate* denotes working together. Because health care encompasses the care by nurses, physicians, and other health professionals (e.g., dentists, social workers), all professional health care workers "collaborate" in the general sense of the word. They do this to provide a broad spectrum of efficient and effective care for their clients even when they are functioning in their independent professional practice modes.

| PLANNING—PHASE III

The third phase in the nursing process is planning. As this discussion begins, consider some general notions about the nursing process. The assessing, analyzing, and diagnosing aspects, as described earlier, may sound laborious. In actuality, nurses perform and record a fairly complete assessment and care plan when the client enters an agency. In most instances, however, they perform the nursing process briefly. For example, while listening to the client, the nurse is assessing, analyzing, and diagnosing. Likewise, planning, implementing, and evaluating may take only moments. This approach to the nursing process occurs many times through the course of providing care to a client. Often, the data and care plan are not written down immediately. Although certain aspects are recorded later, even these will be a synopsis of the actual interaction. Thus, and most importantly, the nursing process becomes primarily a way of thinking.

Planning, implementing, and evaluating are sometimes grouped together as the therapeutic or action portion of the nursing process. To begin with, one aspect of planning is projecting the realization of achievement. Together, the nurse and the client identify outcomes that are reasonable and relevant, choose among alternative interventions, and implement the plan.

Iyer and colleagues stated, "planning involves the development of strategies designed to prevent, minimize or correct the problems identified in the nursing diagnosis. . . . [This component] consists of four stages:

1   Setting priorities
2   Developing outcomes
3   Developing nursing orders (measures or interventions)
4   Documentation"
    (1986, p 114)

Bower stated, "Planning nursing care for people in a constantly changing milieu [environment] demands that the nurse be able to analyze, synthesize, and organize an incredible amount of data . . . Nursing care planning . . . is a process that requires a systematic and comprehensive approach" (1982, p 10). She stated also that nurses must "preserve the individuality of the person or family, assess health needs, establish priorities in nursing care, determine nursing interventions, and refer persons to appropriate resources" (1982, p 10).

In addition to this description of the planning phase, several other thoughts can be included. First, planning occurs as the result of a systematic data collection and nursing diagnosis, and follows naturally from these primary activities. Second, in keeping with this text's philosophy, the notion of health and strengths will also be added to the planning phase in the following discussion. Thirdly, both definitions suggest that the nurse does the planning. Although this may happen in certain instances, the goal is client participation in the planning phase according to his or her ability. The notion of the client's active role may be confusing at first. For clarification, consider that the nurse does not necessarily stop the thinking process to consult the client. Moreover, the nurse, coming from a knowledge and experience base, does planning that the client could not be expected to do. Essentially, there are a variety of ways to plan with clients, the most important of which is to listen when developing a plan. A clinical illustration at the end of this chapter demonstrates these ideas.

Goals and Expected Outcomes

Goals or *expected outcomes* are predictions of what the person hopes to attain given his or her strengths and needs. Goals are developed to maintain and promote strengths and move toward problem solving and decision making. The person's particular wishes are considered equally with the knowledge base of the nurse. As goals are developed, expectations of how the client will look, act, or feel are stated for the purpose of evaluating the outcomes. Goals can be adjusted to meet changing needs. The criteria stated below provide guidelines for constructing goals.

Goals Are Written in Behavioral Terms and Individualized to Suit the Person Who Expects to Attain the Result

Goals are constructed to reflect the person's, rather than the nurse's, behavior. For example, stating a goal, "the person will maintain . . . ," or "the person will demonstrate . . ." clearly identifies the person as the one who will achieve the result. Thus the client goal becomes person-centered. The nurse's goal is to facilitate the client in that venture.

Goals Are Written Using Measurable Terms with Outcome Criteria

Use of action verbs will demonstrate for both client and nurse that outcomes have been attained. Examples include: state, verbalize, demonstrate, recite, gain, lose, smile, or exercise. Consider the goal, "the person will state his or her new low-sodium diet from memory." This is a start, but does not include the time frame criterion. If the client is hospitalized, the goal might be: ". . . state his or her diet by discharge." However, if there are other goals to attain that go beyond this one, such as the client learning to choose the correct foods from the daily menu, then the time frame may be different. For example, "the client will state his or her new diet from memory within 1 week after instruction begins." Then, "the client will choose the correct foods for a low-sodium diet from the daily menu by discharge."

Other examples of criteria-referenced goals include the following:

- The client will state that his or her pain has decreased within 2 days after beginning use of relaxation techniques.

- The client will demonstrate ability to take his or her own blood pressure by discharge.
- The client will maintain his or her blood pressure within the current range (150/90 to 130/80).
- The client will maintain his or her ability to achieve a restful sleep.
- The client will smile three or four times a day.
- The client will walk in the hall 2 days after surgery.

Some goals cannot be structured easily within a time frame. For example, "The client will verbalize feelings of increased safety and security" provides one means of measurement with the action word "verbalize." The time frame, however, is missing. Nursing interventions are planned — avoiding a time frame for the present — to help the client feel safer, and eventually to verbalize those feelings. When the goal is affective, or feeling related, the nurse begins where the client is. Then, following some success, a time frame for further achievement is planned.

Goals Are Written as Short-Term and Long-Term

Goals are written to reflect plans for a short period of time or for a more extended period. *Long-term goals* often refer to a broader accomplishment which, although eventually realistic, can only be attained through a series of smaller steps. For example, "the client will lose 50 pounds over the next 12 months." *Short-term goals* reflect smaller steps that can be pursued one a time. They demonstrate achievement, provide encouragement, and suggest ways to attain the long-term goal.

Consider the following short-term goals suggested to meet the long-term goal of a 50-pound weight loss.

The client will

- identify his or her weight as a problem,
- state his or her wish to lose weight,
- verbalize knowledge of good basic nutrition,
- plan with the nurse a diet relevant to his or her needs,
- lose 1 pound a week beginning in 2 weeks.

To make these goals clearer, a time frame could be added, particularly after the first two goals have been achieved, thus, note the time frame suggestion of 2 weeks to attain the other goals before the client begins to lose weight. Perhaps after assessment, 2 weeks seems to be a realistic time period for the overall plan to begin. Specific time frames for the first few goals are omitted, however, to provide some freedom, but further evaluation may suggest a need for readjustment of the goals, and also the addition of a time frame. Continued plans for weight loss can also be developed.

Consider the following goals for Mrs. Carol, the client discussed in earlier sections:

The client will

- continue to express her feelings regarding sense of fear, abandonment, and grief.
- maintain a positive client-nurse relationship.
- perform own basic hygiene by 3 days after surgery.
- establish a plan to decrease fatigue.
- state that she feels safe when asked by the nurse.
- state differences between herself and family members who have died from similar disease.

To summarize, goals are planned with the client and reflect both his ability and readiness to work toward attaining his plans. Goals are written in measurable terms according to the behavior of the client. Goals may be both long- and short-term and are evaluated and revised as necessary.

| IMPLEMENTING — PHASE IV

Implementing refers to accomplishing or fulfilling. Implicit in this notion is the attainment of certain planned goals making implementation the active rather than the mental portion of the nursing process. Implementation may otherwise be known as nursing measures, nursing actions, or nursing interventions.

Nursing Interventions

Nursing interventions, nursing actions, or nursing measures are the steps taken to help the client attain the stated goals, and are directed toward promoting or maintaining health. They are planned using the person's strengths and are implemented to mobilize those strengths toward self-care capabilities. Nursing interventions are derived from

- Scientific knowledge associated with the biophysical and behavioral sciences
- Nursing theory based on research
- Past nursing experience.

Interventions can be categorized as *diagnostic* and *therapeutic* as indicated in the following examples.

Diagnostic Interventions

Diagnostic interventions are nursing actions that help the nurse and the client better determine the needs and the course of events in a given situation. They are also interventions in the sense that they help maintain the safety of the client during the observation or monitoring that must occur. Examples of diagnostic interventions include the following.

- *Observe* — consider such aspects as nonverbal behavior, skin color changes, progress in ambulation, and response to medication.
- *Inspect* — examine a wound for signs of infection.
- *Monitor* — check vital signs on a regular schedule, test urinary glucose and acetone four times a day, weigh the client daily.
- *Percuss* — determine changes in condition.
- *Listen* — obtain data to detect changes in voice tones either for cues to respond in a specific way or for clues to a person's needs, concerns, or wishes; auscultate (listen with a stethoscope) to determine changes in condition.

Refer to Table 8–4.

Therapeutic Interventions

Therapeutic interventions are nursing actions planned to maintain strengths and treat problems. Examples of therapeutic interventions include the following.

- *Listen* — provide opportunities for the person to verbalize; sit with and talk to the person; use touch and acknowledge strengths.
- *Problem solve.*

- *Support physiological needs* — assist persons with activities of daily living as needed; irrigate wounds and change dressings; encourage fluids to prevent dehydration; provide interventions for pain relief.
- *Educate* — provide specific health information as needed and appropriate.
- *Plan* — plan a diet with the client, a stop-smoking regimen, or a program of family discussions to improve relationships.
- *Refer* — assist the person to find other professionals, services, or facilities to help with his or her needs.
- *Meet basic needs.*
- *Support developmental task resolutions.*

Effective Interventions

Assessing and planning, although they represent formal phases within the structure of the nursing process, require approaches that are suited to the needs of the individual person. As mentioned in our discussion of the holistic person in Chapter 4, all of a person's subsystems are interrelated, with the healthier parts contributing to overall coping efforts. When coping becomes ineffective, energy may be borrowed from stronger subsystems, causing them to become weaker. If too much energy is drained away, feelings of hopelessness and helplessness may occur. The result may be a perceived loss of control and a diminished sense of self-esteem.

Use of a framework on which to base interventions will often increase their effectiveness. The concept of caring, as described in Table 8–15, is one such framework. When using this approach, the nurse first works toward a trusting relationship with the client and then gradually assists the person to maintain or recover control over his life. Suggested interventions for achieving control within this trusting relationship are listed in Table 8–16. As the client experiences more control, the nurse helps him establish goals, using a conscious effort to support and promote the client's strengths, thus elevating his or her self-esteem. Gradually, the client develops a more positive orientation, that is, an ability to project himself or herself into the future. As the client feels more hopeful, the cycle of trust, control, goal development, self-esteem, positive expectations, and hope repeats itself, resulting in greater control and less dependence on others.

Iyer and associates stated, "implementation is the initiation of the nursing care plan to achieve specific outcomes" (1986, p 177). Implementation indicates that the nurse and the client together have put the plan into action. "Implementation is the actual giving of nursing care. It is nursing therapy or nursing treatment, each of which is the giving of nursing care. . . . Implementation of the nursing care plan contributes to comprehensive care because the plan considers the biopsychosocial aspects of the client" (Marriner, 1979, p 127).

Implementation is a complex undertaking. Certain activities — such as providing oral hygiene or teaching the side effects of particular drugs — are obvious interventions, while other nursing actions — such as providing support — are less clear. The notion of giving support is a conglomerate of many interventions that must be identified individually so that the nurse has specific direction. Encouraging verbalization, identifying strengths, and assisting with problem solving are some examples of giving support. Using a theoretical framework will assist the nurse to develop interventions with a conscious and purposeful approach to decision making. Maslow's Basic Need Theory and the Concept of Caring that is derived from the linkages of several theorists are just two examples of such frameworks.

TABLE 8-15
THE CONCEPT OF CARING

Interventions	Definitions
Develop a trusting relationship	**Trust**—the assumption that another is responsible and honest and has integrity; the belief that we are safe with another; the ability to take risks concerning another person, a pet, or an inanimate object such as a car; the ability to act without fear of the outcome; a mode of positive expectation and hope
Assist the person to maintain or recover control over his life.	**Control**—the act of exercising restraint or direction over some thing or person
Assist the person to establish goals	**Goal**—the aim or end toward which effort is directed
Assist the person to develop higher self-esteem	**Self-esteem**—the individual's personal judgment of his or her own worth obtained by analyzing how well his or her behavior conforms to the person's self-ideal; the frequency with which the person's goals are achieved will directly result in feelings of increased self-esteem
Assist the person to develop a sense of positive expectations and hope.	**Hope**—expectation of something desired; confidence (trust) in another person, event, or outcome; promoting the promise of advantage or success
	Hopelessness—despondency, despair, abandonment of self to one's "fate"; inability to mobilize resources to cope; the sense that nothing can help, that the situation will never improve.
	Despair—the state of believing that one has no further control over a situation, an event, or even of one's life
	Helplessness—weakness, dependence, ineffectiveness; inability to mobilize resources; being without hope
	Impoverishment—the state of feeling, in some measure, helpless–hopeless, sad, and fatigued, and often hostile and bitter; one's self-esteem is low and problem-solving skills are minimal

(Swain MA, Erickson H, Tomlin E, et al: Personal communication concerning research project: Health promotion among diabetics: Comparing nursing systems. Department of Health, Education and Welfare: Division of Nursing, Grant No. NV00658-03, September 1978–September 1981)

TABLE 8-16
INTERVENTIONS TO ASSIST THE CLIENT IN REGAINING CONTROL

- Help the person recognize and recall his or her strengths.
- Respect the person's ability and right to make decisions about his or her care.
- Support the decisions the person makes and gear your interventions toward helping him or her carry out his or her plans.
- Explain all nursing actions to the person and ask for his or her suggestions on how to proceed.
- Use the person's ideas about his or her care and provide the person with appropriate information so he or she can make safe decisions.
- Acknowledge the person's accomplishments and express your respect. Remind the person of other successful problem solving he or she has done.
- Listen to the person's statements of how he or she feels. The person knows better than anyone else what those feelings — both physical and psychological — mean.
- Provide opportunities for the person to perform activities as he or she is capable.
- Use a positive approach which indicates your expectation that the person will become increasingly able to take care of himself or herself.

Consider the following interventions for Mrs. Carroll.

- Use interventions from Table 8-5, Table 8-15 (The Concept of Caring), and Table 8-16 (Interventions to Assist the Client in Regaining Control).
- Provide opportunities throughout the day for client to explore thoughts and feelings.
- Suggest how client is different from father and sister-in-law.
- Help client reminisce about past with husband.
- Plan a daily program with periods for rest and activity.
- Monitor blood pressure, pulse, and respirations after periods of activity or when client expresses fatigue.
- Help client determine which activities tire her and suggest ways to conserve energy.

| EVALUATING — PHASE V

Evaluating is, in part, appraising by an authority. The nurse may be viewed as the authority in a given situation because of theory base, past experience, and assessment skill. The client, however, is the authority on his particular strengths and needs. Therefore, implicit in this interpretation of evaluating is the collaboration of the nurse and client, each using his or her particular authority to decide together on future directions of care.

Evaluating and revising represent that phase of the nursing process in which the person's strengths, needs, and goals, along with the planned interventions, are reassessed and revised as necessary. Iyer and colleagues stated: "Evaluation is defined as the planned, systematic comparison of the client's health status with the outcomes" (1986, p 237). In other words, the stated goals or expected outcomes are used as a standard for evaluating the degree to which the person has improved his health status.

Evaluation begins with implementation of the nursing care plan. Throughout the delivery of care, the nurse considers the effectiveness of the plan in helping the client achieve his or her goals. If, for example, the client is working on a weight reduction plan but continues to overeat, the nurse reassesses the situation and a more relevant plan is developed. Interventions may be better suited to the client's resolution of trust and control issues than to diet planning. Or, if the client is ready to move through a care regimen more quickly than usual — for example, able to ambulate, do daily self-care activities, begin fluids — the nurse adjusts the usual plan to accommodate the client's adaptation.

Although this discussion of evaluating as a phase in the nursing process has focused on the individual person and his or her attainment of health-directed goals, evaluation can also be applied in a broader sense. Evaluation can be used to determine the quality of health care delivered in an agency or to judge the performance of health-care personnel, either through self-evaluation or the peer-review process.

Another important aspect of the nursing process is its interactive nature, as indicated earlier. Erickson and associates "view the nursing process predominantly as an ongoing, interactive, interpersonal relationship that includes use of the formal scientific mode of thought" (1983, p 105). These authors indicated that a formal step-by-step process is not necessarily followed, but rather, from the moment of contact between nurse and client, the nurse is "analyzing while listening, intervening, and evaluating; evaluating while intervening, analyzing and listening — in short, doing the nursing process (as a general problem solving) in her head while simultaneously giving [implementing] care" (p 105).

Little and Carnevali helped with this notion by stating: "The concept of the nursing process has several general properties. This pattern of thinking and behaving

1   is cyclic and recurring;
2   may be carried on with awareness, or almost automatically;
3   can be learned in terms of skill and speed;
4   may be carried out with varying speed ranging from almost instantaneous thinking to protracted deliberation;
5   integrates priority setting and feedback mechanisms into every step
6   is dependent upon the effective use of a body of knowledge
7   involves verbal symbols (words)
      (1976, p 11).

The clinical illustration in the box is offered as an example of the planning, implementing, and evaluating phases of the nursing process.

Clinical Illustration

At midnight, the hospital telephone operator phoned the nursing unit stating that our patient, Betty Drayton, had called the switchboard. Betty said that she needed help but the nurses would not answer her light. I thanked the operator and went to Betty, whom I knew well. I approached her and said, "Betty, how can I help?" She brightened momentarily when she saw me but then began to cry. "Those nurses, they were so awful tonight. They would never come when I called. They're mad at me; everyone is mad at me because I wouldn't go to exercise class today and I wouldn't walk. But I don't want to do anything but go home." I responded, "The nurses feel that these activities will help you get home faster. They worry about you and get frustrated when you don't follow the plan."

I had sat down on her bed rather than in a chair, putting my hand on her arm, because I knew that Betty needed the closeness and acceptance this would indicate. Listening to her, I remembered that she had raised many children, and had been extremely tired and psychologically impoverished prior to her surgery. She had stayed in intensive care longer than usual and had relied on having her own nurse. I had worked with her occasionally and knew that her special need was to be taken care of. If she had perceived that she was being ignored, she would experience a deficit in her love and safety needs. I also thought she was struggling with issues of trust and autonomy (Erik Erikson, 1963). For example, because she mentioned going home, I asked her how she might help herself get ready. She thought a moment and then said, "Well I suppose I could do all those things they wanted me to do today, but *I* want to decide that for myself instead of always being told what to do." I asked her how she might do that. Again she thought and then stated that she would get up in the morning without being told and start her own care. She was hesitant about being independent but her need to go home was becoming greater than her need to be taken care of in the hospital. I affirmed her strengths by supporting her statements and telling her I thought she was planning well for herself. I also assessed her blood pressure, pulse, and respirations to be certain that her restlessness was not related to a physiological change. I told her that I was not assigned to her during the night, but would be across the hall and she should call me if her nurse was busy.

The whole interaction took about 7 minutes. Using the nursing process, I moved back and forth among the five phases as we talked. From a theory base linking physiology with Maslow, Erikson, and nursing knowledge, I considered her physiological, belonging, safety, and esteem needs. I used her health-oriented statement that she wanted to go home to help her deal with her need for autonomy, or more control over her own activities. I let her know that I would be available if she needed me so that she would feel safe and have some of her sense of trust restored. I followed this up by smiling and waving as I passed her room for awhile until she fell asleep. I was able to evaluate my plan and nursing interventions as I saw that she stopped crying, began smiling a little, and announced that she would take a walk before she tried to sleep. In addition, I observed that she arose early in the morning and began her care. I believe that this transformation occurred in a short time because I focused on her rather than on her disease, or annoying behaviors.

| CONCLUSION

Nursing process is a scientific problem-solving method whose goal is the promotion of self-care abilities. Nursing process may be divided into five phases: assessing, diagnosing, planning, implementing, and evaluating. Diagnosing, was emphasized heavily because of the national attention focused on it. Aggregation, although not usually identified as a phase of the nursing process, involves synthesizing the results of nursing interventions to make predictions about the most effective approach for a given situation. Aggregation provides an important strategy for theory development.

The assessing phase involves collecting data about a person's health status to identify needs and strengths. A number of tools such as observations, interview, and palpation assist data collection. Assessment was presented as purposeful and involving establishing trust and maintaining confidentiality. Data can be organized in many different ways and from a variety of theoretical perspectives, and an overview of data collection frameworks indicated the many kinds of data used to provide holistic care. When analyzing data, the nurse draws on norms from basic sciences, humanities, and nursing to assist in recognizing patterns in the data; in turn, these conclusions are validated with the client to determine strengths and needs.

Nursing diagnoses, the outcome of the diagnosing phase and the result of data analysis, can take many forms. Diagnoses, according to NANDA and from a more holistic perspective, were discussed. The importance of using client strengths and involving the client in setting goals and planning care were considered.

The implementing phase was discussed as nursing interventions or measures designed to achieve the goals. This action step encompasses many obvious nursing procedures and treatments and less obvious interventions to build trust and demonstrate caring. Evaluating was indicated as important both as the final phase of the nursing process and throughout the other phases as the nurse interacts with the client and on his behalf.

The use and continued reinforcement of the nursing process stimulates the development of nursing research and theory and thus promotes nursing's growth as a profession.

| STUDY QUESTIONS

1   Describe a health-care situation from your experience in which identifying a person's strengths would have assisted the problem-solving process.

2   Suppose your friend, a medical student, asks you what nursing diagnosis is all about. Using the ideas from this chapter about purposes of nursing diagnoses and client strengths as a component of nursing diagnoses, outline the points you would list to answer this question.

3   Suppose your friend who is majoring in business asks you what nursing is all about. Using the ideas from this chapter about the nursing process, outline the main points you would use to answer this question.

| REFERENCES

Abdellah FG, Beland IL, Martin, et al: Patient Centered Approaches to Nursing. New York, Macmillan, 1960

American Nurses' Association: Nursing: A Social Policy Statement. Kansas City, MO, American Nurses' Association, 1980

Benner P: From Novice to Expert: Excellence and Power in Clinical Nursing Practice. Menlo Park, CA, Addison-Wesley, 1984

Bernzweig EP: The Nurse's Liability for Malpractice, A Programmed Course, 3rd ed. New York, McGraw-Hill, 1981

Bower FL: The Process of Planning Nursing Care: Nursing Practice Models, 3rd ed. St. Louis, CV Mosby, 1982

Campbell J, Finch D, Allport C: A theoretical approach to nursing assessment, J Adv Nurs 10:111–115, 1985

Carnevali DL: Nursing Care Planning: Diagnosis and Management, 3rd ed. Philadelphia, JB Lippincott, 1983

Carnevali DL, et al: Diagnostic Reasoning in Nursing. Philadelphia, JB Lippincott, 1984

Carpenito LJ: Nursing Diagnosis: Application to Clinical Practice. Philadelphia, JB Lippincott, 1987

Chinn PL, Jacobs MK: Theory and Nursing: A Systematic Approach, 2nd ed. St Louis, CV Mosby, 1987

Donnelly GF, Sutterley DC: From the Editors. Top Clin Nurs 5:vi, 1984

Dumas R, Leonard RE: The effect of nursing on the incidence of postoperative vomiting. Nurs Res 12:12–15, 1963

Durand M, Prince R: Nursing diagnosis: Process and decision. Nursing Forum 5:50–64, 1966

Engel G: Grief and grieving. Am J Nurs 64:93–98, 1964

Erickson HC, Tomlin EM, Swain MA: Modeling and Role Modeling: A Theory and Paradigm for Nursing. Englewood Cliffs, NJ, Prentice-Hall, 1983

Erikson EH: Childhood and Society, 2nd ed. New York, WW Norton, 1963

Gordon M: Nursing diagnoses and the diagnostic process. Am J Nurs 76:1276–1300, 1976

Gordon M: Nursing Diagnosis: Process and Application. New York, McGraw-Hill, 1982

Gordon M: Manual of Nursing Diagnosis. New York, McGraw-Hill, 1985

Hagey RS, McDonough P: The problem of professional labeling. Nurs Outlook 32:151–157, 1984

Henderson V: The Nature of Nursing. New York, Macmillan, 1966

Hurley ME (ed): Classification of Nursing Diagnoses: Proceedings of the Sixth Conference. St. Louis, CV Mosby, 1986

Iyer PW, Tapfich BJ, Bernocchi-Losey D: Nursing Process and Nursing Diagnosis. Philadelphia, WB Saunders, 1986

Jones PE: The Revision in Nursing Diagnosis Terms. In Kim MJ, Moritz DA (eds): Classification of Nursing Diagnoses: Proceedings of the Third and Fourth National Conferences, pp 196–202. New York, McGraw-Hill, 1982

Kennison B: Nurses and Patients: The Clinical Reality of Sickness. Doctoral dissertation, University of Michigan, 1983

Kim MJ, Moritz DA (eds): Classification of Nursing Diagnoses: Proceedings of the Third and Fourth National Conferences. New York, McGraw-Hill, 1982

LaMonica EL: The Nursing Process: A Humanistic Approach. Menlo Park, CA, Addison Wesley, 1979

Little DE, Carnevali DL: Nursing Care Planning. Philadelphia, JB Lippincott, 1976

Marriner A: The Nursing Process: A Scientific Approach to Nursing Care, 2nd ed. St. Louis, CV Mosby, 1979

Marriner A: The Nursing Process: A Scientific Approach to Nursing Care, 3rd ed. St Louis, CV Mosby, 1983

Maslow AH: Motivation and Personality, 2nd ed. New York, Harper & Row, 1970

McCain RF: Nursing by assessment—not intuition. Am J Nurs 65:82–84, 1965

Mundinger MO, Jauron G: Developing a nursing diagnosis. Nurs Outlook 23:94–98, 1975

Orem DE: Nursing Concepts of Practice, 2nd ed. New York, McGraw-Hill, 1980

Piaget J: The Psychology of Intelligence. Totowa, NJ, Littlefield, Adams, and Co., 1973

Popkess-Vawter SA: Strength-oriented nursing diagnoses. In Kim MJ, McFarland GK, McLane AM (eds): Classification of Nursing Diagnoses: Proceedings of the Fifth National Conference. St Louis, CV Mosby, 1984

Rogers M: An Introduction to the Theoretical Basis of Nursing. Philadelphia, FA Davis, 1970

Roy SC (ed): Introduction to Nursing: An Adaptation Model, 2nd ed. Englewood Cliffs, NJ, Prentice-Hall, 1984

Roy SC: Roy's adaptation model. In Parse RR: Nursing Science: Major Paradigms, Theories, and Critiques. Philadelphia, WB Saunders, 1987

Shamansky SL, Yanni CR: In opposition to nursing diagnosis: A minority opinion. Image: J Nurs Scholarship 15:47–50, 1983

Swain MA: Curriculum Development. The University of Michigan, School of Nursing, 1973.

Thomas MD, Coombs RP: Nursing diagnosis: Process and decision. Nurs Forum 5:57–64, 1966

Westfall UE: Nursing diagnosis: Its use in quality assurance. Top Clin Nurs 5:78–88, 1984.

Yura H, Walsh MB: Nursing Process, 3rd ed. New York, Appleton-Century-Crofts, 1978

Yura H, Walsh MB: Human Needs and the Nursing Process. New York, Appleton-Century-Crofts, 1978

Yura H, Walsh MB: Human Needs 2 and the Nursing Process. Norwalk, CT, Appleton-Century-Crofts, 1982

Yura H, Walsh MB: Human Needs 3 and the Nursing Process. Norwalk, CT, Appleton-Century-Crofts, 1983

9 | INTERPERSONAL COMMUNICATION IN NURSING

KEY WORDS	After completing this chapter, students will be able to:
Accurate observation Active listening Assertiveness Communication Congruence Connotation Denotation Empathy Interview Nonverbal language Process recording Trust Verbal language	Explain the importance of effective communication to quality nursing care. Contrast helping relationships with social relationships. Describe the four roles of the nurse in a helping relationship. Describe the components of empathy. Identify effective and ineffective communication techniques.

This chapter introduces the nature and application of interpersonal communication in nursing. The material is appropriate to nurses regardless of practice setting, specialty area, or job title. Helping relationships within the nursing profession take several forms with the nurse playing many different roles either separately or in combination. Important and challenging roles related to interpersonal communication are in keeping with nursing's professional emphasis on health. These roles include direct administration of physical care, advocacy on behalf of clients, psychosocial support, and health education and counseling. They require the nurse to combine problem-solving and communication skills and act as a therapeutic listener and resource liaison.

Locked in each person is a wealth of unique experiences, strengths, feelings, and values. Effective **communication** is the master key that unlocks such human resources, enabling a nurse to understand, to care, and to help another person. The person, in turn, learns that the nurse does understand, does care, and will assist him or her. Such resonance between two persons, in this case between nurse and client, underlies a helping relationship and a most rewarding profession.

Interpersonal communication is both a science and an art. As a science, it requires disciplined study of concepts and practice of technique to gain certain skills. As an art, it requires the fusion of the nurse's self with creativity, insight, and practice in order to achieve style. The distillation of art and science into a personal style of interaction is neither automatic nor innate; study and practice are required to develop one's own skill and interpersonal style.

Human communication is a complex process in which two (or more) persons exchange messages and derive meanings. Effective communication occurs when persons exchange messages and derive a mutual understanding of the intended meaning. The rationale for the importance of communication in nursing was captured by Watzlawich and colleagues (1967) in a general classic principle of communication: a person cannot *not* communicate. When the behavior (verbal or nonverbal) of a person (nurse or client) is perceived by another, communication occurs.

NURSE-CLIENT INTERACTIONS AS HELPING RELATIONSHIPS

Most nurse-client interactions occur within the context of helping relationships in which a nurse "has the intent of promoting the growth, development, maturity, improved functioning, improved coping with life" of the client (C. Rogers, 1961, pp 39–40). In a traditional helping relationship, a client might identify a health problem or illness and seek help from a doctor; the doctor might then order nursing services to assist the client. Examples include counseling in pain management, sexuality, ostomy care, nutrition, management of illness at home, grief and loss resolution. Today, more clients are seeking nursing care directly in times of crises. Nurses, too, are offering services more directly to prevent a problem or illness and to maintain the health of the client, the family, and the community. Thus, helping relationships may be client-initiated or nurse-initiated.

Characteristics of Helping Relationships

All helping relationships have the same intent and share certain common characteristics. As professional helpers, nurses exemplify the following characteristics:

- Awareness of self and values
- Ability to analyze own feelings
- Ability to serve as a model
- Altruism
- Strong sense of ethics
- Responsibility

Genuineness and unconditional acceptance of the other person are essential qualities for those who wish to help persons become healthier in mind and body. In exploring what it means to help another human being, counselor and behavioral science researcher Laurence Brammer describes most distressed persons as deprived, ignored, isolated, or deficient in knowledge or skill, rather than as diseased or ill. This fact often surprises nurses who enter the field to work with "sick" persons and subsequently learn the enormous needs of all deprived persons for nursing services. Brammer outlined the characteristics of an effective helper as follows.

- *Awareness of self and values.* The nurse needs to be able to answer "Who am I? What do I believe? What is important to me?" in order to help another person answer those questions. A certain level of insight precedes the use of a most important tool in nursing, the "use of self" as a care-giver.
- *Ability to analyze own feelings.* Nurses as helpers gradually learn to recognize and cope with their own feelings of joy and grief, power and anger, accomplishment and frustration.
- *Ability to serve as a model.* To show another person the route to health, a nurse necessarily maintains a certain level of health — in mind, body, spirit, and life style.
- *Altruism.* Nurses characteristically convey a sense of altruism, that is, they receive self-satisfaction from helping people in a humanistic way.
- *Strong sense of ethics.* Nurses strive to make the best possible judgments based on high principles of human welfare.
- *Responsibility.* Two dimensions of responsibility are inherent in nursing: taking responsibility for your own actions and sharing responsibility with others (1979, p 16).

Professional Versus Social Relationships

A successful helping relationship between nurse and client represents a different order of interaction than that which occurs in a friendship. This difference is not because of any superiority in the nurse but because of the mutual trust and the responsibilities for assisting others that characterize professional relationships. Although many elements of a professional relationship are warm, friendly, and social in nature, there is an underlying purpose in helping relationships that is beyond mutual enjoyment. The nurse's purpose is to enable the person to adapt to changing life circumstances in as healthy a way as possible, and the nurse empowers the person to maximize his or her strengths to achieve personal potential. Table 9–1 outlines the essential similarities and differences in the two types of interactions. Many nurses are convinced that clients must like them and that a successful relationship is a friendly one. This attitude, while popular, is neither possible nor advisable in most helping relationships. The effective nurse avoids developing "favorite" patients toward which he or she is extremely affectionate, as well as negative stereotypes of clients. With either extreme, the nurse would lose the objectivity necessary to give quality care.

Helping Roles

The nurse helps the client by acting in one or a combination of the following roles:

- Direct administration of physical care
- Advocacy on behalf of clients
- Psychosocial support
- Health education and counseling

TABLE 9-1
A COMPARISON OF SOCIAL RELATIONSHIPS AND PROFESSIONAL HELPING RELATIONSHIPS

	Social Relationships	Professional Helping Relationships
Impetus	Mutual need satisfaction and experiential sharing	Client need or concern
Goal orientation	Usually no definite goals	Always goal oriented and purposeful
Commitment	No stated responsibility to continue the relationship if problems occur	Responsibility to problem solve difficulties encountered
Acceptance	No expectations made of accepting the other person; acceptance qualified	Helper accepts the client as he or she is; unqualified acceptance
Judgment	Value-based judgments are made to determine compatibility	Value-based judgments may occur, but mutual awareness and sharing of such perception is essential
Assistance	Voluntary assistance may be offered or refused	Obligation to provide assistance or resources for client to assist himself or herself
Trust	Develops voluntarily, dependent on shared experiences and values	Helper obliged to build mutual trust
Confidentiality	No explicit obligation, although the degree of intimacy determines confidentiality	Helper operates under ethical duty of confidentiality to divulge knowledge only to responsible parties with client consent
Limits of interaction	Flexible to meet needs, interests, and convenience	Defined in advance, renegotiated to meet client needs or helper availability
Mutual understanding	Voluntarily sharing understanding	Obligation to use effective communication to understand client needs

(Adapted and expanded from Gold HG: Therapeutic relationships — Social relationships. Unpublished manuscript, University of Michigan School of Nursing, Ann Arbor, 1973)

Direct Administration of Physical Care

This is the traditional and time-honored role of the nurse. In the 1970s, this helping role evolved from one of performing service for others to one of assisting others to regain or retain the ability to care for themselves. Nurses provide direct assistance for those clients who are temporarily or permanently unable to care for themselves. Obviously examples of such clients include: dependent children; adults whose self-care abilities are altered by surgery, chronic or acute disease; and the frail elderly. The majority of relatively healthy persons retain responsibility for their own health care and use nursing help as they perceive a need. Helping means that control remains with the client.

Advocacy on Behalf of Clients

The growing complexity of and rapid changes in the health-care delivery system make the client's search for satisfactory answers and solutions more difficult. Nurses perform an invaluable service by searching out the available solutions on behalf of the client as a consumer. In this way, the client can make informed decisions in meeting his or her own needs. Sometimes the client becomes both the patient himself or herself and his or her family. For example, an elderly woman caring for her bedridden husband at home may need to arrange a variety of direct-care personal services, including those of the visiting nurse and relief for herself as caregiver. Or, perhaps this same woman needs the nurse's intervention with family members to examine the seriousness of a health situation in order to effect solutions to unfinished family business.

Psychosocial Support

The often-abused phrase "psychological support" includes a variety of methods by which the nurse sustains the emotions, the morale, the culture, and the spirituality of a client, Communication skills of empathy and assertiveness are essential to this kind of support. Nurses learn to react to the stress behavior of clients and generally, when clients show signs of distress, nurses act to comfort and support them. In such situations, skills of problem solving and anticipatory crisis intervention prepare the client by describing what to expect in a stressful situation and by providing sufficient information for him or her to make informed decisions and maintain self-esteem and self-control.

Social support is usually found among such individuals and groups as one's friends, co-workers, neighbors, community organizations, and church congregation. Either physical absence or inability to participate may interrupt these networks. Often, the nurse can help re-establish contacts by suggestion or direct intervention.

Health Education and Counseling

The effective nurse motivates a client to learn, grow, and change his or her health behavior as needed. The nurse's role as a health educator and counselor depends on the ability to facilitate — not dictate — another person's growth. Nurses teach clients as if to say, "Here is some information. Use whatever seems helpful. I will support you in your decision." This basic approach to teaching adults can be altered appropriately when dealing with more dependent or unstable clients. The role of the nurse as health educator will receive special elaboration in Chapter 10, which is devoted to the learning-teaching interaction.

At any given time, a practicing nurse is likely to be enacting several of the above roles simultaneously. Teaching a new mother about infant care involves constant psychosocial support of her mothering abilities, as well as health education and counseling. Care of a dying person may include advocacy of death with dignity, along with physical care and psychosocial comfort to the dying person and his or her family. The four helping roles of the nurse overlap constantly in caring for, and caring about, people.

DEVELOPING NURSE-CLIENT RELATIONSHIPS

Helping relationships as dynamic interpersonal processes do not automatically exist, but grow much the same way a garden grows. Careful preparation of growth conditions are a necessary first step. The progressive caring, feeding, and supportive direction given in a growth phase help any plant and any relationship to be self-sufficient and productive. Skillful nurses, like skillful gardeners, redirect disabled life back toward health, being ever careful not to neglect, oversupply, or destroy it in the process. Both gardeners and nurses eventually enjoy the satisfaction of a harvest, the closing of one growth cycle and the beginning of another. Throughout, there remains a mystical quality in the growth of a plant, the growth of a person, and the growth of a helping relationship.

Trust

Growth in the interpersonal process is dependent on the development of mutual trust. **Trust** evolves when one person risks his or her own self-esteem, seeks support from another, and finds it. The helper fosters trust, not dependence, by making and keeping commitments, sharing responsibilities with the client, and ensuring confidentiality. "We cannot morally encourage disclosure about values, attitudes, and behavior unless we are certain that we can guarantee confidentiality" (Benjamin, 1976, p 54).

Few qualities of the helping professional are as essential as confidentiality. Imagine the damage to a growing, trusting relationship should a client discover that a nurse has inappropriately spread personal communications. It is unlawful, unethical, and in many cases a breach of contract with the employment agency to breach confidence. Sharing information that is vital to the health and safety of the client with other responsible caretakers is essential; however, the client has the right to be informed of a nurse's need to share vital information with others. Note-taking and other types of recording should never be the focus of an interaction, as in, "Hold it, I didn't get all of that down." Secretive note-taking destroys trust, while asking the client's permission to take notes and sharing them with him or her acknowledges the client's control over the information. It is important to remember that trust flows through any successful helping relationship.

Three Phases of Growth in Nurse-Client Relationships

In a growth process, helping relationships are divided into three phases:

1 *Opening (or initial)* — introduction and preparation of the personal growth conditions take place in this phase. In the opening phase of the relationship, the underlying goal of both persons is to adapt to each other and establish trust.
2 *Working (or developmental)* — this second phase of a relationship fosters growth and change, problem solving, and decision making. Throughout the working phase, both nurse and client strive to maintain trust during stressful decision-making and problem-solving encounters.
3 *Closing (or terminating)* — the closing of a successful relationship can be considered a harvest of mutual satisfaction between nurse and client. The closing phase requires both persons to redirect trust, often by referral to another care-giver or by agreement that the client is self-sufficient again.

These flexible phases form a chain of interactions, ending at a level higher than began.

Guidelines for Successful Helping Relationships

Since successful helping relationships do not occur automatically, teaching communication skills is now an important part of any nursing curriculum. As Norris reminded us, "The curricular trend which acknowledged communication content as basic to nursing assessment and intervention in all areas of practice was a significant advance in nursing education"

(1986, p 106). Aspiring nurses learn appropriate approaches to developing helping relationships as suggested by the following guidelines for the various phases.

Opening Phase

During the opening phase of a successful professional relationship, both nurse and client prepare to work together by establishing a contract, so to speak. In opening a helping relationship, the use of contracts, as suggested, will help the client (and nurse) adapt to a new relationship and to changes in the relationship.

Contracts may include formal statements such as those used by Steckel (1980) in her interventions with persons with diabetes. Usually, however, they are informal agreements that set the limits for several important aspects of the interaction. Consider the following examples:

1 How often will the nurse and client meet?
   Example: "I will be the nurse caring for you on the day shift all week."

   or

   "I will be the primary nurse responsible for your care. Even when I'm not on the nursing unit, I can usually be reached by telephone if you need to talk with me."

2 What will be the purpose of the meetings?
   Example: "I will be the nurse helping you to plan for the care of your child at home. I will stop by each afternoon for a few minutes so we can work together."

3 How will the confidential information be handled?
   Example: "For me to be most helpful to you, I will need to have you tell me how you honestly feel about caring for your husband at home. Also, what information about your feelings, if any, do you want me to share with your daughter?"

4 What will be the terms for closure of the relationship?
   Example: "I will expect you to let me know when you think you can manage on your own."

One characteristic of the opening phase of many relationships is testing behavior, a common prelude to trust. Each person establishes a sense of security in the relationship by testing the limits set by the other. This usually is an adaptive behavior to see if the other person means what he or she says. For example, the hospitalized client may express insecurity by calling the nurse repeatedly; this behavior may reflect the client's difficulty in believing that the nurse is concerned with his or her needs and care even when the nurse is not directly visible to the client. Clients whose life experiences or ethnic backgrounds are different from the nurse's will test the nurse's willingness to understand them, sometimes with queries such as, "How can you know what it's like?" The nurse who replies, "I know just how you feel," may be believed only if an honest example follows: "I've had a similar thing happen to me."

Testing behavior can be a direct indication of the amount of security and trust in a relationship; as interpersonal trust grows, testing behavior subsides. A clear indication of movement into the working phase of a relationship is the cessation of testing behavior. However, the issue of trust is a larger issue than trust in the nurse-client relationship. The nurse recognizes the persons who have not resolved developmental tasks of trust versus mistrust may be genuinely unable to trust the nurse. Reasons for mistrust may be deep-rooted and have little to do with the nurse's interpersonal skills.

Working Phase

At the point of completing a contract with the client, the nurse moves the interaction into the working phase by beginning the helping process. The working phase is the part of the relationship in which helping and growth occur, whether the nurse gives direct care, counseling and teaching, or psychosocial support. The care given centers on the client's needs and problems. Therefore, one of the most useful tools of the working phase is problem solving: the systematic process of identifying, clarifying, and resolving troublesome situations. Abdellah and colleagues (1960) recognized the need for nurses to use a basic structure for solving difficult clinical problems, regardless of the type of setting. This process — that is, the nursing process — is rooted in the scientific method.

Problem solving is widely adaptable to all nursing situations. At times, identifying the exact nature of the problem can be difficult and time consuming, requiring that the problem solver turn the problem around to view it differently or emphasize another part of a complex problem. In working with a difficult family situation, for example, a nurse may begin to question whether the sick member of the family is really the source of the problem, or whether other members of the family, the community, or the environment are really the cause.

It is imperative, however, that the nurse not become involved in problem hunting to the extent of interrogating or otherwise forcing clients to "Tell me your problem!" Many troubled persons, if they do recognize their own concerns or problems, may not be able to verbalize them.

As nurses adopt the concepts of self-care — that is, helping others to help themselves —they recognize that helping the client to solve his or her own problems, whenever possible, is preferable to problem solving for the client. Therefore, the following process of helping the client solve problems is recommended.

1   Explore what concerns the client has about his or her past, present, or future health situation.
2   Use client-centered communication to identify the exact nature of the problem from the client's perspective.
3   Explore with the client what he or she has already tried to do to resolve the problem.
4   Explore what the client sees as possible alternative approaches to the problem now.
5   Explore what the client sees as positive and negative consequences of each alternative he or she proposes.
6   Explore what the client sees as barriers preventing him or her from taking action.
7   If the client is not able to suggest any approaches to his or her problem, the nurse may now suggest new approaches.
8   Explore the consequences and barriers the client sees inherent in your suggested approaches.
9   If several approaches are suggested, help the client to decide which would be most appropriate for him or her to try first.
10 If the client indicates readiness to take action on his or her problems, provide

the client with the information, materials, and support he needs to begin. If the client hesitates or shows unreadiness, return to Step 6 to explore the barriers.

11 After the client tries a new approach, schedule contact with him or her to learn the outcome and to reinforce any progress. If new problems arise, begin again with Step 1 to explore the concerns. If negative consequences occur, help him to deal with them as constructively as possible

(Webb E: Helping the Client to Problem Solve. Unpublished manuscript, Wayne State University College of Nursing, Detroit, 1976).

This client-centered process of assisting clients to solve their own problems builds self-esteem and independence in the client. This approach can be adapted to many nursing situations, even when the client is very ill or debilitated, helping him or her to control decisions about his or her own health. At times, progress may be slow, especially in long-term relationships. Testing behavior may recur as a signal of frustration, unmet needs, or wavering trust.

Closing Phase

Closing gestures are very likely to determine the client's perception of the entire interaction and, thus, his or her willingness to enter future helping relationships. Successful closing is planned in advance in order to provide time for adapting to the loss. It attaches value to the preceding interaction. The challenge is to focus on the client's achievement as a point of departure for possible future achievements.

Interactions of long duration may end in small celebrations or gift giving. Sometimes patients or their families leave gifts of fruit or candy for a group of health-care workers as a token of their appreciation. Occasionally, a patient or family may single out a particular individual for special remembrance. Although some nurses may be more comfortable than others in receiving gifts, Gordy (1978) pointed out the necessity of examining the meaning of the gift when deciding to accept it. Gifts may represent gratitude, guilt, or some other more personal and less obvious intent. One such small token made a lasting impression: one patient, who was dying of cancer, joined in wedding shower festivities with a dimestore gift of a cheery plastic orange-shaped juice container.

Testing behavior during closing may be an attempt to hang on to the nurse. Testing behavior is a common manifestation of separation anxiety, an insecure feeling of loss occurring at the end of meaningful relationships. In an attempt to protect themselves and adapt, clients may withdraw as if to say, "I'll end this relationship before you leave me." Working through loss can be a growing experience and thus a positive behavioral sign. A realization of waning interaction time often prompts client (and helpers) to intensify the relationship near the end and signs of grieving and loss reaction may appear. Just as the opening and each working step is planned, the closing is anticipated, planned, and enjoyed as the fruit of a successful relationship.

INTERPERSONAL COMMUNICATION PROCESS

Elements of a Human Communication Process

The interdisciplinary study of human communication combines the fields of biophysics, physiology, psychology, sociology, anthropology, and ecology. Indeed, these sciences form the basis of a nursing perspective on communication and the educated nurse may use all of them to communicate effectively with clients as persons.

Communication has been described as a process, a continuous circular flow of energy. Most models of the communication process contain the following elements: source (also known as stimulus), message, transmitter, and receiver (also known as response). David Berlo (1966) described the human factors of sociocultural influence, environment, communication abilities, attitudes, and knowledge that modify the process. Later communication scientists have added the element of feedback to complete a circular pathway of communication (Fig. 9–1). When a message proceeds in one direction from the source to the receiver, it is termed a *one-way communication*. A one-way communication neither expects nor encourages a response from the passive receiver. When the flow of a communication includes a feedback loop, it is termed *two-way communication*. The receiver is expected and encouraged to participate actively in the exchange. A traditional lecture, for example, is one-way; the question-answer period afterward is an attempt to establish a two-way dialogue. Effective nursing interactions are two-way communications involving both client and nurse as active participants.

Mass, Intrapersonal, and Interpersonal Communication

The field of human communication may be divided into three components: mass communication, intrapersonal communication, and interpersonal communication. Although each is a complex process, the three vary in scope. Mass communication is the transmission of messages to a large audience of receivers. The modern media communicate information efficiently to the largest possible groups of receivers. Intrapersonal communication, in contrast, occurs largely within the single individual when the mind or the body interprets messages for the person. **Interpersonal communication** is the exchange of messages between two (or a small group of) persons. Effective interpersonal communication requires, in addition, the understanding of the meaning in such messages. The foundation of effective nursing lies in effective interpersonal communication.

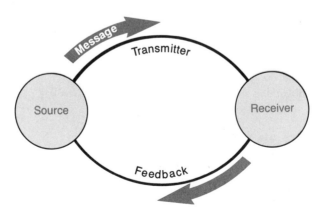

Figure 9–1   The communication process.

Interpersonal Process Applied to Nursing: A Theoretical Perspective

Entire theoretical systems for nursing are based on the interpersonal process as an interaction and have been detailed by such nurse scientists as Peplau (1952) and Orlando (1961). According to Meleis (1985), the interaction theorists represented a school of thought in nursing theories that was preceded by needs theorists such as Henderson and followed by outcome theorists such as Roy. Meleis' analysis helps to clarify the place of the interpersonal process in nursing over time and in concert with the evolution of nursing theory. The approaches of these and other theorists are highlighted in Table 9–2.

The so-called needs approach associated with certain nurse-theorists, however, is not to be confused with the basic needs approach of Maslow discussed in detail in chapter 4. Rather, the needs of Henderson were more concerned with physical activities of daily living than with growth needs. Therefore, nurses who practiced from this needs approach were primarily physically busy with preplanned activities carried out for the patient, and their communications could be expected to be related primarily to such activities.

The interactionists, influenced by humanistic psychology, facilitated the person based on situational circumstances and were increasingly concerned with psychosocial aspects of nursing care. One might expect the communications of these nurses to be especially sensitive to client-centered needs of the moment.

The outcome theorists were primarily concerned about how the nurse could regulate the system to foster healthful adaptation. They tended to be more future rather than present oriented and communication could be expected to reflect such goals.

Bandler and Grinder (1975) have developed a theory of neurolinguistic programming (NLP) from the sciences of linguistics and psychiatry. NLP postulates that American culture and language exhibit three patterns of language use: kinesthetic, auditory, and visual. Most individuals tend to communicate most comfortably in one of these modes rather than the others. One challenge for the nurse, then, is to assess which pattern a given client uses most and apply that knowledge to establishing interpersonal communication.

As nursing extends its theoretical base, the availability of varied communication

TABLE 9–2
SELECTED EXAMPLES OF THEORETICAL APPROACHES TO INTERPERSONAL PROCESS

Theorist(s)	Approach
Nurses: Henderson	Needs approach — not to be confused with basic needs approach of Maslow. Communication related primarily to preplanned physical activities carried out for the patient.

Interactionists:
  Peplau, Orlando
Humanists:
  LaMonica,
  Watson
	Interaction-humanistic approach: assisted person based on situational circumstances; often concerned with psychosocial aspects of nursing care, especially sensitive to client-centered needs of the moment, quality as process.

Outcome theorists: Roy	Approach is future-oriented with nurse regulating interpersonal process and other variables to foster healthy adaptation as outcome, quality as outcome.

Others:
  Bandler and
  Grinder
	Neurolinguistic programming approach. Approach assesses dominant pattern of language use: kinesthetic (movement), auditory (hearing), visual (sight). Interaction acknowledges pattern client uses most.

strategies increases. Weidenbach, who contributed much to nursing's theoretical foundations in the 1960s and 1970s, also wrote about matters of everyday importance to all nurses. Her book in collaboration with Falls was titled *Communication: The Key to Effective Nursing* (1978). Pluckhan (1978) focused primarily on the intrapersonal [within] dynamics that must be an integral part of any interpersonal [between] communication model. The centrality of communication to nursing is evident in the title of her book, *Human Communication: The Matrix of Nursing.*

The skillful practitioner will let the nature of the client and the situation determine when it is appropriate to focus most on needs, interaction, outcomes, or some other future scientific approach. All of the above theoretical perspectives suggest, however, that there is a range of internal and external variables that modify the nurse-client interaction and affect communication.

Variables Affecting Communication

Internal Variables:
Biophysical, Psychological, and Sociocultural

Within each individual, certain forces facilitate, while others disrupt, the ability to communicate effectively. The level of consciousness affects verbal expression: the unconscious person must communicate his or her needs by body language and depends on a care-giver to interpret the needs correctly. Other biophysical variables hindering communication are: sensory losses, such as hearing and visual impairment; motor impairments; and any biochemical imbalance that causes confusion, especially drug intoxication. In contrast, a biophysical variable that aids communication is muscular coordination, which develops with the growing child into more and more effective speech and motor expression. Humans of all ages, however, can learn to overcome physical barriers to communication.

Anxiety also affects the ability to communicate. And what some observers might view as a client's selective inattention or choice not to hear a message may be something quite different. For example, sometimes the client may not be able to make such a choice. Rather, perhaps the client cannot — at this time — give evidence of absorbing the message. Later, when he or she is able to act, the previously unattended to message may come into conscious awareness to be used.

The entire realm of perception — the interpretation of stimuli — influences communication. Each human mind learns to perceive stimuli in certain patterns, influenced by personal values and attitudes. A typical example relates to age perception: the adolescent calls anyone over 30 "middle-aged" and anyone over 50 "old." The 60-year-old perceives himself as "middle-aged," referring kindly to the "old" man of 80 down the street. Thus, our perceptions are molded by our psychosocial experiences in life.

Sociocultural variables in communication present both obvious and hidden forces. Spoken communication obviously succeeds better if both persons speak in the same language; differing dialects and word connotations of other cultures may prove to be hidden disrupters of understanding. Nonverbal communication also varies across languages and cultures. For example, direct eye contact is viewed as sincere in the American culture but may be viewed quite differently in other cultures (e.g., Native American, Asian).

Also hidden are individual values, which can block one's ability to understand the other's message. If a nurse values a stoic response to pain, for example, she may not even be able to listen to the whimpering complaints of a client after surgery or be aware of the reason for her negative feelings.

External Variables: Environment

All interpersonal communication occurs within the context of the surrounding environment as discussed in Chapter 5.

Anyone who has tried to concentrate on a lecture while sitting in an uncomfortable chair amid construction noise knows how the environment can hinder communication. This is another opportunity to provide an environment conducive to psychosocial support, as described earlier in the chapter. Rather than memorizing rules of environmental structure, such as furniture arrangement, the nurse develops a finer sense of assessment by using empathy in evaluating the physical environment: "If I were frightened or embarrassed in coming to this agency, how would I respond if interviewed in the waiting room? behind a curtain? in a private room?"

Application of Maslow's hierarchy of needs to interpersonal relations would suggest that the individual might not be ready to communicate highest-level concerns without some provision of environmental comfort and security. Before beginning interactions with a client (especially lengthy ones), the nurse assesses his or her comfort level and security feeling through questioning and observation. Physical comfort is augmented by such measures as body positioning, supplying drink or food, supplying pain medication, rearranging furniture, and controlling room temperature and ventilation.

Security, in this case a feeling of psychological comfort, results from specific relaxation techniques, respect for territoriality, and provision of privacy. The crucial element of confidentiality in interpersonal relations depends directly on the provision of as much privacy as possible. In addition, a private atmosphere lessens distractions to both nurse and client and diminishes interruptions that may connote disinterest. Minimizing distractions can maximize the chances of effective interactions.

TYPES OF COMMUNICATION
LANGUAGE

Humans communicate meaning to each other through the use of language: patterns of behavior designed to influence others. These patterns of behavior are learned responses and are culturally determined. Communication scientists have distinguished two types of communication behavior: verbal language, which conveys meanings through words, and nonverbal language, in which means other than words are used. For the purpose of study, we first will consider each of these languages separately. Then, to view man as a holistic being, we will examine how persons combine verbal and nonverbal languages.

The nurse must first comprehend the verbal and nonverbal components of a client's message to analyze the combined meaning of both. Likewise, the client will seek to understand the nurse's meaning by examining verbal and nonverbal language.

Verbal Language

Consider the dollar bill: a rectangular piece of crinkled paper, it has very little significance until someone assigns meaning to it. In this case, the U.S. Treasury has assigned a value of 100 cents to it; other countries value the dollar differently in comparison to their own currency standards. A dollar bill is a symbol of some worth, a symbol exchanged to meet the needs of individuals.

In a similar way, a word possesses very little significance until assigned a meaning

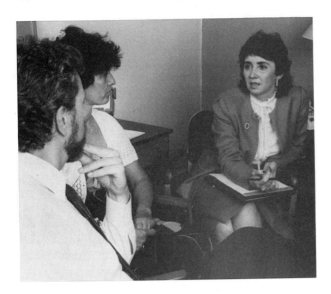

Communication is an essential nursing skill.

within a cultural or subcultural group. A word is a symbol of meaning that a person exchanges to meet his needs. Use of **verbal language**, then, is a symbolization process in which words are chosen as representative of an intended meaning. Commonly, the terms *verbal* and *oral* are used interchangeably and inaccurately: verbal language is the larger concept encompassing all use of words, both oral (spoken) and written.

Oral communication serves as the most common vehicle of deliberate interchange among persons. As such, the spoken word is subject to many misunderstandings. Nurses should remember this in their oral communication with clients. For nurses, the importance of both speaking and listening is sometimes underestimated.

In a study "to discover the specific oral communication skills necessary for success in nursing, and those skills most in need of improvement, according to Directors of Nursing . . . communication skills associated with listening were most important and in greatest need of improvement" (Wilmington, 1986, p 291).

Written communications are of a higher order, being more formal and permanent than oral communications. Although nurses orally transmit much information about client care, professional and legal responsibility for providing excellent care requires documentation in written form. The need for nurses to develop effective writing skills is crucial. Written care plans not only transmit important information to other health-care team members, but they are also legal documents. Nursing publications convey creative and innovative nursing to even wider circles of practitioners and students.

Word differences among subcultures may be subtle but significant. A person who believes he or she understands the language of another may discover that words, although identical in sound, differ in their meaning from one subculture to another. For example, the word "bust" is pronounced the same but quite likely interpreted differently by a sculptor, a fashion designer, and a drug addict. Words, then, are deciphered in context. Indeed, humans search for the meaning of words in the context of sentences or conversations; taking words or phrases out of context typically leads to misunderstanding.

The health professions, as a subculture, have created a language that changes the context of many common words. The use of such professional jargon increases the chance of misinterpretation between client and professionals. Consider this example: "You're NPO after midnight and you should void 2 hours post-op." The nurse has knowledge of technical terms that may be unfamiliar to the client. The challenge is to establish a common language level by deciphering the technical words for the client and educating him about their meaning.

The meaning of words has two dimensions: denotation and connotation. **Denotation**, a standardized meaning, is derived from a cultural consensus on the usage of the term. In contrast, subcultural usage of a word determines its **connotation** or implies a judgment of its attributes. The noun *nurse*, for example, denotes a person giving care to another in need; various connotations of the word include "handmaiden," "professional," and "manager."

Nonverbal Language

Symbols and actions other than words make up **nonverbal language**. Numerous studies have shown that nonverbal behavior expresses intended meaning, especially feelings, more accurately than does verbal behavior (Galloway, 1971). Yet, nurses sometimes ignore clients' nonverbal expressions. Nonverbal language is culturally determined. To interpret the meaning of a body movement or gesture without consideration of cultural context is equivalent to stereotyping. A client may wish to call the nurse by pet names such as "honey" or "dear," for example, which represent long-standing cultural behavior. Labeling this behavior as rude and condescending is inaccurate.

In clinical practice, the nurse encounters many clients who are unable to use verbal language: the infant and growing child not yet developed in speech, the comatose accident victim unable to speak, and the depressed person not yet ready to speak. The practitioner must use astute observation skills in order to understand the needs of these clients. For example, Hollinger (1986) highlighted the importance of touch as a nonverbal communication technique with elderly clients whose access to other nonverbal communication may be diminished with age. Pediatric nurses may use unconventional techniques to convert children's feelings and nonverbal responses to verbal language (Whaley and Wong, 1985).

Sight

Behaviors in the nonverbal language that are observed by sight include those of facial expression, gestures, and body postures, as well as physical appearance. The finely coordinated muscles of the face often give the most subtle indication of meanings.

One of the nurse's first observations is the client's eye contact and eye movements. In American culture, eye contact conveys an open, sincere approach to another person. Averted eyes may signal disinterest, diversion, or humility, and often may raise tension in the interaction. In the extreme, however, a fixed and glaring gaze also serves to increase the anxiety of another, as if he or she were being scrutinized. Several barriers, such as surgical masks, hospital equipment, or telephone communication, prevent open-eye contact in clinical situations. The nurse removes a barrier when sitting down to speak to children or to a person in a wheelchair or bed; such a simple action establishes eye contact and avoids the authoritative position of towering over the client.

Posture conveys meanings of interest and disinterest, of alertness, and of withdrawal.

Sometimes the client who curls into a fetal position may communicate withdrawal: "Leave me alone." The fetal position may also be a protective behavior signaling, "Take care of me."

Other observations made by sight include those of muscle tension and rapid-breathing patterns that are characteristic of anxiety. However, each individual manifests anxiety with his or her own pattern of nonverbal behavior, such as chain smoking, nail biting, pacing, and rocking. The nurse's ability to observe and validate such characteristic signs of anxiety increases the probability of understanding the client's meaning.

Appearance speaks of many traits. Let us examine the meaning of professional appearance. Nurses and other health professionals in faded blue jeans typically do not match the client's perception of professionals, thereby jeopardizing credibility and trust, while a clean and neat appearance, uniformed or not, connotes such credibility immediately.

Appearance can give the perception of sexual invitation — for example, clothes such as tight slacks or short skirts can provoke sexual response. Some would say that such apparent sexual invitation can occur without the nurse's specific intention, while others would contend that since the potential effect of such appearance is known to the nurse at some level of awareness, the behavior is arguably unprofessional. In either case, the client's reaction is merely an expression of unmet needs, such as for affection or touch.

Color has language all its own. White hospital uniforms connote cleanliness; the recent popularity of colored and patterned uniforms or regular clothes seems to connote nontraditional values among younger nurses. Use of brightly colored graphics provides stimulation in children's playrooms and hospital rooms that are otherwise stark and sterile.

Nonverbal Sounds

The skilled nurse trains the ear to observe speech sounds, because how something is said is as important as what is said. What is not said may be more important still. The skill of active listening involves listening for nonverbal vocalizations such as sighs, cries, and voice inflections accompanying words. Voice pitch, hesitations, and utterances, usually in combination with facial expressions, impart feelings of excitement, surprise, confusion, sarcasm, and mistrust. Such feelings can be heard by perceptive ears.

Silence as a nonverbal behavior holds a range of possible meanings, from boredom to contemplation, anger to introspection. Clients who are silent during an interaction may cause anxiety in nurses. Yet, silence can be a useful communication tool as it gives clients time to organize their thoughts and experience feelings prior to expressing them. The nurse's silence can convey recognition of individual worth, the importance of being in interaction through silent presence, and the willingness to be present without the need to control a situation verbally. A quiet presence, and perhaps a simple nonverbal clasp of hands, can convey caring beyond words and in a way that the person can quietly accept.

Touch

Nursing is a touching profession: the intimate nature of many nursing tasks requires that caring be transmitted by touch. And yet, nurses have been cited as avoiding touch with seriously ill and aged clients. Touch is as essential for the elderly as for the newborn. The ability to reach out and touch a client may be more common in some cultures than in others. Although a nurse may prefer to know the person better before touching him or her, the nature of many short-term nursing interactions precludes lengthy introductions. In one study, hospital patients receiving spontaneous touch from nurses perceived that the nurses showed genuine interest in them within a very short time (McCorkle, 1974). For nearly two decades, Kreiger's name has been synonymous with therapeutic touch in nursing. Krieger believed that therapeutic touch or the laying on of hands transfers and mobilizes energy resources, and that by therapeutic touch, the nurse transfers energy to the client as well as mobilizes client energy (Krieger, 1975).

Space

Touch may intrude as well as soothe, and the observant nurse decides how and when to touch based on each client's response. Threatening touch represents intrusion into the personal space of another. Personal space can be envisioned as a bubble surrounding each individual and forming a part of his personal, portable territory. Though we often joke about personal space among friends, this concept can have real professional significance.

Territoriality, or the human's instinctive drive to protect his or her space from intrusions, provokes defensive behavior by the person suffering intrusion. A client may become angry should the hospital nurse touch articles on "his" or "her" bed. In turn, nurses can become defensive when clients or other professionals enter "their" workspace. Ardrey (1966) claimed that possession of territory fulfills three of the human being's most basic needs: identity, security, and stimulation. Nurses who are aware of the territorial needs of clients can use the concept of territoriality to enhance communication. Carl, an 11-year-old child with Down's syndrome, underwent open-heart surgery and was required to spend many days in the recovery unit. When he awoke and found a large poster of his hero, Hulk Hogan, taped to the ceiling above his head, he knew he was in a safe place.

Anthropologist Edward Hall created the term "proxemics" to mean the use of space in interpersonal relationships. Space, or distance between communicators, is an extension of the concept of touch. Hall described four distances for interactions:

1   Intimate distance (up to 18 inches) for privileged touching
2   Personal distance (18 inches to 4 feet) for interaction with well-known persons
3   Social distance (4 to 12 feet) for impersonal business
4   Public distance (over 12 feet) for formal speaking
    (Hall, 1966, pp 109–120)

Nurses are granted intimate distance with a majority of clients and should maximize this privilege by deliberately maintaining this closeness. The nurse who pulls her chair out from behind her desk to talk with the patient and spouse increases the likelihood of an intimate and meaningful exchange. Some nurses fear touch will arouse sensual feelings in clients. But the mature and secure nurse learns to overcome this concern, learns how to increase the client's own self-esteem through touch, and promotes the use of therapeutic touch—such as massage—for relaxation, pain relief, and sound sleep.

Time

Closely related to spatial communication is the concept of temporal communication: the use of time and timing behavior to transmit meaning. American middle-class time orientation values the accomplishment and performance of tangible tasks. In nursing, sitting quietly with a client is sometimes considered not doing anything. Other cultures, notably the Navaho Indians and Japanese, value highly the vigil of sitting with a distressed person. Much of American culture stresses a "here-and-now," present orientation or an upward-bound, future orientation to time. This explains a sometimes unwelcome tendency to insist that very ill or disabled persons look ahead optimistically. We can help the dying person to find satisfaction in his or her past by moving away from a future orientation ourselves.

Other considerations of time involve the length and timing of messages, and the effective communicator will know and not exceed the attention span of listeners. Nurses working with children modify treatments and activities to shorter, more frequent sessions to avoid restlessness. Avoiding interruptions, another element of timing, assists in sending a complete message and prevents frustration and misinterpretation. Cultural variations in time perception need validation, for example, although some cultural groups value punctuality, others do not; this could lead to misinterpretation when tardiness occurs.

Congruence: Matching Verbal and Nonverbal Behavior

In order to comprehend the holistic person, the nurse observes both verbal and nonverbal behavior and combines these to analyze the meaning. This analysis searches for **congruence** between verbal and nonverbal behavior:

Congruent: "I appreciate your help" (direct eye contact, soft smile).
Incongruent: "I appreciate your help" (eyes averted, muscles tense).

Especially with distressed clients, the verbal behavior will often be incongruent with nonverbal behavior. Whereas congruence can be interpreted as an indication of open, trusting communication, incongruous messages signal the need for exploration of needs and feelings not expressed. The nurse mobilizes skills of empathy and validation to understand the client's conflicting messages and in this way maintains an open, trustful interaction.

ACHIEVING EFFECTIVE COMMUNICATION

Use of Self

Even experienced nurses strive to improve three abilities in order to become more effective communicators:

- *Knowledge* — increased understanding of communication dynamics,
- *Insight* — improved self-awareness of strengths and weaknesses,
- *Sensitivity* — sharpened perception of other's needs (Pluckhan, 1978, p. 18).

The term "use of self" represents the nurse's ability to integrate all three of the above abilities to produce successful interactions. Understanding the dynamics of the underlying communication process, its characteristics and variables, helps prevent communication problems. Nurses also learn how best to assist others when they become more aware of their own values and behaviors. Candidates for nursing often have a basic sensitivity to others; developing and expressing that sensitivity is a challenge throughout nursing practice. Nurses bring themselves, their experiences, perceptions, and prejudices to their helping relationships. The nurse who also develops a solid knowledge base, self-awareness, and sensitivity brings valuable resources indeed to the helping relationship. Whereas knowledge is gained by disciplined study, sensitivity develops by mastering empathy.

Achieving Empathy

Empathy is the ability to enter into the life of another person in order to perceive his thoughts and feelings (Benjamin, 1976, p 47). The nurse attempts to understand the clients' lives, their problems, values, feelings, and meanings, "to sense the client's private world *as if* it were your own but without ever losing the 'as if' quality" (C.R. Rogers, 1957, p 99). Nurses who can separate the client's problems from their own avoid emotional burnout; these nurses offer empathy instead of sympathy.

"*I'm so sorry for you. I know just how awful it must be . . . it's too bad.*" Few client's need this awkward compassion. Empathic understanding, which consists of active listening, accurate observation, empathic response, and validation, is much more helpful:

"*This must be hard for you.*"

"*I would be very frustrated if this were happening to me.*"

"*I had the same kind of surgery and I remember how much it hurt to cough.*"

"*I can suggest some of the things that have helped our other patients with a similar problem.*"

"*Other patients with this problem often tell us . . .*"

Active Listening

Active listening is the cultivated skill of deriving meaning from the words or nonverbal expressions of another. While hearing refers to the passive reception of sound waves by the ear, listening encompasses active concentration and perception of another's message using all the senses. Because humans communicate their needs through verbal and nonverbal behavior, the nurse employs sight, hearing, touch, and smell to listen actively. Hein (1975) advocated that the nurse listen for themes — patterns of communication behavior — in order to assess another's needs. Common themes expressed by others include the following.

- Self-effacement (attempts to reduce one's significance)
- Poverty of resources needed to cope with a present stress
- Self-centeredness ("*help me*"), indicating insecurity
- Wellness or strength to deal with stress (often overlooked in our search for problems)
- Loneliness, creating despair
- Loss manifested in grieving behavior
- Humor, a coping mechanism of tension release

Accurate Observation

Accurate Observation, the companion skill to active listening, involves not only looking at the client, but also identifying crucial facts about his or her nonverbal behavior. Knowing what to observe and recognizing how you observe are both essential.

How easy it is to jump to conclusions about what we observe and to offer solutions prematurely! Instead, nurses learn to differentiate an observation from an inference or conclusion, in order to prevent a misunderstanding. For an observed behavior, any one of several conclusions may be valid.

Observation

A woman wears a diamond ring on the third finger of her left hand.

Possible Inferences

The woman is married or engaged.

The woman likes diamonds.

The woman has inherited an heirloom ring that fits her third finger.

The nurse who jumps to conclusions — *"I see you are married"* — risks embarrassment and misunderstanding. Stating observations, not inferences — *"I see you wear a diamond"* — avoids communication breakdown.

Empathic Response

After careful listening and accurate observation, a nurse responds to the client's message with a verbal, nonverbal, or combination response. Touch is a powerful and effective response to another person; it is often part of an empathic response. Nurses are privileged to hear intimate, painful, and moving accounts of the stress in others' lives. Successful empathic responses, or feedback, tell the client that the nurse is attempting to understand not only the client's situation but also his feelings and values.

Kalisch (1973) identified five categories of nurse empathic functioning. A modification of this approach suggests the following three levels of empathic response that nurses use:

Level 1. Responding to situations (least effective)

Level 2. Responding to feelings (more effective)

Level 3. Responding to values (more effective)

At Level 1, the helper responds to the situation, the facts and events stated by the client.

CLIENT: *"I was so upset and disappointed that I had to have another operation."*

NURSE: *"You had to have another operation?"*

This response only restates the client's situation. Such a response is helpful to focus the interaction, but it is not considered an effective empathic response until it reflects feelings and values.

Level 2 responses can reflect feelings that are either stated openly or implied.

CLIENT: *"I was so upset and disappointed that I had to have another operation."*

NURSE: *"You became upset and disappointed when you heard you would need surgery again? Maybe frightened, too?"*

Such responses state the clients' feelings, helping them to cope with these feelings by sharing them.

Level 3 responses reflect a deep awareness of another's values, of what is really important to him or her. Usually, a helper is able to perceive a client's values after a trusting relationship has been established.

CLIENT: *"I was so upset and disappointed that I had to have another operation."*

NURSE: *"It's important to you to be at home with your family . . . ?"*

Using data the nurse has about the client, she perceives that this client's underlying value is being with the family. In questioning the client about this, a helper completes the empathic understanding by using validation.

Validation

It is necessary to gain some feedback from the client to know whether the empathic response is an accurate perception.

NURSE: *"And is it important to you to be at home with your family?"*
CLIENT (NODDING):   *"We really can't afford a baby-sitter for the entire 5 days I'll be gone . . ."*

The client affirmed her value of being with her children and raises her true concern of expense.

At times, our empathic responses are not accurate, and the client corrects our understanding.

CLIENT: *"Frightened? No, I've been through this before. I'm just angry that I got an infection the last time I was in this hospital!"*

Validation completes a feedback loop, making empathy a two-way communication.

Other Communication Techniques

Nurses learn that there are many effective and ineffective communication techniques. With formal instruction and practice, they learn both to differentiate between these and to develop an effective personal style. Additional techniques useful in maintaining a client-centered interaction include the following:

- Thoughtful use of silence
- Stating observations (*"You look sad today."*)
- Reflecting and paraphrasing client's stated or implied feelings and values (*CLIENT: "I don't know what to do next."* NURSE: *"You're frightened and confused."*)
- Summarizing (*"So, from what you've told me, you feel confident about managing this new diet plan."*)
- Seeking clarification (*"Tell me what you meant when you said you couldn't go on like this."*)
- Explaining procedures, expectations, etc.

Nurses also learn the pitfalls of

Reassuring falsely (*"Everything will be okay."*)
Moralizing, preaching, and advice giving (*"You really shouldn't . . ."*)
Stating their personal value judgments *"I think smoking is a bad personal habit."*)
Criticizing and ridiculing (*"Your plan is ridiculous."*)
Denying client-perceived problems (*"Your situation isn't that bad . . ."*)
Responding defensively (*"I was only trying to help."*)

Some techniques, like questioning, can be effective if appropriately used. Exploratory [what] questions that invite a response beyond *"yes"* or *"no"* are effective for most adults. For instance, *"Tell me about your family,"* rather than, *"Are you married?"* Children or confused elderly persons, however, may be better able to respond with a simple *"Yes"* or

"No." Similarly, harsh, insensitive, or multiple questions by a nurse may confuse, frustrate, or anger patients. Client questions may be direct requests for information or indirect requests for the nurse's empathic response.

Some effective communication techniques, such as humor and daring to be yourself, receive minimal attention in formal nursing literature. Both techniques may be effective as the following examples illustrate.

Sullivan and Deane explained: "Shared healthy humor is positively experienced and mutually enjoyed by the originator and the receiver. Helping the institutionalized elderly make use of humor in mastering the challenges of aging is a caring behavior in the nurse" (1988, p 23).

Ufema shared a view about how being yourself can be effective in communicating with dying patients:

> Our ability to make choices is part of what makes us human. Helping the dying patient have a voice in deciding the quality of the remainder of his life can give you some sense of success in working with him.
>
> How to talk to your dying patient? Be yourself, be honest and open, and remember that death isn't the enemy.
>
> Not recognizing our common humanity is. (1987, p 46).

Interviewing—Putting It All Together

Communication theory and skills have one purpose: producing an effective interview between nurse and client. Health **interviews** are either information-gathering interviews or helping interviews (or sometimes both):

- *Information-gathering interviews* are those in which the nurse seeks information from a client in order to plan or deliver nursing care.
- *Helping interviews* (also called *therapeutic interviews*) are those in which the nurse tries to help another to problem solve, plan for the future, cope with stress, etc. Chapter 8, discusses how nurses identify health needs and plan, administer, and evaluate nursing care. Interviewing is essential to that process.

Unfortunately, the connotation of interview has evolved to mean cleverly forcing the other person to confess—such tactics cannot promote trust in a helping interview. Nor is the monotonous, bureaucratic approach of "I just have a few (dozen) questions" acceptable. Successful interviewing uses a healthy balance of verbal and nonverbal behavior, empathy and assertive responses, and client-centered techniques, each chosen specifically to promote trust.

Assertive Communication

Learning to communicate effectively with other persons requires that several interpersonal skills be mastered. **Assertiveness**, a proactive problem-solving and coping behavior, is a verbal communication skill that states one's own rights positively without infringing on others' rights. Effective use of assertiveness prevents interpersonal misunderstanding and solves the inevitable conflicts that do arise.

Interpersonal communication styles can be described as either passive, assertive, or aggressive. The passive communicator abdicates his or her own rights, while the aggressive communicator infringes on the rights of others. The challenge for the assertive nurse is to develop a style of interaction that neither passively accepts nor aggressively attacks other persons.

Assertive behavior has five purposes.

- To let another person know your feelings and thoughts (simple assertion).
- To identify and acknowledge another's needs (empathic assertion).
- To call attention to a specific situation (confrontative assertion).
- To express appreciation to another (soft assertion).
- To identify to another person where you agree and disagree (persuasive assertion). (Bakdash, 1978)

The use of assertive behavior reflects a mature level of self-confidence. A competent and confident nurse chooses to use assertive behavior rather than passive or aggressive behaviors in interpersonal conflicts. Many nurses who would not feel comfortable being totally passive or terribly aggressive have found that they can use assertive behavior to communicate their own needs (Simms and Lindberg, 1978). The assertive nurse takes responsibility for his or her own actions, seeks workable compromises, clearly expresses her own needs, and avoids defensive outbursts and silent smoldering. The following example contrasts passive, aggressive, and assertive responses.

CLIENT: *"Nurse, this soup tastes terrible and it's cold; I won't eat it."*
NURSE A *(passive)*:   *"Okay. Give it back to me."* (silently thinking, *"Why does everyone complain to me?"*)
NURSE B *(aggressive)*:   *"Well, it's not my fault. You'll have to speak to the dietitian. I can't help you."*
NURSE C *(assertive)*:   *"That's disappointing. You can either have it warmed up or substitute something else. Which do you prefer?"* (workable compromise)

Assertive responses require significant practice because many persons must unlearn habitual passive or aggressive behavior before learning more effective assertive behavior. To help a client become more assertive, the nurse first helps him or her acknowledge his or her rights as a consumer of health-care services. As an advocate for the client, the assertive nurse protects the client's rights to privacy, confidentiality, and full understanding of the care received.

As nurses develop increasingly assertive styles, they learn to respect and protect the rights of others, including clients and colleagues. They also use assertive behavior to speak responsibly about what nursing can contribute to health care for today and the future.

Evaluating Communication

Just as evaluating is on ongoing activity within the nursing process, it is also an ongoing activity within the communication process. Both the nurse and client benefit from informal evaluation which may be simply an indirect question such as, *"Let me see if I understand what you are saying."* During a serious study of interpersonal communication, a technique called **process recording** may take a written form similar to that illustrated in Table 9–3. In this more formal analysis, actual verbal and nonverbal interaction is carefully recorded and analyzed.

Using a tool such as process recording, nurses may validate their communication techniques with professional peers. Beginning nursing students may present such process recordings to faculty members and clinical instructors for constructive critique.

TABLE 9–3
NURSING PROCESS RECORDING

Client	Nurse	Analysis
I'm just not satisfied with this x-ray film.	You're dissatisfied that the results of this test are negative?	Nurse uses reflection to paraphrase or mirror the client's stated or implied feelings and values. The nurse attempts to pinpoint the reason for the client's feelings.

Barriers to Effective Communication

A number of common barriers are associated with the biophysical, psychological, sociocultural, and environmental variables that affect communication (Table 9–4). When evaluating communication, the nurse evaluates the extent to which such barriers may be present. Many of these and other similar barriers are under the nurse's control. Some personal barriers (e.g., sociocultural value) pertain as much to the nurse as to the client. Person-centered care will be attentive to such barriers and provide relief to the fullest extent possible. The nurse who breaks confidences both creates a barrier to effective communication and

TABLE 9–4
BARRIERS TO EFFECTIVE COMMUNICATION

Biophysical

Unmet basic needs: oxygen and gas exchange, food, fluids, elimination, rest, comfort, sexual fulfillment
Level of consciousness
Sensory losses, for example, hearing or visual impairment
Motor impairment, for example, speech or writing
Biochemical imbalances, for example, drugs, alcohol

Psychological

Unmet basic needs: safety, security — anxiety and fear, love and belonging, esteem
Ineffective listening and selective inattention
Perception

Sociocultural

Values
Illiteracy
Past experience
Unfamiliar language including differing dialects and word connotations

Environment

Noise
Uncomfortable temperature, ventilation, lighting
Positioning of communicators
Interruptions

threatens the helping relationship. Inaccurate assessment of the client's developmental state or personal situation may also create barriers. If the purpose of an interview or interaction is not clear to the client or if a client feels his or her strengths and priorities have been ignored, communication may seem futile. The nurse who is sensitive to any discrepancies between verbal and nonverbal communication may suspect such potential barriers exist. Willingness or invitation to receive feedback from the client about the situation may forestall the development of barriers.

When evaluating communication, the nurse can also reflect on whether the suggested techniques for achieving effective communication are being used consistently. Therapeutic and nontherapeutic techniques are both summarized and compared and contrasted in Table 9–5.

| CONCLUSION

This chapter has presented communication as both an art and a science essential to effective nursing. The nurse-client relationship represents a special helping relationship with inherent responsibilities and rewards. Effective communication is important during direct administration of physical care and psychosocial support, and during advocacy for clients. Effective communication is also one of nurses' most effective tools for assisting persons to adapt to life changes.

TABLE 9–5
THERAPEUTIC AND NONTHERAPEUTIC TECHNIQUES

Therapeutic	Nontherapeutic
Active listening	Selective or inattentive listening
Accurate observation, stating observation	Stating inference
Empathic response from modeling client's world	Sympathy voiced from perspective of nurse's world
Therapeutic touch	Impersonal distancing
Maintaining confidences	Betraying trusts
Creative use of self	Impersonal interaction
Thoughtful silence	Resistive or fearful silence
Reflection	False reassurance
Restatement	Advice
Summarization	Moralizing Approval or disapproval messages Criticism and ridicule Threats or defensive responses

Well-chosen questions:
  Open-ended except "why?"
  Indirect
	Questions overused: rapid fire, demanding yes or no answers, direct and harsh queries

| STUDY QUESTIONS

1   How do helping relationships differ from social relationships?

2   From your own personal perspective, what are the biophysical, psychological, sociocultural, and environmental variables that particularly influence communications between nurses and clients?

3   What are your strengths or unique personal skills that might influence your interpersonal communication?

| REFERENCES

Abdellah G, Beland IL, Martin, et al: Patient-Centered Approaches to Nursing. New York, Macmillan, 1960

Ardrey R: The Territorial Imperative. New York, Atheneum, 1966

Bakdash DP: Becoming an assertive nurse. Am J Nurs 78:1710–1712, 1978

Bandler R, Grinder J: The Structure of Magic. Palo Alto, CA, Science and Behavior Books, 1975

Benjamin A: The Helping Interview. Boston, Houghton-Mifflin, 1976, 1981

Berlo DK: The Process of Communication: An Introduction to Theory and Practice. New York, Holt, Rinehart & Winston, 1960

Brammer LM: The Helping Relationship: Process and Skills. Englewood Cliffs, NJ, Prentice-Hall, 1979, 1985

Galloway CM: Non-verbal: The language of sensitivity. Theory into Practice 9:227–230, 1971

Gordy HE: Gift giving in the nurse-patient relationship. Am J Nurs 78:1026–1028, 1978

Hall ET: The Hidden Dimension. New York, Doubleday, 1966

Hein E: Listening. Nursing '75 5:93–102, 1975

Hollinger LM: Communicating with the elderly. J Gerontol Nurs 12(3):9–13, 1986

Kalisch B: What is empathy? Am J Nurs 73:1548–1552, 1973

Krieger D: Therapeutic touch: The imprimatur of nursing. Am J Nurs 75:784–787, 1975

McCorkle R: Effects of touch on seriously ill patients. Nurs Res 23:125–132, 1974

Meleis AI: Theoretical Nursing: Development and Progress. Philadelphia, JB Lippincott, 1985

Norris J: Teaching communication skills: Effects of two methods of instruction and selected learner characteristics. J Nurs Ed 25(3):102–106, 1986

Orlando I: The Dynamic Nurse-Patient Relationship. New York, GP Putnam's, 1961

Peplau H: Interpersonal Relations in Nursing. New York, GP Putnam's, 1952

Pluckhan ML: Human Communication: The Matrix of Nursing. New York, McGraw-Hill, 1978

Rogers C: On Becoming a Person. Boston, Houghton-Mifflin, 1961

Rogers CR: The necessary and sufficient conditions of therapeutic personality change. J Consult Psychol 21:95–103, 1957

Simms L, Lindberg J: The Nurse Person, New York, Harper & Row, 1978

Steckel SB: Contracting with patient-selected reinforcers. Am J Nurs 9:1596, 1980

Sullivan JL, Deane DM: Humor and health. J Gerontol Nurs 14(1):20–24, 1988

Ufema JK: How to talk to dying patients. Nursing '87 (17)8:43–46, 1987

Watzlawich P, Beavin J, & Jackson D: Pragmatics of Human Communication. New York, WW Norton, 1967

Weidenbach E, Falls CE: Communication: The Key to Effective Nursing. New York, Tiresias Press, 1978

Whaley LF, Wong DL: Effective communication strategies for pediatric practice. Pediatr Nurs 11:429–432, 1985

Wilmington SC: Oral communication—instruction for a career in nursing. J Nurs Ed 25:291–294, 1986

10 | LEARNING AND TEACHING

KEY WORDS	After completing this chapter, students will be able to:
Affective learning Behavior modification Behavioral objectives Behaviorism Cognitive learning Health education Learning – teaching Psychomotor learning Teaching	Describe the learning – teaching interaction as a problem-solving communication process. Recognize behavioristic, cognitive, and humanistic approaches to learning. Describe how the nurse functions as a health educator. Describe the various steps of the teaching-learning interaction in the context of the nursing process. Differentiate behavioral objectives in the cognitive, affective, and psychomotor domains. Describe learner-centered methods of meeting learning needs.

Learning – teaching is an important subconcept of professional nursing. Learning involves a change in behavior and implies adaptation to an environmental situation. If nurses believe that persons grow, adapt, and develop to fulfill human potential as Maslow suggests, then learning is really the process of becoming. As such, learning is less an occasional or episodic activity and more a matter of ongoing change. Nurses need basic knowledge about how their clients learn, which they use both to understand their clients as persons and to understand how learning is sometimes focused to meet immediate health needs.

Theories about learning come from psychology and are applied in education through the practice of teaching. Much of the knowledge about how to teach clients comes from the interdisciplinary study of human communication. Because "person" is the recipient of nursing care, person is the origin and source of health-care needs that nurses address through teaching. Just as client needs determine the care nurses give, it is client learning needs that determine what teaching nurses do. Therefore, the learning – teaching interaction is a nurse-client interaction that requires both effective interpersonal skills and the problem-solving skills of the nursing process. We emphasize learning, that is, put it first, because learning needs precede and determine teaching. Also, placing learning first emphasizes what the client is "doing," learning. Using this logic and emphasis, the nurse is facilitating client learning—a form of health adaptation. When teaching, nurses incorporate interpersonal communication skills as nursing action within the nursing process. Thus, teaching occurs primarily during the implementation (i.e., intervention) phase of the nursing process.

Facilitating learning is a nursing intervention that assumes greater importance as persons take more responsibility for their own health. It is through facilitating client learning that the nurse can function as an influential health educator. Clients need information to make informed choices, control their health situations, and mobilize their strengths. Clients may also need to learn new behaviors, new activities, and different feeling responses to internal and external stressors. Nurses individualize teaching just as they individualize other interventions. A learning need corresponds to other nursing diagnoses; it can be a problem to be solved or a strength to be augmented. To facilitate learning, nurses will use all their nursing-process and interpersonal communication skills. Therefore, what clients learn is in part an evaluation of nurses' teaching abilities and also of their sensitivity to basic and higher-level needs.

THEORIES ABOUT LEARNING

Many theories about learning attempt to explain the phenomenon. We still have much to discover about why learning occurs as it does. Psychologists who support various learning theories offer different explanations of how learning occurs. Instead of considering various theories as being in conflict with one another, it is often more useful to regard them as focusing on different aspects of learning or behaving. As Reilly suggested, numerous theories are rooted in various assumptions about humans, the nature of knowledge, and the process by which persons learn (1975, p 2).

An eclectic approach to learning, which the authors advocate, presumes that no one learning theory is more correct than another. An eclectic approach leads one to select from various theories, using whatever fits best from each source while being alert to the inconsistencies of different theories. For our purposes, we shall divide learning theories according to whether they emphasize behavior, cognition or thought processes, or a humanistic-holistic view of the person. A brief discussion of the various types of learning theories will enable us to compare and contrast them.

Behavioristic Learning Theories
Conditioning

Behaviorism represents learning as a process of making connections through association. Its origin is the conditioned response. This technique, developed by Ivan Pavlov (1849–1936) with his salivating dogs, was more concerned with neurology than psychology. Behaviorism itself was founded by John B. Watson (1878–1958). The contemporary proponent of conditioning is B. F. Skinner (1904–   ), the father of behavioral technology. Skinner concentrated on the role of reinforcement in establishing conditioned or desired responses. As Carpenter explained in *The Skinner Primer*, "the central principle of learning . . . refers to the fact that an act becomes more frequent when it is followed by a positive consequence" (1974, p 32). Although Skinner's principles of reinforcement were developed in the animal laboratory with pigeons, they can be applied to the control of health-related behavior by means of behavior modification programs.

Behavior Modification

Behavior modification has been widely used to control smoking and also to achieve socially acceptable behavior in a variety of institutions. **Behavior modification** involves a carefully planned schedule of positive reinforcement when desired behavior occurs. This reinforcement may involve tokens, approval, or praise from a significant person. The reinforcement must be perceived as positive by the learner as well as the teacher.

As persons with health problems become aware of how behavior modification works, they may choose to provide their own meaningful reinforcement. For instance, they may use biofeedback techniques to reduce stress and promote relaxation. The consumer movement in health care has had the important effect of bringing health information and reinforcement under client or internal control. For example, expectant mothers choose natural childbirth and husbands become helpers in reinforcing healthy birthing behaviors.

Nursing Implication

The nurse possesses much information that the client could use to manage his or her own health behavior. Contrary to the way many people understand behavior modification, the learner's response, not the teacher's stimulus, is the key to behavior change. Additionally, for reinforcement to operate in any setting, the learner must believe that what is to be learned will help meet a particular need. Consider the following example, the situation of Mrs. Williams.

> Mrs. Williams, age 40, is some 50 pounds overweight and was recently diagnosed as being hypertensive. She admits to being somewhat concerned about her high blood pressure. Her mother was hypertensive and died of a stroke as a young woman. Until recently, Mrs. Williams did not know that decreasing her weight could possibly also decrease her elevated blood pressure. With the help of her nurse, Mrs. Williams discovered that she is eating a balanced diet but that her caloric intake exceeds her energy expenditure. Given this information, Mrs. Williams' response has been to maintain a reasonable food intake and increase her exercise. A definite weight loss and steadily decreasing blood pressure have provided reinforcement for her to continue the diet and exercise response for several months. Note that her response brought reinforcement that influenced behavior.

$$\text{Response} \longrightarrow \text{Reinforcement} \longrightarrow \text{Future Behavior}$$

The initial step for the nurse is to shape learning by reinforcing—preferably in a positive manner—the adaptive behavior observed in the client-patient. This reinforcement can be done without knowing either what goes on inside the person or exactly why. It is also possible and appropriate to use the natural setting and the client's response, rather than worrying about contriving artificial stimuli. Any possible stimulus the nurse might contrive —such as a size 7 dress or pictures of a slim teenager—would probably be far less effective than the very real stimulus of her mother's fate, which Mrs. Williams chose for herself once she had the necessary information. Because behavioral conditioning focuses on the response of the individual learner, the nurse recognizes that instruction, teaching, or facilitation— just like other nursing interventions—must be individualized to be most effective.

Cognitive Learning Theories

Cognitive learning theorists include the Gestalt psychologists—for example, Max Wertheimer and Kurt Lewin—and developmental psychologists like Piaget. The Gestaltists were concerned with insight, namely the "aha!" experience. This insight involves a perceptual reorganization that allows ideas to combine in such a way that $1 + 1 = 3$ rather than the usual 2. Another way to say this is that insight makes clear the relationships of puzzle pieces to each other, so that the puzzle makes sense. Nurses often do see persons gain sudden insights into complex and puzzling health situations, as the Gestaltists theorize.

Developmental psychologists' important contribution to learning has been a better understanding of age-linked stages of cognitive development. This has led to teaching children at their appropriate stage of development rather than as small adults. For example, a pediatric nurse may apply Piaget's theory and use a three-dimensional model to teach a school-age child about his heart function. The nurse knows that the concept of heart as pump is insufficiently developed in the elementary-school student to be understood through a verbal explanation. The cognitive development of a child at this age is at the stage of concrete operations rather than formal thought. Developmental readiness is a key factor of many cognitive approaches, as is individual readiness expressed as motivation.

Humanistic Approaches to Learning

Humanistic approaches to learning are a rather recent development growing out of humanistic or "third force" psychology. Humanistic approaches to learning emphasize the affective or feeling responses toward learning. This focus remains a prime consideration, even if what is to be learned is new knowledge or a motor skill.

A humanistic approach is sometimes also called existential or phenomenological. *Existential* is a term rooted in philosophy and concerned with a person's subjective

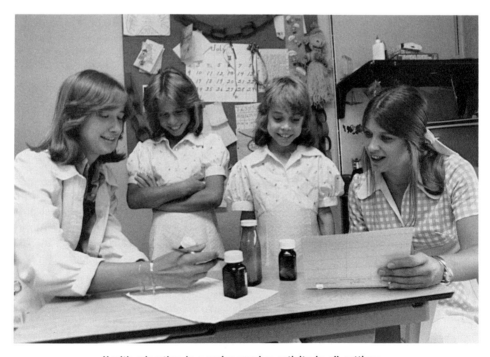

Health education is a major nursing activity in all settings.

awareness of his or her existence. The existential perspective is a self-deterministic view. The term *phenomenological* refers to a concern for what is happening in the here and now. From an existential perspective, behavior is dealt within the present. There is neither the Freudian concern for the past nor the behavioristic emphasis on shaping future behavior.

The humanistic viewpoint emphasizes the importance of the person's view of self, the human being's unique human potential as a learner, and learning as a product of the person's perception. A hallmark of the humanistic approach is the belief that the human being has a basic drive toward health and self-actualization.

Humanism and Holism

The humanistic view of learning is particularly pertinent to a holistic philosophy of health care, that is, one that focuses on the whole person. The rationale for such an approach is rooted in the belief that understanding one's health problems is essential to adapting to those health problems and moving toward health and self-actualization. This view also assumes that where no health problems exit, a person still learns to manage his or her health care to promote continued and heightened well-being. Although each person is unique, the common basic needs shared with fellow humans provide the basis for learning needs common to all persons if they are to achieve self-actualization.

Abraham Maslow (1970) and Carl Rogers (1961) represent theorists who advocate humanistic approaches to learning. Their concepts and principles have a special relevance for nursing.

Maslow's humanistic approach and hierarchy of needs suggest a way to prioritize nursing interventions so that physiological needs are met first, followed by safety and security needs, love and belonging needs, esteem and self-esteem needs, and ultimately growth needs. In Chapter 8 we have made other applications of this hierarchy to the prioritizing of various nursing interventions. Much of traditional nursing care has involved meeting the physiological needs that an ill person was unable to meet for himself or herself. Increasingly, nurses are also focusing their care functions toward promoting and maintaining health and assisting clients to meet growth needs that foster self-actualization. Nurses are also assisting clients to use their own strengths or self-care abilities.

Another humanistic psychologist and teacher who was especially concerned about personalized approaches to the learner was the late Carl Rogers. He contended that "independence, creativity, and self-reliance are all facilitated when self-criticism and self-evaluation are basic and evaluation by others is of secondary importance" (Rogers, 1969, p 163).

Common Beliefs Among Learning Theories

The nurse using an eclectic approach to learning should understand the common beliefs among various learning theories. Table 10–1 summarizes some of these common beliefs and also suggests the approaches emphasized by each theoretical perspective. Using these ideas, along with a basic knowledge of persons as unique individuals and the nursing process, the nurse is ready to consider the many learning needs of clients.

Because the human process of "becoming" is open-ended, there are always learning needs to be identified. Whether a particular learner is willing to address these is another but important consideration, as is the reason for the client's interaction with the health-care

TABLE 10-1
COMPARISON OF BELIEFS COMMON TO MAJOR THEORIES ABOUT LEARNING

Common Beliefs	Approaches		
	Behavioristic	Cognitive	Humanistic
Learner is the focal point of the learning process	Rate of learning differs	Structure needed differs	Significance of learning differs
Learning is a multisensory process	Motor output activity emphasized	Thinking process emphasized	Feelings about learning dominate.
Readiness of the learner is important	Reinforcement must contribute to meeting need learner is ready to address	Developmental readiness is a key factor	Readiness is willingness to experience the "here and now"
Learning is doing	Action of learner starts the chain of reinforcing events that shape behavior	Doing or activity is mental or intellectual	The most significant doing is experiencing with the whole person, that is, feeling as well as thinking
Learner establishes personal significance of learning	Will determine whether reinforcement is seen as positive or negative. Whatever client learns or however he or she behaves is meaningful to him or her	Knowledge gained is perceived by learner as helping him to adapt	Process of learning to learn may be as important as what is learned
The learner needs feedback	Feedback provides information, validation, correction, reinforcement, and confirmation of self-worth as well as ability		
	Result of action influences future action		Person-to-person nonjudgmental feedback of great significance
			Feedback conveys unconditional positive regard for other person as unique and valued individual

delivery system. A ready, active, and motivated learner is essential for any learning process to be successful. Each learner decides how much he or she is willing to invest in coping or mobilizing resources. What the nurse suggests the learner "do" must be acceptable to him or her at some level if it is to receive serious consideration. Can the nurse really assure that the client will feel better, be happier, or live longer? When a client seems to make a maladaptive choice, the nurse assumes the client's frame of reference to understand his rationale.

The nurse who strives to make learning meaningful to the individual increases the chances that a nursing intervention of teaching will be effective. For the client to value the nurse's teaching expertise and seek it again and again, he or she will need to perceive the learning process and its outcome as positive. As health-care professionals, nurses have many opportunities to facilitate client learning, both in carefully planned and extemporaneous ways. Of course, other important considerations include time and resources of both the client and agencies of health-care delivery. Now that we have examined the interpersonal process of learning, we are ready to explore the process of effective teaching.

LEARNING-TEACHING INTERACTION AS PROBLEM-SOLVING PROCESS

The learning-teaching interaction is not only a communication process but also a problem-solving process. As indicated so many times in previous chapters, the nursing process is the problem-solving process of professional nursing. It is logical, therefore, to approach the learning–teaching interaction within the context and organization of the nursing process. This means the steps of the learning–teaching interaction parallel those of the nursing process:

- Collecting data (assessing)
- Determining what the assessment means for this client at this point in time (analyzing)
- Using the data to identify strengths and to state learning needs (identifying problems)
- Clarifying behavioral objectives (formulating goals)
- Identifying appropriate interventions
- Using teaching methods or strategies (implementing interventions)
- Evaluating both learning and teaching
- Evolving a learning-teaching philosophy and synthesizing learning theory (aggregating)

Collecting Data to Assess Learning Needs

Assessing the person's strengths and biophysical needs, including growth and development needs, enables the nurse as teacher to identify problems and learning needs that are truly personalized. Assessing learner needs should include the following steps of assessment:

- Use of empathy to anticipate learning needs
- Assessing level of knowledge, skill, and attitude
- Assessing level of comprehension
- Assessing readiness to learn (motivation)

Beyond the basic learning needs, individual learning needs are difficult to predict. An effective nurse-client relationship is crucial to detecting these individual needs. Without open, sensitive, two-way communication, a nurse never learns what the client wants and needs to learn.

The assessment of a client's current understanding, skill, or attitude communicates this message: "You are a competent person; you are capable of learning and adapting; I will help you build on what you already know and do." Consider what message is conveyed to a client when the nurse does not "start where he or she is" but reteaches what he or she already knows. Consider also the total breakdown of the helping relationship when the nurse begins teaching far beyond the client's understanding.

Beginning with the hypothesis that all clients are capable of learning and comprehending, the effective nurse-educator sees the challenge as that of discovering how best to facilitate client comprehension. Typically, data on stage of growth and development or on level of vocabulary give a rough indication of potential comprehension. But, the possibility exists for the nurse to stereotype levels of comprehension based on social class, occupation, age, or years of formal education. Inbred perceptions of poor people, unskilled workers, older people, or unschooled clients label them "unable to comprehend" before they have a chance to prove otherwise. Nurses avoid such stereotyped labels. Instead, they recognize the value in full, lifelong learning experiences acquired informally and independently through many crises and changes.

Finally, in assessing a learner's readiness to learn, educators speak of a "teachable moment": a period of time in which a learner is receptive and ready to listen, to adapt, to learn. Ideally, then, teaching should be timed to take advantage of a learner's "teachable moments" so that learning occurs more readily.

These moments can often be anticipated. Indeed, the entire concept of anticipatory crisis intervention is derived from the fact that before a predictable crisis—for example, childbirth—a client is open and receptive to learning and growing. Prehospitalization teaching also attempts to promote leaning before a crisis.

In contrast, many other receptive or teachable moments occur spontaneously, informally, and suddenly. Nurses and students sometimes tend to view teaching much too formally, missing many of the constant and unlimited opportunities for informal learning–teaching. A crucial assessment skill is the ability to recognize the client behaviors which are indicative of learning receptivity. Such client behaviors include direct and indirect questions and other information seeking behavior. Some examples might be: some regular exercise, which indicates an awareness of the contribution of exercise to health and possible interest in expanding this activity; breast self-examination, indicating willingness to learn other protective measures such as increasing dietary fiber; reading lay books about health-related matters.

Analyzing the Learning–Teaching Situation

Analyzing the learning–teaching situation involves determining what the assessment means for this client at this point in time. The teacher tries to assess the learner's motivation—the drives, present or future—that would facilitate learning. When a nurse-educator perceives no motivation for learning, it is possible to induce motivation by sustained psychological support. It is important to remember, however, that dealing with other perceived needs may indeed be more important. Remember also that factual information alone is a necessary but not sufficient motivator to change. Therefore, simply telling a person the changes he or she must make in his or her diet will rarely prompt the person to do so, unless he or she is able to express what this change in life style means to him or her as a person.

This is the time to analyze motivation. What is the prime motivation for continuing the learning–teaching process: the needs of the client to learn or the needs of the nurse to teach? Now is also the time to analyze expectations. What are realistic expectations of the learning–teaching interaction? Consider the press of other needs and also the time and other resources available. As clients are sicker and hospital stays are shorter, this analysis becomes more important. Nurses must make the most of their time to facilitate client learning if indeed that is a priority. Taylor suggested the following:

- Start your teaching on admission.
- Teach at every opportunity.
- Set realistic goals for your patient.
- Include the family in your teaching plan.
- Use teaching aids and group instruction.
- Document what you teach
  (1987, p 20–21)

Based on the data collected about the person and other pressing needs, the nurse will analyze whether a suggestion such as group instruction will be effective and efficient for this particular situation.

Stating Learning Needs

Once the nurse identifies data indicative of a client's learning need, the question arises, "How do I work these data into the nursing process?" The answer is found in the following test: "If the assessment demonstrates a learning need, then begin a learning-teaching process within the nursing process."

In other words, proceed to state a learning problem or need, set mutually acceptable learning goals, enact teaching interventions, and evaluate progress.

Typically, a learning need can be stated as a problem in a variety of ways, for example:

- Limited knowledge of prescribed medications
- Anxiety caused by limited ability to perform one's own personal care

Such problems, as with any problem statement, should be validated with the client or family if at all possible: "I wonder if you'd like more information, or if you'd like to talk about this procedure you'll have tomorrow?"

Clarifying Behavioral Objectives

At this point in the learning–teaching process and within the nursing process, goals are formulated to direct the interventions that follow. These will clarify the expected outcomes of teaching or facilitation of learning. Specifically, learning goals are called **behavioral objectives**. *Behavioral* learning objectives are statements of what the client will do or say as evidence of learning. Such behavioral learning objectives describe the intended outcome of learning, stating the performance expected of the learner as a result of teaching (Mager, 1962). They state measurable behavior changes, such as the ones listed at the beginning of each chapter in this text. Standard format reads, "The learner will . . ."

Because learning occurs in three domains, behavioral learning objectives are stated within each domain:

- Cognitive
- Affective
- Psychomotor

Cognitive learning objectives use verbs demonstrating results of thinking processes: "The client will state how salt affects his blood pressure."

Affective learning objectives reflect the client's feelings, attitudes, and values: "The client will express her reactions to her mastectomy scar."

Psychomotor learning objectives state actions and skills: "The client will demonstrate clean technique in changing his dressing."

The nurse who communicates effectively with the client will have the necessary information to assist in writing realistic and meaningful objectives and in deciding which learning priorities are important for the client.

Identifying and Implementing Teaching Interventions

An incredible number of teaching interventions exist, some traditional, some innovative. How do you choose teaching methods and materials? Various interventions — or teaching methods — can be effective if chosen to match the client's learning needs and behavioral learning objective: the most creative lecture will not reach psychomotor skill; clients can learn effective expression if there is an opportunity to vent feelings. (Teaching may also be required for them to learn how to vent.)

Again, it is important to remember that the whole point of implementing teaching interventions is to communicate information that will enable clients to change their knowledge, feelings, attitudes and values, or psychomotor action and skills. In fact, Redman defined teaching itself as a special type of communication that is carefully structured and sequenced to produce learning (1984, p 8). Teaching uses basic communication skills such as active listening, empathy, helping responses, and assertiveness. The client who needs to learn how to change a colostomy drainage bag wants the nurse to understand what it means to him or her to do such a procedure. Similarly, the nurse may be called on to teach other than technical aspects of care. The client who wants to learn how to express his or her needs more openly seeks a signal from the nurse that he or she also recognizes this client priority as an important component of care. Other skills of supporting and crisis intervention are interwoven.

Further consideration of the learner's ability, developmental stage, cultural values, and past experiences aids the choice of teaching methods. Each client's reading ability, visual and hearing ability, and interest level differ. The nurse chooses reading materials appropriate to the reading level of the client and compensates for sensory losses when teaching. Common problems of ineffective teaching result from methods below or beyond the client's developmental stage. In a recent study, Streiff asked whether clients understand nurses' instructions. Sadly, she found that "the majority of study participants (54.7%) read at levels that did not allow them to comprehend any of the patient education materials available at their site of primary care" (Streiff, 1986, p 48).

Children's education progresses with their levels of concentration, abstraction, and coordination. Knowledge of growth and development is applied when teaching children about health. In contrast, children's materials are not appropriate in teaching adults, however dependent they may be. When teaching, nurses rely on general guidelines for matching teaching methods to client needs. Very many such guidelines have been written, most of them concentrating on the nurse. The learner-centered guide to teaching methods presented in Table 10–2 provides a contrast. This guide proposes that the nurse can

TABLE 10–2
LEARNER-CENTERED GUIDE TO TEACHING METHOD

Learning Need	Method
If a person needs to learn:	The nurse can facilitate learning by using:
Awareness of self, own attitudes, and values	ive exercises, questionnaires, values-clarification activities
Awareness of others' situation, attitudes, and values	Roleplaying, interacting with others with similar conditions or strengths or problems
Awareness of own behavior	Reverse role-playing, audio or video playback, analysis of interactions
Basic factual information	Lectures and discussion, reading, self-directed media programs
Concepts and relationships of ideas	Reading, discussion, models and graphics
Application of concepts to practice	Opportunity for guided practice
Manual skill	Skill practice, demonstration – return demonstration, programmed learning
Relating to others	Group discussion, play groups, roleplaying, counseling
Self-expression, self-confidence	Group discussion, creative arts (music, art, movement), positive reinforcement, role modeling
Decision making, priority setting	Make decisions and receive feedback
Adaptation to life style change	Counseling, self-help and mutual help groups, contracting

facilitate learning by focusing on what the learner or client needs to learn, rather than on what the teacher or nurse wants to teach. Additionally, the methods in the guide require some form of communication or interpersonal interaction, either "live" or using previously prepared communication materials.

Ever more creative teaching methods evolve constantly. The use of artistic expression in composition, movement, music, and drama has developed particularly in mental health settings. Relaxation methods of controlled breathing, hypnosis, meditation, biofeedback, expressive exercise, and introspection prevail in learning stress reduction, self-control, and pain relief. The ever-increasing use of audio and videotapes for self-instruction in health-care settings, home, school, and the workplace has expanded health teaching immeasurably. All these methods and many others are available for nurses to employ in teaching. There are also many traditional library resources to assist nurses' teaching and facilitation of clients' learning. One such book, *Teaching in Nursing Practice: a Professional Model* (Whitman and associates, 1986), seems particularly well suited to beginning nurses.

Beginning nurses (including students) are also more likely than experienced nurses to use a teaching plan that is actually written out. Such a plan may be in a form similar to the one included in the following example (Table 10–3). Just as with nursing process record-ing, the written teaching plan provides an opportunity for feedback from peers and experts.

TABLE 10-3
SPECIFICS OF A TEACHING PLAN FOR MRS. ROBINSON

Learning Need	Behavioral Objective	Intervention
Cognitive—limited knowledge of altered respiratory status	Mrs. R. will verbalilze alterations in respiration and appropriate interventions for these	Explain briefly how respiratory function is compromised by surgery, anesthesia, and pain. Explain what intervention is necessary. Demonstrate procedure for coughing and deep breathing.
Affective—feelings of helplessness after surgery	Mrs. R. will verbalize decreased feelings of helplessness and therefore be receptive to learning	Spend time with her even when she does not talk. Help her vent feelings of helplessness. Listen carefully to facilitate development of trusting relationship. Acknowledge and reinforce all positive, growth-oriented behaviors. Assist her to view herself as a total person rather than focusing on limitations. Assist both person and family to express their feelings to each other.
Psychomotor—decreased muscle function as a result of surgery, anesthesia, and pain medication	Mrs. R. will maintain clear lungs and will gradually increase mobility from a few steps to regular hall ambulation	Assist with coughing and deep breathing q 1–2 hr while awake and q 3–4 hr during sleep hours. Assist with ambulation q.i.d. until able to proceed without assistance. Help her walk a bit farther each time.

Evaluating Learning

If, indeed, the nurse has developed a learning–teaching process within the nursing process, the evaluation component flows logically from the goals and interventions. Just as evaluation is an important component of the nursing process, it is an equally important component of the learning–teaching process.

We can refer again to the brief example in Table 10–3 to provide an illustration for evaluating learning. Note that the learning needs and corresponding behavioral objectives span all three domains of learning: cognitive, affective, and psychomotor. All three objectives require different ways of evaluating to determine what was learned. For the cognitive or knowledge objective, the nurse will want to evaluate what the client "knows" as a result of the learning–teaching interaction. There are many nonthreatening ways to create situations in which the client can demonstrate his or her knowledge. Based on this information, the nurse will determine whether or not this objective has been meet. The evaluation of affective objectives requires creating the climate and opportunity for voicing feelings. This in turn suggests both that feelings will be expressed and that this expression will be in the direction (decreased helplessness) intended. In this example, the positive or satisfactory evaluation of psychomotor objectives requires that the client demonstrate both the coughing and ambulating (walking) behaviors.

Imagine that an evaluation of a teaching plan for Mrs. Robinson reveals the following: objectives 1 and 2 were both met; however, we conclude that objective 3 — the psychomotor objective — was only partially achieved. From oral and written reports, it is evident that Mrs. Robinson ambulates when assisted or reminded but does not take the initiative to ambulate unaided although she is physically able to do so. As a result of this evaluation, our nursing plan may be as follows:

- Continue to provide gentle reminders of the need to increase ambulation.
- Acknowledge and reinforce efforts to increase ambulation.
- Plan part of the time spent with Mrs. Robinson to include ambulation.
- Allow additional quiet time together when she can express other feelings or concerns.

Teaching skill develops over time and with practice. While observation of other teachers helps the novice learn methods and techniques, each teacher must employ creativity to develop an individual style. With each teaching experience, a way to learn is to ask these questions:

- How would I improve this session the next time I teach it?
- Did the client meet his goals, i.e., the behavioral learning objectives?
- If so, what are the factors leading to his success?
- If not, what happened to prevent this accomplishment.

Although it is possible to measure the client's learning when using behavioral objectives, it is nearly impossible to predict what long-term influence the nurse may have had on the client or how a single individual may have motivated his or her future learning, for only the learner determines what will be learned. Durbach and co-workers made this same point: "We must also consider whether our quest for measurable learning outcomes really encourages the kind of evaluation of learning and teaching that is most helpful to clinicians and patients. . . . Behavioral objectives tend to favor the concrete and measurable over the abstract and subtle" (1987, p 88).

Facilitating client learning is what the nursing intervention of teaching is all about. Teaching usually involves a learning facilitation that has many dimensions. Often the more formal didactic presentation or lecture-demonstration is our initial thought about how to teach. With more attention to the matter, many of the learner-centered methods in Table 10–2 may occur to us.

THE NURSE AS A HEALTH EDUCATOR

Health Education

In 1976, President Gerald Ford signed into law the National Consumer Health Information and Health Promotion Act, defining six activities of consumer health education:

1   Inform people about health, illness, disability, and ways in which they can improve and protect their own health, including the more efficient use of the delivery system.

2 Motivate people to want to change to more healthful practices.

3 Help people to learn the necessary skills to adopt and maintain healthful practices.

4 Foster teaching and communication skills in all those engaged in educating consumers about health.

5 Advocate changes in the environment that will facilitate healthful conditions and healthful behavior.

6 Add to knowledge through research and evaluation concerning the most effective ways of achieving these objectives (Somers, 1978).

Concepts of clients' rights, advocacy, consumerism, health behavior, adaptation, communication, and research pervade this law.

All health professionals share responsibility for health education, that is, facilitating another's learning to live and adapt in the healthiest possible style. Nurses are important health educators. Health is, after all, nursing's primary domain, and nurses outnumber the members of any other health profession. Nurses are also with clients 24 hours a day in hospitals where a great deal of teaching occurs.

The ability of persons to learn health promotion and preventive practices, to learn to manage illness, and to learn to care for themselves and dependents underlies the health of the nation.

Health Education Activities

Health education activities span the entire range of health care: prevention, maintenance, recovery, and rehabilitation. The nurse-educator who teaches school children basic health habits helps them to learn illness prevention. Assisting an older person to regulate and monitor several medications exemplifies health maintenance teaching. Nurses teach preoperative and postoperative care to hasten recovery from surgery and, equally important, to shorten hospital stays, while nurses working in hospice programs teach dying persons and their families how to adapt to death. Because increasing the cost effectiveness of health care is a national priority, it is important for nurses to document their health education activities that contribute to these efforts.

Health education, then, is a life span activity that includes many types of professionals, many levels of health care, and many locations. As interest in sports and physical fitness, healthy nutrition, and aging increases, relatively unexplored areas for health teaching become obvious.

Health Education Categories

The scope of health education activities spans the following categories, each succeeding group representing a slightly narrower focus:

- Community health education
- Occupational health education
- School health education
- Group health education
- Family health education
- Client/patient education

In their broadest form, immunization campaigns and stop-smoking media campaigns, for example, attempt to teach large communities of persons. Health teaching done in businesses, industries, and schools attempts to maintain healthy workers and students. Such teaching may be concerned with helping persons to make their health needs known or helping them to learn strategies for resolution of lifelong developmental tasks. When focused on groups of persons, families, and friends, health teaching promotes mental and physical health of colleagues, parents, and children. Persons who are ill receive care and teaching in both formal and informal education sessions. Such teaching may instruct about how to increase functional abilities given personal limitations.

Although nurses have focused traditionally on client and family teaching, the opportunities increase yearly for teaching throughout the broad scope of the categories listed above and across the entire life span. The efficient use of teaching opportunities will need to increase also. With increasing severity of illness and decreasing length of stay in traditional hospital settings, traditional means of delivering health teaching could be caught in the squeeze. Facilitating client learning in the optimal way will be a challenge to all nurses' effective communication, nursing-process skills, creative teaching methods, and use of modern instructional technology.

Very early in a nursing program, students gain a wealth of experience in health teaching. Anyone with interests in health, teaching, and communication may find nursing offers unexpected opportunities.

CLINICAL EXAMPLE SYNTHESIZING COMMUNICATION AND LEARNING–TEACHING PROCESS

Nurses often have the opportunity to combine their skills in communicating and teaching in ways that create remarkable results. The following clinical example provides such an illustration. In this example, the nurse communicated with and taught both the client and his spouse. The communication was effective and the learning of both was confirmed as the illustration validates.

Mr. and Mrs. Johnson are a couple in their late 50s who had recently been married. They had known each other many years before, but Mr. Johnson had previously been married to someone else; Mrs. Johnson had never married. After they had met again, they decided to marry, but continued to live apart for several months while they arranged to combine their two homes and financial situations gradually.

During this period, shortly following their marriage, Mr. Johnson began having urinary difficulties caused by prostate problems and entered the hospital for surgery. He came to the state where his wife was residing so that she could be closer to him and assist in his convalescence. After the surgery, he had difficulty urinating and finally had to begin a program of intermittent self-catheterization (ISC), that is, using a drainage tube to empty his bladder. Mr. Johnson seemed unable to do this at all, so the nurses did the catheterization procedure for him at the beginning. Mrs. Johnson was very upset because she felt her husband was highly nervous and would never be able to do this himself. Furthermore, she stated that she could not do it for him. The nurses noted that Mr. and Mrs. Johnson were very shy with each other and, while they seemed to have a warm and affectionate relationship, they had apparently not developed much intimacy. Having to deal with this very intimate problem seemed to leave them baffled and overwhelmed.

In addition, the physicians were eager for Mr. Johnson to leave the hospital because of economic issues. Since he was technically able (medically) to leave the hospital, the insurance reimbursement might be doubtful if he stayed longer. Thus, communication, learning–teaching, and economics were the challenges faced by the primary nurse over the next 2 days. It may seem surprising that she was able to help this couple work through the problems they had, improve their own communication and begin work toward a more intimate relationship, learn a somewhat difficult procedure, and leave the hospital in record time. This is what she did.

1. The nurse spent time with the husband and wife separately, assessing their needs and listening to their fears and concerns. Although she was gentle and very patient, she quietly helped them to understand that ISC would be necessary for a short time. She explained that they would have support and that a nurse could visit them at home for awhile to answer their questions. However, she also told them that the visiting nurse would not be available to do the catheterization procedure.

2. The nurse did the catheterization procedure several times with the husband and wife together and had them watch. Gradually, she had first one, and then the other, take over parts of the process. Although at times she found the situation exasperating, she remained composed and talked them slowly through the procedure. She had to be firm and insist, particularly with Mr. Johnson, that he stay focused and give his attention to the immediate situation. Eventually, they both were able to do the catheterization procedure. The nurse also reminded Mr. Johnson that his wife was only to do the procedure when he was very tired, or occasionally for a break. She emphasized that this was his responsibility. She also told the couple that Mr. Johnson should continue trying to empty his bladder normally and probably would be able to do so within a few days after returning to a more comfortable environment.

3. Evaluation came when the nurse was able to see Mr. Johnson sucessfully demonstrate ISC. However, another way of evaluating was to hear what Mrs. Johnson stated to the head nurse. She said that the nurse's kind and gentle manner, along with a certain firmness that finally made them see the need to learn the procedure, was the reason that they had been successful when she (Mrs. Johnson) had never thought it possible. The nurse had given support, helped them feel less shy with each other, and provided good instruction for their learning.

In addition, by facilitating the discharge of Mr. Johnson at an earlier date than was thought possible, the nurse dealt with the economic issues as well.

| CONCLUSION

The learning–teaching interaction was singled out as a special application of interpersonal communication and problem solving, and teaching was approached as the facilitation of client learning. Nurses will use all their interpersonal communication skills and knowledge of learning theories to facilitate learning within the nursing process framework. Nurses, as "health" professionals, must assume considerable responsibility for educating their own clients and for the nation's health education.

| STUDY QUESTIONS

1   Define teaching and learning. How do they differ? What is the primary focus in a nurse-client, learning–teaching interaction? Give a rationale for your answer.

2 What are your strengths or unique personal skills that might influence the learning–teaching process?

3 How can teaching methods be adapted for adults? Children? Elders?

4 Write an original behavioral objective for each of the learning domains:

  a Cognitive — thinking,

  b Affective — feeling,

  c Psychomotor — action or skills

5 Describe how knowledge of Maslow's hierarchy of needs might help you assess a learner's motivation.

| BIBLIOGRAPHY

Carpenter F: The Skinner Primer. New York, Free Press, 1974

Durbach E, Goodall R, Wilkinson K: Instructional objectives in patient education. Nurs Outlook 35(2):82–83, 88, 1987

Mager R: Preparing Instructional Objectives. Palo Alto, Fearon, 1962

Mager R: Preparing Instructional Objectives, 2nd ed. Belmont, CA, Pitman Management & Training, 1984

Maslow AH: Motivation and Personality, 2nd ed. New York, Harper & Row, 1970

Redman BK: The Process of Patient Education, 5th ed. St. Louis, CV Mosby, 1984

Reilly DE: Behavioral Objectives in Nursing: Evaluation of Learner Attainment. New York, Appleton-Century, 1975

Rogers C: On Becoming a Personal. Boston, Houghton-Mifflin, 1961

Rogers C: Freedom to Learn. Columbus, OH, CE Merrill, 1969

Somers A: Promoting health, consumer education and national policy. Nurs Digest 6:1–11, 1978

Streiff LD: Can clients understand our instructions? Image 18(2):48–52, 1986

Taylor RA: Making the most of your time for patient teaching. RN 50(12):20–21, 1987

Whitman NI, Graham BA, Gleit CJ, et al: Teaching in Nursing Practice: A Professional Model. Norwalk, CT, Appleton-Century-Crofts, 1986

11 | NURSING ETHICS AND LEGAL ASPECTS

KEY WORDS	After completing this chapter, students will be able to:
Accountability	**Describe basic human rights.**
Bioengineering	**Describe a person focus for bioethics.**
Bioethics	**Identify examples of personal bioethical issues that are of**
Documentation	**particular concern to you.**
Liability	
Licensure	**Identify major ethical issues confronting nurses, other health**
Litigation	**professionals, and society.**
Malpractice	**Describe accountability.**
Nursing standard	
Policy	
Psychological	
competence	
Reasonable care	
Rights	
Values	
Values clarification	

This chapter introduces you to some of the many ethical and legal aspects of nursing and health care. Ethical issues and legalities of health care are subjects of comprehensive nursing books. Obviously, this discussion will be only a cursory introduction, presenting some of the more common ideas, terms, and concepts that are relevant to nursing practice. For specific legal advice, nurses consult lawyers or primary sources of legal information. Similarly, difficult ethical issues stimulate a need for interdisciplinary consultation, discussion, and consideration of varying ethical viewpoints. The field of bioethics is growing rapidly both in scope and prominence. Nurses need to be well informed about its development and involved in shaping the relationship between bioethics and nursing practice.

As Davis and Aroskar wrote, "Moral philosophers beginning with Socrates, Plato, and Aristotle have for centuries attempted to answer the two major questions of ethics: What is the meaning of right? of good? and, what ought I to do?" (1978, p 20).

The lay use of the term *moral* generally means conforming to the rules of right conduct defined by a particular social group. Morality is one type of social regulation of behavior. For some issue areas, morality and law are similar. In other areas, considerably more variation in conduct is culturally influenced. For example, before the revolution in socially acceptable sexual conduct, sexual morality was equated with virtue or chastity, especially for females. Though laws have changed little, a return to more restrained sexual behavior has been culturally influenced by the concern for AIDS.

Ethics is a discipline involved with good and bad, moral duty, obligation, and values. Ethics is also concerned with social and political philosophy and the philosophy of law. Only in the last decade has biomedical ethics been a well recognized discipline. Because biomedical ethical issues have implications for other life and health sciences, we prefer the term **bioethics** to designate those health issues of an ethical nature that concern nurses.

The professional use of the term *ethics* implies a high standard of moral quality of professional practice. Accepted practice standards of one's peers are professed in occupational codes of ethics as for nursing, medicine, law, etc. (See Chapter 2 for the Code for Nurses.) Ketéfian identified a dimension of moral behavior for nurses called "professionally ideal moral behavior" which was defined as "professionally valued and ideal nursing behaviors that are congruent with the principles expressed in the Code for Nurses" (1987, p 13).

Although bioethical issues are of social and economic significance, the person is the focus for our initial consideration of ethical issues and their implications for nurses.

The concept of client autonomy is a recurring theme of ethical issues. Autonomous means independent and self-governing. Autonomous describes an essential quality of "person" as well as a type of behavior. The autonomous person can be described as being rational and unrestrained. This indicates that the person is self-governing and independent regarding his or her decisions and activity. As Mappes and Zembaty (1981) stated, the fully rational person has a number of abilities related to formulating and achieving personal goals.

Persons who are not aware or rational may be unable to demonstrate autonomous behavior. However, autonomy remains an essential quality of their person, that is, a part of human character, integrity, and holism, and preserving that autonomy becomes a concern for nurses as professional care-givers of such persons. When clients are not independent regarding either decisions or activity, nurses intervene. Nurses help persons do those things that they would do unaided if they had the necessary strength, will, or knowledge. They do this in a manner that enables the client to be as independent or autonomous as possible.

To be sure that they do not impose their personal goals on clients, nurses need to develop self-awareness about their own continuous growth and development. Self-awareness also helps to guard against exercising any personal need to control or have inordinate authority over others. Whenever students or graduate nurses find themselves labeling clients — calling them "stubborn," "uncooperative," or "noncompliant" — it is instructive for them to take stock of their own expectations and behaviors. These situations are common warning signals that a power struggle may be developing; they are particularly inappropriate and suggest that nursing is not being practiced from a perspective that values clients' abilities for self-care and autonomy. The nurturance or nursing of these self-care powers is the ultimate goal of nursing judgments and action. Some would actually call this the nurturance of autonomy — a state of knowing and freely exercising persons' actual reality-based choices.

Many persons who seek the services of health professionals may rightly or wrongly believe that their autonomy is threatened because of their dependency on others for care services. Ill and hospitalized persons are likely to believe themselves constrained even when they are aware and rational.

Two particular constraints that may be of concern are lack of ability and coercion. An example of the former constraint is the elderly person who lacks the strength to resist heroic lifesaving measures. Constraints on a person's autonomy can sometimes be justified to prevent public or private harm, to benefit the individual or others, to prevent offensive behavior in public, or to prevent self-harm (Mappes and Zembaty, 1981, p 11). Fatherly interference with a person's autonomy is a form of control called *paternalism*. Although we usually think of paternalistic interference as compromising or constraining the rights of clients, it may not be intentionally limiting and often goes unrecognized.

| VALUES

The concept of values is a basic notion underlying both the scholarly discipline of ethics and the practical application of ethics in a profession. In Chapter 4, the idea of values was introduced as a characteristic of persons that both makes them unique and defines the beliefs they share with other persons. A **value** is a belief or custom that frequently arises from cultural or ethnic backgrounds, family tradition, peer group ideas and practices, political philosophies in one's country, and educational and religious philosophies with which one identifies. Values, therefore, help explain similarities and differences between individuals and groups.

Values are often based in intangibles rather than in fact and may be so strongly held as to be worth dying for, for example, honor, freedom, family. Values are powerful motivators of behavior. To determine persons' values, we can observe how they use their personal and material resources. The following questions are examples of those we might ask: How does each care for his or her physical body, use time and money, and relate to other people?

We commonly use the term *value* in such a way that it is attached to the person rather than the thing valued. Things or ideas generally valued by many people — such as health and friendship — come to be labeled as valuable in and of themselves. Hence the use of adjectives to describe cultural, scientific, and humanitarian values.

Development of Values

Values are both simple and complex and vary in the degree to which they are believed to be important by the person. Because values are learned, they parallel other learned behavior, taking shape in early life and being influenced first by early care-givers and family. Later, peer experiences, formal learning, and societal institutions shape values. As people become more autonomous in behavior, they act on not only those values personally held, but also on those they understand to be acceptable to the larger social system of which they are a part. The more important values become part of a personal moral conduct. At this point in our discussion of developing values, it is appropriate to consider a prominent theoretical approach to moral development as proposed by Kohlberg (1987).

Moral Developmental Approach to Ethical Issues

Moral development begins with the transition from instinctive thought to a higher form of thinking based on logic. The work of Kohlberg (1987) presents a hierarchical organization for understanding moral development. (Fig. 11–1).

This representation is somewhat similar to both Maslow's hierarchy of needs and

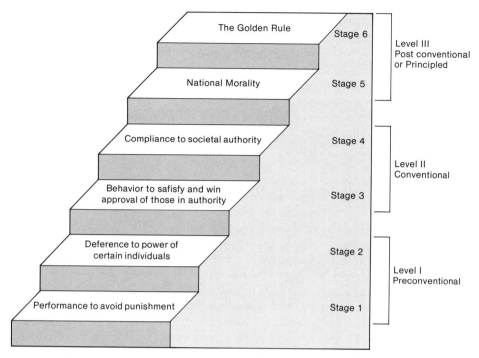

Figure 11-1 Hierarchy of moral development (according to Kohlberg).

Piaget's stages of cognitive development (see Chapter 4.) Kohlberg's three-level model helps one to relate individual moral growth to an accepted pattern of moral development for persons in contemporary American society. This model further divides moral development into six stages—two in each level—as detailed in the following discussion. Not every person achieves the highest level of moral functioning, just as not all persons achieve self-actualization as described by Maslow.

Level I moral development (preconventional) occurs in early childhood with the beginning of value development. At this age, the self is completely dependent on adults for nearly all aspects of existence from physical needs of food and shelter to other needs such as safety and love. In the first stage of level I, moral behavior becomes equated with performance to avoid punishment. Deference to the power of certain individuals in an unquestioning way characterizes the second stage of this level. At this age, the child accepts the labeling of behavior by significant others, whether they be parents or care-givers. We can use this model to understand the children's behavior in the much-publicized child molestation accusations against a California child-care center several years ago. Given these stages of moral development, it is not surprising that the preschoolers involved were not vocal about alleged incidents. The children believed their behavior to be good or bad as labeled by the adults in authority. This is more obvious after the fact and when viewed from Kohlberg's theoretical perspective.

Level II development (conventional), according to Kohlberg, occurs at a time when children are moving from concrete operations to the formal operations of adult thought.

This shift enables persons to envision various hypothetical alternatives relating to issues. The transition to formal thought occurs at different ages for different individuals, and, for some persons, the cognitive shift precedes the moral development growth by several years.

In stage 3 of level II, the norm for interpersonal rules is still that behavior which satisfies individuals in authority and wins their approval. One can imagine that a child in the health-care system who is at stage 3 may be reluctant not to do as asked, even if frightened, angry, or hesitant for other reasons. In stage 4 of level II, where compliance to societal authority becomes a more accepted mode of behavior, reluctance to ask questions may have a different etiology.

Level III development (postconventional or principled), the challenging of conventional morality, is an adolescent characteristic. Stage 5 of this level is sometimes called the stage of national morality and has been identified as the governmental morality that affects national health-care policy. The legalistic orientation that characterizes this stage is directed toward rights and obligations expressed in contracts between professionals and parties being served. This last level of moral development is also labeled the autonomous or principled level. Principles apply not just for their law and order values, but because they express society's consensus about what is right. Stage 6 of level III moral development goes beyond a circumscribed national view and pertains to humankind in general. This stage has also been characterized as applying The Golden Rule.

For most nurses, the initial socialization to professional values occurs during late adolescence or early adulthood. At this point, many persons may not have reached closure of their personal moral developmental process. Thus, adding professional responsibilities complicates coping with ethical issues. It is usually comforting to students to realize that professional faculty understand this developmental process and, further, that they are eager to assist students in making this transition. Growth beyond Kohlberg's stages of conventional morality makes one sensitive to universal ethical and moral principles as well as to the value of unique persons and their differing views.

As Davis and Aroskar stated:

> Nurses could form a consensus and move actively to Kohlberg's 6th stage — that is, the principled thinking orientation — and actively practice the principle of respect for the individual person. What changes would have to be made in the bureaucratic structure and organization of work for this principle to be honored in patient care? Who should bear the costs? (1983, p 83)

Values Clarification

Moral judgments in both personal and professional life are made in relation to values, not facts. Because any person holds individual and shared values, both clients and nurses hold wide ranges of values. Given this reality, it is apparent that very often nurses and their clients will hold dissimilar values. Dissimilar values can contribute to misunderstanding or serious conflicts. If nurses are going to give person-centered care, they will need to find ways to accommodate these differences. This accommodation must be achieved both for the sake of their clients' health care and also for the sake of nurses' own personal and professional well-being. Understanding one's own values can be a first step that helps a nurse to identify, understand, and learn strategies that accommodate these differences. As Steele and Harmon stated, "The goal of values clarification is to facilitate self-understanding" (1983, p 1).

Values clarification, is as the name suggests, clarifying what values are important to a person. It is a self-awareness process that not only identifies what values are "me," but also asks the individual to prioritize or rate different values to determine which are most important. This detailed self-assessment gives a more complete picture of one's total individual value system.

Values clarification exercises can be oriented toward both personal and professional values. Questions in personal values clarification exercises might include the following examples.

- Name five things that are most important to your life today.
- List five goals you would most like to achieve in your lifetime.
- How did you spend your time last week? Divide the time into 5% blocks for major activities. Compare how this time allotment relates to the things you think are most important and the goals you hope to achieve.

Questions nurses might ask regarding professional goals include

- How much do I value nursing as a commitment to a lifelong career of learning and competence?
- Do I like to care for some kinds of clients and not others?
- Do I prefer healthy to ill? young to old? physical to psychological disabilities?

A first step in accomplishing exercises like the preceding is to reflect on such questions privately. A second and more enlightening step is to participate in values clarification activities with nurse peers, other health professionals, and laypersons outside the health professions.

Many specific reasons exist for nurses to examine their value systems.

- Some inconsistencies in personal values are not apparent until consciously examined.
- Some inconsistencies may cause problems if conflicting values are caught in the decision-making process.
- Personal values may conflict with certain professional practice responsibilities.
- Examining values can guide ethical choices in professional practice.
- Values clarification contributes toward functioning at a higher level of moral reasoning.

As Steele and Harmon stated:

Values clarification can result in personal growth, in establishing values which are consistent, and in helping in the decision-making process. It is one strategy for making practitioners more humanistic and it fosters the art of professional practice. . . . It also gives direction for the assessment of clients' values. It provides direction for planning and implementing individualized nursing interventions which incorporate the nurturing and caring behaviors of the profession. (1983, p 16)

| A Person Focus for Bioethics

A person focus for the bioethics of concern to nurses makes logical sense because persons are indeed the recipients of nursing care. While nurses care for persons both as individuals and in groups, they do so in ways that are always mindful of individual dignity, values, and rights. Because of this immense concern for individuals, not only by nurses but by other professionals and clients themselves, the concept of autonomy is a recurring theme of ethical issues.

Rights of Person and Group

The term **rights** has an ethical connotation as well as a legal definition. As Davis and Aroskar wrote, "Rights as entitlements are claimed to privacy, to life, to die, to a healthy environment, and to health. Special rights of various groups, such as children, the mentally retarded, and pregnant women, are also claimed" (1983, p 68).

The idea of personal rights is clearly related to concern and respect for the individual member of the society. Who gives, monitors, and protects which rights and for whom is not so clearly defined. Claims about rights might be viewed as assertions or demands intended to influence and change social and legal boundaries of health-care policy. For example, some claim the right to health itself while others argue that access to health care is the issue.

The concept of individual rights becomes an issue or problem when the values of individuals or rights of individuals conflict. Individual persons (clients, client, and caregiver) may have conflicts. Or situations may arise where an individual is in conflict with the rights of society: for example, a psychotic person capable of injuring others. Conflicting rights are illustrated by persons' rights to confidentiality in conflict with the public good and society's rights in reporting gunshot wounds, venereal disease, and child abuse. Similar but less obvious conflicts might include persons' rights to engage in behavior that interferes with gaining or maintaining health. For example, substance abusers, the overweight, drunk drivers, and persons refusing to wear seat belts or motorcycle helmets inflict a potential economic burden on society for their care. Recently, some women have alleged discrimination against their health rights; specifically, they find the male domination of the medical profession and control of health-care policy to be offensive.

The issue of individual rights is also buried in larger health-care issues which will be discussed later in this chapter. For example, the burgeoning cost of the Medicare system has created a crisis. The diagnostic tests, drug treatments, and high technology that have revolutionized health care have accounted for one third of the rise in cost of the Medicare program in recent years. In this example, the right of certain individuals seeking high technology for extraordinary care — for example, dialysis and transplant — threatens the right of society to fund a system of ordinary basic care for the elderly and the poor. As this decade begins, federal legislation addresses the problem of catastrophic illness. It is possible that ordinary basic care will receive appropriate attention, too.

Perhaps the best known declaration of rights is that published by the American Hospital Association (1970). This Patient's Bill of Rights served to raise the consciousness of both clients and health-care providers (see Table 7–7). Some see this declaration as a well-meaning document without a mechanism for enforcement. Others charge that the statement does no more than pay lip service to an ideal and is thus a mockery. Certainly the stated rights offer a moral challenge to health-care providers to act in the spirit of the intent. Documents which declare the rights of other specific groups also serve to raise consciousness. These documents include the following:

- Declaration on Rights of Mentally Retarded Persons, United Nations, 1971
- Declaration on Rights of Disabled Persons, UN General Assembly, 1975
- Declaration on the Rights of the Child, UN, 1979

- Therapeutic Bill of Rights. In Kittrie NN (ed): The Right to Be Different, pp 400–408. Baltimore, John Hopkins University Press, 1971
- The dying person's bill of rights. Barbus AJ: Am J Nurs 75:99, 1975

The above are only some of many such documents. Others speak to a range of special interest groups including pregnant women and senior citizens.

Personal Bioethical Issues

A person focus for bioethics emphasizes that there are a number of bioethical issues that are concerned with the essence of persons along a continuum from conception to death. Many of the life-and-death bioethical issues center on the underlying question: "When is a person not a person?" Names like Louise Brown (the first test tube baby) and Karen Quinlan (a long-term comatose young adult) remind us of this underlying question about the nature of person. An ad hoc committee of the Harvard Medical School (1968) proposed that irreversible coma, rather than the cessation of vital functions, be the criterion for death. Their decision became timely when improved resuscitation and life-support measures maintained the lives of many who otherwise would have died. This action acknowledged the loss of personhood and, incidentally, made lifesaving transplant organs more readily available.

Exploring the nature of ethical dilemmas may help you to understand moral values different from your own. To some professional nurses, the ideas of test tube babies, termination of life support systems, and abortion on demand are particularly distressing. The following discussion is an introductory sample of issues along the continuum from conception to death. Issues cluster at the beginning and end of life, with remaining concern focused on the *quality* of the intervening life. These issues involve conception, pregnancy, the rapidly developing area of high-technology neonatal care, bioengineering in its many facets, the psychological competence of persons, and the termination of life. Although these topics are presented here in the context of person as client-patient, some implications for nurses as care-givers are also raised.

Pregnancy

The issues of pregnancy are related to its facilitation, prevention, and normalcy. For most of history and in most parts of the world today, the dominant issue has been how to prevent pregnancy, childbirth, and overpopulation, rather than how to facilitate new life. Even today, the facilitation issues are mostly the concern of members of an affluent minority seeking the benefits of modern science in curing their childless state. The delay in marriage and childbearing of upwardly mobile women seeking career independence will undoubtedly cause this issue to become more prominent in this group. Some women are postponing attempts at pregnancy until an age when fertility has naturally decreased. Many of these women do not fully realize the possible implications of their decisions. The need to be in control of their lives has led to their independence; the same need has also likely made them believe that infertility happens only to other people.

While science has made great strides in facilitating pregnancy, the ability to induce fertility without the likelihood of multiple births is less well controlled. For health-care providers and society at large, the issues concerning multiple births are related to the very demanding and extremely expensive care which multiple premature births require. Hospital bills of several hundred thousand dollars are commonplace for each pregnancy episode which may or may not yield a desired outcome for the client. Newly perfected in vitro techniques are diminishing the chance of unwanted multiple births. However, a technique that aborts some among several fertilized eggs also raises additional ethical issues, and so does the ability of a mother without ovaries to conceive from donor eggs.

Prevention issues center around how to avoid conception or intervene afterward to prevent live births. The control of reproduction is both a personal issue and a societal issue. The encompassing ethical questions concern both overpopulation and the allocation of scarce resources. The control of reproduction ranges from permanent sterilization, to temporary contraceptive measures, to abortion. All of these methods create ethical issues for at least some clients and some health-care providers. Sterilization raises such issues as personal autonomy, societal control, and tampering with the human genetic pool. Contraceptive issues include access to pregnancy control related to age, religion, and economics. Traditionally, women have been held responsible for birth control, which probably accounts for lack of research on male birth control and only recent acceptance of vasectomy. Now, male sterilization — widely available through such a simple procedure as vasectomy — raises questions of contraceptive responsibility (his or hers). Male sterilization also gives men opportunities for more visible and permanent participation in pregnancy control.

The sexual revolution among young people, especially teenagers, forces the issues of teenage contraception into the open for both the public and health professionals. The introduction of more permanent contraceptive devices, such as intrauterine devices (IUDs), has blurred the issues between contraception and abortion since the mechanism of interference with pregnancy is one that occurs after conception. Long-term medical contraception with the pill raises ethical issues of solving one health-care dilemma (unwanted pregnancy) and creating others, ranging from weight gain to serious cardiovascular complications including stroke.

In all manner of pregnancy prevention, the issues of autonomy, right, and coercion are prominent. These issues share the common foundation, "What is the essence of persons?" In allowing abortion, the Supreme Court favored the view of a fetus as biological life and not a "person" before the age of viability. The Court also reaffirmed the rights of a woman to autonomy and control of her own body. Interestingly, although men have recently assumed greater responsibility in controlling pregnancy, the Supreme Court view basically disregards any paternal rights.

Perspectives about abortion range from conservative to liberal, from the extremes of prolife to complete freedom of choice. Additional intermediate perspectives relate to saving maternal life and providing relief in cases of rape and potentially defective children. Because nurses are called on to be both care-givers and counselors, a clear understanding of one's own personal values and religious beliefs is necessary to make decisions about professional involvement in abortion issues. For a full discussion of this and other personal bioethical issues, the reader is referred to *Bioethical Decision Making for Nurses* by Thompson and Thompson (1985).

Recent issues surrounding conception and pregnancy are revealed in the press as unprecedented in a variety of ways, including the following.

- What is a woman's right to use a sperm bank's holding of her dead husband's donation?

- What should be the fate of preserved embryos conceived by parents now deceased?
- What should be the role of surrogate pregnancy in rescuing products of unwanted conception?
- What should be the care of an anencephalic (without viable brain tissue) infant whose organs would benefit others?

Neonatology

Many of the issues related to neonatology have their origin in issues of pregnancy and contraception related to potential or known defective offspring. The ethical issues in this area have grown with the burgeoning technology of modern health care, which has the potential to rescue not only premature infants but viable products of abortion and miscarriage. Again, the positions vary about what is appropriate care for both potentially normal and defective neonates. They range from conservative to liberal views and from ordinary to extraordinary means. An extraordinary intervention perspective maintains that if a life can be saved, it should be. On the one hand are the prolife, right-to-life advocates and on the other hand, the freedom-of-choice advocates.

While a person-centered perspective might tip the scale toward a quality of life ethic and away from a mere life view, many questions would still remain.

- If the answer is not to save lives at all costs, then what is the answer about which lives to save? Who decides?
- What is the role of the parents? Of health professionals? Of society at large?
- What economic costs are reasonable and who should bear them?
- What research is justifiable?
- What are other rights of the neonate regarding the quality of his or her life?
- How do you give person-centered care in instances when the medical decision is to rescue a severely compromised infant or when the withholding of basic needs—such as food—becomes an issue?

In 1988, the ANA's Committee on Ethics released Guidelines on Withdrawing or Withholding Food and Fluid. Especially in instances like infant care, the Committee concluded that it is the moral and professional responsibility of nurses and others to determine whether providing food and fluid is in the person's best interest. The Committee further concluded that in almost all cases such a decision should be made if doing so provides comfort.

At first glance, it may appear that modern medicine and its technology have been the sole reason for increased neonatal survival. However, the role of highly skilled nurses with advanced education should not be overlooked. Neither should the increased ethical burdens borne by around-the-clock care-givers—such as nurses—go unnoticed. Increasingly, nurses are assuming more proactive and collaborative involvement in ethical decision-making processes for their clients-patients. Nurses are also asserting themselves among peers to receive the collegial support that sustains care-givers in such demanding situations.

Bioengineering

The issues of **bioengineering** begin with genetic screening and counseling. They range from manipulation of genes and embryos to organ transplants and artificial replacement of body parts. Over the years, genetic counseling has evolved from intervention after infant death or defect to preconception screening. Genetic screening involves testing population groups for genetic problems. The ethical issues of screening include privacy, confidentiality, and individual versus societal rights. Truth telling, human experimentation, informed consent, the potential for political evil, and the conflict between medical and religious viewpoints are also issues. Gene therapy is thought to have the potential for good or evil. For good, it might replace a defective gene with one that is healthy, while for evil, it might create animal-slave mutations. There is also some fear that DNA experimentation will create killer bacteria or human clones.

Artificial insemination with donor semen might be considered an early form of bioengineering even though conception took place in vivo (in life). The clear intent was to conceive a normal child by carefully selecting the donor. Within recent years, the element of engineering has increased as fertilization now takes place within the laboratory in vitro (in glass). The growing blastocyst is then transplanted to the mother. The engineering element is also in evidence when one considers the laboratory failures that preceded the success.

Organ and body part replacements are both natural and mechanical. Generating natural organs for transplants can impinge on rights of donors. The enormous cost of transplants, both natural and mechanical, adds additional issues related both to resource allocation and who will pay. Transplants of organs such as kidneys and the replacement of joints such as knees and hips are becoming commonplace. Their success rates and less serious ethical issues have made them quite acceptable. Heart transplants, however, continue to be fraught with both technical and ethical problems. To donate one of two kidneys to a close relative is a sacrifice of sorts. It is, however, quite another circumstance for one human life to be lost in order that another be saved. And, the idea of keeping donors alive until their organs are harvested may be unpleasant to many persons in spite of the potential lifesaving benefits. Recent cases of anencephalic (without brain) babies who were kept alive to donate other healthy organs illustrate the point. This practice gained considerable publicity partly because of the prominent medical center involved. It is clear that, whatever the future holds, the ethical issues related to bioengineering successes and failures will only increase.

Psychological Competence

In a person-centered approach to nursing care, the person in his or her biopsychosocial spiritual totality is, as indicated earlier, the recipient of nursing care. The psychological status of the person includes his or her cognitive functioning or thinking, his or her affective functioning or emotional feelings, and also his or her behavioral or psychomotor functioning. **Psychological competence** then refers to ability to function adequately in all these areas. Personal bioethical issues spanning a wide range contain at least some element of psychological competence related to these cognitive, affective, and behavioral domains.

Apart from the broader issue of competence to be considered in relation to "informed consent," mental retardation is perhaps the most often cited topic involving ethics and the cognitive domain. From a person-centered perspective of nursing care and health promotion, the label "mental retardation" is unfortunate given the varying degrees of functional ability that remain for the persons so stigmatized. About 3% of the general population is so classified. The causes of mental retardation can be divided between genetic and acquired.

The former category is illustrated by Down's syndrome (a chromosomal disorder) and Tay-Sachs disease (a disturbance of lipid metabolism). Acquired mental retardation can occur prenatally with maternal afflictions and in the neonatal period or in childhood from such varied causes as the aftermath of infections, poisoning, or social deprivation (Davis and Aroskar, 1978, pp 159–166).

Regardless of the cause of retardation, the rights of mentally retarded individuals to humane and adequate physical and psychological care become an ethical concern for nurses. These rights guide nurses' assessment, analysis, planning, intervention, and also their evaluation of nursing care. Providing for mentally retarded persons in the community rather than in institutions both highlights and blurs the assistance needed. Assistance may be needed to secure their rights of family living and appropriate educational and employment opportunities. And, at times of hospitalization, special concerns arise for client education, informed consent, and research participation.

Ethical issues related to diminishing cognitive competence may also arise during serious illnesses or with the care of elderly clients. Nurses, as around-the-clock care-givers, make around-the-clock observations. They are often aware of confusion and diminished mental skills that other episodic care-givers do not notice. This diminished cognitive competence may affect decision making and informed consent. Often nurses are also the first professionals to note when the label of confusion is inappropriately applied to clients. Such labeling may pose serious ethical dilemmas by interfering with client autonomy. Erroneously assuming that persons are unable to make decisions may violate their basic rights and deprive them of the control that they could assume for their care and behavior.

Persons with a wide range of psychiatric and mental health problems may pose other ethical dilemmas for nurses. Many such persons have temporary or permanent disturbances in all areas of psychological functioning: cognitive, emotional, and behavioral. The principles guiding ethical decision making in the care of such clients support persons as individuals, emphasize remaining strengths regardless of functional deficits, and recognize the basic human needs shared in common with all persons.

The question of what degree of participation clients with psychological dysfunction can and should have in determining their care is a common and complex one. Mental health reform has emphasized voluntary treatment and humanization. The questions remain about whether behavior change by psychosurgery, behavior modification treatments, or psychotherapy meet primarily the needs of individuals or the collective needs of health professionals and society. As Wasserstrom wrote, "Rather the fundamental point is that required disclosure of one's thoughts by itself diminishes the concept of individual personhood within the society" (Mappes and Zembaty, 1981, p 113). As Mappes and Zembaty stated, "what the concern for privacy protects is information which is deemed by the culture to render the individual unusually vulnerable and exposed. It is information which if known to others, except in special contexts, is unusually capable of causing injury to the person involved" (1981, p 115). The concern for privacy, of course, extends far beyond the care of the psychologically impaired. However, because the threats of coercion against those who are psychologically impaired can be subtle, ethical nurses are challenged not to let these subtleties escape them. Nurses are assuming more proactive involvement in psychotherapy and increasing their potential for influencing ethical decisions in this realm of health care.

Death and Dying

Most persons in our society die in hospitals, nursing homes, or other institutions where nursing care is given. The related ethical issues concern both the process of dying and the actual event of death itself. Not the least of the associated ethical dilemmas is the lack of a precise definition or agreement about what death is. A major turning point regarding the definition of death came from the irreversible coma or brain death definition proposed by the Ad Hoc Committee of the Harvard Medical School in 1968. The several determinations which were to be made only by a physician included the following.

1 Unreceptivity; that is, stimuli produce no response.
2 No movements or breathing during observations made for at least one hour. If the patient is on a respirator, the machine may be turned off for 3 minutes to determine any effort to breathe spontaneously.
3 Absence of reflexes.
4 Flat electroencephalogram (EEG) recorded for a 10-minute minimum and repeated at least 24 hours later without change. (In actual practice, this may be optional, but prudent.)

The above death determination is considered valid in the absence of hypothermia or drug intoxication. In spite of such a definition, it is not surprising that ethical issues continue to surround the cessation of life just as they do the precise beginning of life. Here again, the essence of person remains the underlying question to be answered. A person-centered nursing ethic seeks a consensus decision that involves the person, the family, and health-care providers whenever possible. Such an approach does not preclude weighing the best interests of both the person and society. The questions often become: Is it living or dying that is being prolonged? For whom? And why?

The questions related to death care sometimes seem easier to cope with when persons have already lived a long and full life. The hidden dangers of this view become more apparent as the issues of an aging population, burgeoning technology, and escalating health-care costs become more thoroughly entangled. These dangers remind us of a recent science fiction film in which humans were allotted only a 30-year life span and then targeted for annihilation as part of the social plan.

Two concepts that are associated with death and dying are benemortasia, meaning good or kind death, and euthanasia, also meaning good or pleasant death. The former term is sometimes used in describing the ethics of caring demonstrated especially in the hospice movement. The latter term has been the center of much controversy for years in legal, religious, and ethical discussions.

Euthanasia has been divided into *passive euthanasia*, meaning allowing to die or not interfering with a death process, and *active euthanasia*, which is either killing or actively assisting in the death process. As Thompson and Thompson stated, "The ethical concern is a question of the direct versus the indirect. Direct killing is generally held to be wrong and even called murder. Indirect killing might be called neglect, or an accident, or simply an act of God, or the Natural Law. 'Letting die' is sometimes related to passive euthanasia" (1981, p 187). Additionally, the terms *voluntary* and *involuntary* are sometimes used. With voluntary euthanasia, the client is able to give consent about active or passive means. With involuntary euthanasia, the client, because of his or her condition, is unable to be involved in the decision-making process. These designations lead to four types of euthanasia sometimes described as below.

- Active voluntary — for example, suicide, mercy killing
- Passive voluntary — for example, e.g., refusing treatment
- Active involuntary — for example, mercy killing
- Passive involuntary — for example, letting die

Some ethicists suggest that such labeling is not helpful or clarifying. In reality, many ethical issues arise unlabeled in everyday health care. For example, nurses weigh the ethical consequences of giving pain relief medication which may contribute to a fatal respiratory depression.

The same issue of whether to use ordinary or extraordinary means to support life applies at the end of life as it does at the beginning. Some older persons and their families have proactively responded to this issue by preparing a "living will." Such a document asks health professionals to comply with the person's request for life with quality and death with dignity (see box).

Clients make other attempts to be proactive in meeting the issues of death and dying, including refusing treatment for certain conditions determined to be fatal and participating in hospice movements. Nurses are proactively addressing the issues surrounding death and dying, and are becoming better informed and also confronting feelings and anxieties about death and dying individually and with others. A thorough discussion of the stages of dying is

---

THE LIVING WILL

To My Family, My Physician, My Clergyman, My Lawyer:

If the time comes when I can no longer take part in decisions for my own future, let this statement stand as the testament of my wishes:

If there is no reasonable expectation of my recovery from physical or mental disability, I,

_____

request that I be allowed to die and not be kept alive by artificial means or heroic measures. Death is as much a reality as birth, growth, maturity, and old age: it is the one certainty. I do not fear death as much as I fear the indignity of deterioration, dependence, and hopeless pain. I ask that medication be mercifully administered to me for terminal suffering even if it hastens the moment of death.

This request is made after careful consideration. Although this document is not legally binding, you who care for me will, I hope, feel morally bound to follow its mandate. I recognize that it places a heavy burden of responsibility upon you and it is with the intention of sharing that responsibility and of mitigating any feelings of guilt that this statement is made.

Signed _____ Date _____

Witnessed by: _____

_____

TABLE 11–1
PERSONAL BIOETHICAL ISSUES

Issue or Event	Topic

Pregnancy
  Prevention
  Interruption
  Facilitation
	Contraception
	Sterilization: male and female
	Abortion
	Selective abortion of multiple fetuses
	Artificial insemination
	In vitro fertilization
	Surrogate pregnancy
	Rescue of unwanted products of conception
	Preserved embryos

Neonatology	Birth defects Withholding nutrition Withholding lifesaving interventions
Bioengineering	Genetic screening Manipulation of genes and embryos Organ transplants Artificial organs and joints Eugenics
Psychological competence	Informed consent Behavior modification Psychotropic medication Psychosurgery Mental retardation Paternalism
Death and dying	Truth telling Promise keeping Euthanasia Refusal of treatment

beyond the scope of this chapter. Readers are referred to Elizabeth Kubler-Ross' classic theoretical work, *On Death and Dying* (1969).

Table 11–1 summarizes the various areas of bioethical issues. For each area, several related topics are listed.

| ETHICAL CONFLICTS

Personal and Professional Values

Nurses need to feel comfortable that their personal values are generally compatible with those values associated with the profession. This does not mean that personal and professional values are always congruent. Indeed, ethical conflicts between personal and professional values do occasionally occur. Because of the vast practice opportunities available in nursing, however, most nurses can find a comfortable fit between their personal style and values and professional demands. Considerable variation exists in client populations to be served, settings for practice, and acuity of illness. For example, nurses who might be uncomfortable in abortion situations will choose not to participate in such procedures. The effect of exercising such choice is to avoid the circumstances that are known to cause major

TABLE 11−2
SELECTED BIOETHICAL ISSUES

Issues	Related Questions
Truth telling	Should a patient be told he or she is going to die if the person seems unable to cope? If family members do not want the individual to be told?
Promise keeping	Should a nurse promise not to divulge a patient's awareness of impending death?
Behavioral control or modification	Is patient welfare or staff convenience the intent of control? Are patient priorities considered?
Suicide	Under what circumstances, if ever, is suicide morally defensible? Does the nurse have the right to interfere?
Euthanasia	Is a severely defective newborn better off dead? Should a brain-dead person be considered a dead person? How can a living will preserve the dignity of a person?
Refusal of treatment	What if the nurse disagrees with the person's decision to refuse lifesaving treatment?
Irreversible coma	Is it morally right to hasten the death of a person kept alive by machines in order to transplant vital organs?
Opposing loyalties	Is the nurse obliged to keep hospital beds open if care for individual patients is compromised?

ethical dilemmas regularly. Although such self-selection may forestall major dilemmas, minor ethical issues will invariably remain. Table 11−2 lists selected bioethical issues and examples of related questions.

There are several reasons for including a chapter on ethics in this book. First, readers may learn the nature of the ethical dilemmas and demands in nursing. Perhaps they will also discover that such dilemmas raise very intriguing and stimulating philosophical and practical problems. Such an introduction may confirm that nurses do not have to struggle alone with ethical issues. They can receive professional peer support in trying to resolve such dilemmas.

Whether they recognize it or not, nurses self-select to their profession, a reality that has several implications. Most persons who choose nursing may be described as persons who are broadly interested in people and health; can forego immediate personal gratification to assist another in a caring way; believe in service to humanity; and do not consider monetary gain as the primary motivating factor in selecting a life work.

Client and Professional Values

Nurses bring their personal values to their professional education. The development and clarification of values section presented earlier was included to acknowledge the importance of both clients' and nurses' values. Values clarification, addressed in professional education, can help nurses understand many kinds of potential values conflicts.

Nurses respect client values and choices even when they do not agree with them. This respect is the essence of a principle called *unconditional positive regard*. As Rogers stated in his classic work, "It is an atmosphere which simply demonstrates, 'I care;' not 'I care for you if you behave thus and so'" (1961, p 283). Another important related principle is that behavior has meaning. In other words, what persons are doing at any particular time is serving some useful purpose. That is, it makes sense to them from their model of the world and, further, the behavior reflects values actually held.

Nurses learn to accept that their clients may have religious and cultural values that differ from their own but they guard against imposing their personal values on their clients. Nurses need to recognize where values come from, and recognize and understand their own values as such. Then they can differentiate between their own values and those of their clients.

Values Among Health Professionals

Medicine and nursing have long held varying values for cure and care. This is not to imply that nurses do not value cure nor that physicians are uncaring, rather, it is a belief that "cure as an end it itself" as well as "doctor as the agent of cure" have been values that both attract and hold professionals in medicine. Increasingly, medical care has drifted from charitable and altruistic values to industrial values and services characterized now by product-line marketing and bottom-line cost effectiveness. Again, we can draw on the principle that behavior has meaning. For the most part, American society has tolerated — if not enthusiastically supported — the health-care system favoring cure. If the choice between care and cure could be viewed as an either/or decision, this situation would be more understandable. However, the human being is not physically immortal and technology has limits. Therefore it would seem that a system that supports care and cure more equally would serve more people better over time. Carers and curers can work collaboratively toward that end. This would reduce the care/cure dichotomy between nurses and physicians that has been reflected in their practices.

THEORETICAL APPROACHES TO ETHICAL ISSUES

Theoretical Models

Most traditional ethical theories belong to one of two opposing and mutually exclusive classifications: teleological or deontological. A teleological theory is one in which the ends justify the means. The outstanding example of teleological approach is utilitarianism. The utilitarian approach is sometimes described as advocating the greatest good for the greatest number, or choosing the least evil or least bad outcome. As you might guess, applied medical research supports this theory. The opposite approach in its most extreme form is deonotological theory. Using this theory, the moral right or wrong of an act is considered completely apart from the goodness or badness of its consequences.

Teological and deontological approaches can be illustrated with regard to abortion. In a teleological approach, saving the mother's life justifies taking the unborn life. On the other hand, in a deontological approach, any purposeful termination of life is morally bad; thus the fetus would be spared.

A third traditional approach, sometimes called a moderate deontological approach, is also called Natural Law and derives from the work of St. Thomas Aquinas.

Egoism is another traditional position. The egoist perspective uses self as the measure for right and wrong. Decisions in ethical dilemmas are made in the interest of the self. This means that in nursing, nurses would act in their own self-interest rather than in the interest of their clients. Putting personal needs or comfort before that of clients is generally inconsistent with and contrary to nursing's professional code of ethics. Also, because the self rather than universal principles is the point of reference, this ethical perspective does not provide for moral development as proposed by Kohlberg.

Additional contemporary positions offer modifications of the earlier traditional views. Davis and Aroskar summarized the following approaches as being applicable to nursing.

- Frankena's theory of obligation. This theory is built on two principles.
    - Principles of beneficence: a proactive attempt to do good and not evil.
    - Principle of justice as equal treatment: an attempt to distribute benefits and burdens equally among members of society; fails to specify whether the criterion should be merit, equality, or need.

    If and when the two principles conflict between the priorities of individuals and society, ideally inputs of multiple individuals will yield a consensus.
- Firth's ideal observer theory. This theory requires an all-knowing, impartial moral judge (person or machine) to make decisions that are equal for all and consistent over time.
- Rawls' justice as fairness theory. This theory is built on two basic principles of justice.
    - Each individual is to have the same right to the most extensive system of liberty for all.
    - Social and economic inequalities are to be so that they are to the greatest benefits of the least advantaged and open to everyone under equal conditions of opportunity.
    (Davis and Aroskar, 1983, pp 35–36)

One might reasonably ask, what is the reason for identifying so many ethical approaches when none tell specifically what a nurse should do in any given situation? Perhaps the major reason is to highlight some assumptions that we as experienced practitioners and educators make, and that we hope may influence your approach to ethical decisions.

These assumptions are:

- All nursing practice involves ethical decisions.
- Person-centered care demands a willingness to confront ethical dilemmas.
- Personal and professional values influence ethical decisions.
- Persons (care-givers and clients) can be assisted to achieve higher levels of moral reasoning.
- There is no one "correct" ethical theory.

The questions of applied ethics, that is, what to do in everyday practice, are the questions of most concern to nurses and nursing students. The traditional and contemporary theories of ethics in combination with awareness of personal and professional values and the data of individual situations can assist nurses to develop strategies to cope with ethical dilemmas.

Theories + Values + Situational Data = Coping Strategies

Even religious doctrines, which previously advocated one right ethical answer to life and death issues, are being challenged by scientific technology and the individual assertiveness of clients and health-care providers. Perhaps traditional ethical decision making could be characterized as general ethical approaches of broad and rigid rules applied deductively to specific situations. Increasingly, individual situations are influencing relaxation of old rules through inductive reasoning. However, even personal and societal ethics are subject to swings of the pendulum from conservative to liberal and back again. Recent trends showing the resurgence of conservative influence in health care should be noted.

- The "squeal" rule of the Supreme Court, requiring parents to be informed by health professionals of contraceptive advice to underage teenagers
- An increasing involvement of family (however defined) in health-care decisions
- Renewed interest in the quality, not just high-tech maintenance, of human life

A Practical Strategy for Considering Ethical Dilemmas

With the prior discussion in mind, we suggest a practical approach to ethical decision making as presented in Thompson and Thompson (1985) and modified slightly by the authors. This approach is similar to both the scientific method and the nursing process presented earlier. The nursing process phases corresponding to various aspects of this ethical decision-making approach are indicated in parentheses. The suggested approach illustrates that its various aspects may relate to more than one phase of the nursing process. For example, the steps labeled diagnosis (3 through 6) require a considerable analysis prior to the identification. This approach also illustrates that much of the essential nursing activity is mental thought that precedes and accompanies visible action.

1 Review the situation as presented.
   a Determine what health problems and individual person strengths exist. (Assessing)
   b Identify what decision(s) need to be made. (Assessing, analyzing, diagnosing)
   c Separate the ethical components of the decisions from those issues that can be resolved solely on a scientific knowledge base. (Analyzing)
   d Identify all the individuals and groups who will be affected by the decision(s). (Analyzing, diagnosing)
2 Decide what further information is needed before a decision on a course of action can be made; gather this information from primary sources, if possible. (Analyzing, assessing)
3 Identify the ethical issues involved in the situation as presented. Consider the historical, philosophical, and religious bases for each of these issues. (Analyzing, diagnosing)
4 Identify your own values and beliefs (moral stand) regarding each of these ethical issues and your professional responsibilities indicated by the Code for Nurses. (Analyzing, diagnosing)
5 Identify values, beliefs, and possible rights of other people involved in the situation. (Analyzing, diagnosing)
6 Identify the value and rights conflicts, if any, in the situation. (Analyzing, diagnosing)
7 Discuss who is best able to make the needed decision(s) and identify the nurse's role in the decision-making process: who owns the problem? (Planning)

8 Identify the range of decisions and actions that are possible and the anticipated implications of same to all people involved in the situation. Identify how closely the suggested actions conform to the Code for Nurses. (Planning)

9 If appropriate, decide on a course of action as the nurse in the situation and follow through. (Planning, implementing)

10 Evaluate the results of the action for achieving the client and societal goals. (Evaluating)

11 In retrospect, evaluate and review the results of the actions or decisions and keep them in mind for future situations of this type. (Aggregation)

Nurses may find organizational as well as social constraints to practicing according to the professional code of ethics. For example, the majority of nurses continue to work in hospitals and are under contract to their employers, whereas the code of ethics supports "clients" being the unit to which nurses are primarily accountable. Similarly, social relationships and bureaucratic hierarchies may make adherence to the code and the above strategies difficult. These constraints suggest that nurses under contract may need to negotiate their "right" to perform according to their professional code when they perceive that they are hindered from doing so.

PUBLIC POLICY FOR HEALTH-CARE ISSUES

A **policy** is a purposefully chosen plan of action (or inaction) aimed toward some end. Such a course of action by government is called *public policy*. Policy making can be aimed at various levels of complexity (i.e., micro, subsystem, macro). For example;

- Micropolitics involves few people and has limited impact.
- Subsystem politics focuses on broader policies and may have greater impact, but policy makers still have relative independence in developing and implementing policy. Such subsystem activity recognizes that policy makers within the larger (macro) system have varying levels of interest and expertise regarding different issues.
- Macropolitics focuses on national issues that are broad and have much public interest
  (Kalisch and Kalisch, 1982).

As the Kalisches pointed out, "Decisions pertaining to U.S. health policy have gradually moved into a macropolitical arena over the past thirty years. Limited modifications to health policy still take place on the subsystem level, but major developments in health policy are dealt with at the macropolitical level" (1982, p 80).

Incremental policy making of the past, which tried to remedy issues of access to health care, has brought us to the 1990s with access issues still remaining and health-care cost crises dominating the national scene. What the role of the federal government will be in resolving these crises is a key issue. At one extreme would be an unrestrained market system and at the other a socialized plan for health care. Governmental involvement to set levels of health-care costs according to some pre- or prospective payment plan (rather than paying ever-escalating charges after the fact) is a middle-of-the-road intervention which, although already underway, promises to change shape over time. A major such government intervention was the catastrophic health-care insurance recently added to Medicare.

The development of nursing as a full profession is caught amidst the reform of the health-care system and the conflicting vested interests of other health professionals. The commercial aspects of health care have catapulted it to be one of the nation's largest industries. All of this is happening at a time when a shift to humanism is evident both in society generally and in health care specifically. An example of the latter would be the hospice movement. This shift validates the public desire for person-centered nursing care. But at the same time, economic realities suggest that the delivery of person-centered care by a primary nurse in a traditional manner to a small caseload may not be feasible. What are the alternatives and how will they be determined? As always with finite resources, some difficulties choices will need to be made if the ideal is not economically feasible. Some of the priority setting for nursing care should come from nurses who are informed and able to suggest cost effective nursing care alternatives. Nurses, who understand the foundations, principles, and potential of person-centered care, are the largest group of health-care providers, and must now document nursing care outcomes as economical AND develop new economic and political savvy. Acting collectively, they can influence public policy to support health-care and nursing care alternatives that are humanistic as well as economically feasible.

MAJOR HEALTH-CARE ISSUES NEEDING ETHICAL RESOLUTION

When one reaches a stage of moral development characterized by awareness of universal ethical principles, a tangle of more abstract and larger ethical issues emerges. Although the same or similar questions may have arisen earlier, they assume greater significance when considered from an ethical perspective. Some of these questions are as follows.

- How should burgeoning technology be used?
- How do all citizens get access to health care?
- What should be the quality of health care?
- Who should control health-care decisions?

How Should Burgeoning Technology Be Used?

The burgeoning technology of health care is evident in virtually every hospital: sophisticated university health science center, local division of a large commercial health-care conglomerate like Humana, or a community hospital struggling to provide local service. New technology makes last year's high-tech model of the ever-changing equipment obsolete before it is paid for. Cooperative efforts are beginning and must progress rapidly. These are necessary to determine which center should provide which services. Such planning is mandatory for survival in the conglomerate, corporate world of high-tech health care.

Aside from the ethical issues related to economics, technology has amplified ethical issues related to access and the control of public resources. As always, technology challenges us to make ethical decisions about its use. Some examples, characteristic of this decade of technology, are the following:

- A U.S. president pleads for a liver transplant for a singular infant who is only one of many in similar circumstances.
- A judge orders castrating drug treatment for a convicted sex offender.

Surely such illustrations are just the tip of the iceberg at a time when discussions of the "ethics" of nuclear war are making their way to the professional literature.

How Do All Citizens Get Access to Health Care?

If access to health care is a right of all, inequality of access denies this right to some. Thus, inequality of access becomes an ethical issue. Some of the specific problems related to access are listed below:

1   Access to health care is controlled largely by physicians who traditionally give illness care. If nurses are capable of certain health-care management, are they ethically responsible to try to have this management designated as part of the role of nursing? Nursing would then assume privileges of both control and accountability.

2   Health-care services are geographically clustered. This distribution creates an advantage for the suburban middle class and a disadvantage for many elderly and poor people living in rural or inner-city areas. What is nursing's responsibility and opportunity to serve underprivileged areas?

3   Health-care costs are becoming too expensive. Even persons with moderate incomes can be financially devastated by a catastrophic illness or health problem. Who is ethically responsible?

Nurses and other health-care providers must work together to provide access to both health and illness care, better distribution of services, and affordable health care. The latter means that options other than the most expensive care must be appropriately available. Many persons have used an emergency room for nonemergency problems — such as a sore throat — because it seemed the only service available. Screening in less expensive neighborhood clinics could reduce expensive visits to sophisticated specialty-care facilities. Nurses might assist clients to use health-care facilities appropriately or they might work to make such neighborhood clinics available. In an article titled "Nursing's Window of Opportunity," Maraldo and Solomon wrote, "The greatest problem in health care today — high cost — offers the greatest advantage to nursing" (1987, p 84).

What Should Be the Quality of Health Care?

Quality of health care becomes an ethical issue because quality of health care is related to quality of life. The issues of access and quality are also, of necessity, related. If one does not have access to the system, the chances of receiving quality care are low. From a technological or medical perspective, the quality of health care may be high for those with access. The quality of life is compromised, however, by dehumanizing, depersonalized, and unwanted interventions. Then even those with access may perceive the quality of health care to be low. To provide quality health care and access to all persons is an ethical goal. It would require major reordering of our national social and economic priorities. If we allot fewer health-care resources than needed, how shall we decide who gets quality care?

Who Should Control
Health-Care Decisions?

The concept of client autonomy is a recurring theme in ethical issues. A person-centered nursing perspective affirms the client-patient as the focus of ethical decision making. High-level wellness is both relative and individual. Therefore, the client can be expected to make personal health-care decisions based on what the person, not the professional, defines as his or her concept of health. If the professional accepts this premise, then how the individual client views his or her health care becomes important. The criteria for judging the success of clients' health-care decisions will change also. Effective coping and positive health-care decisions will be acknowledged by health-care professions. Many trends, including the consumerism movement and home care for birth and death, suggest that persons are interested in controlling their own health-care decisions.

Tax dollars ought to support the health-care delivery that persons want and need. Despite the billions of dollars poured into tertiary (i.e., specialized) care, most persons will have only a minimal need for such services during their lifetimes. It is possible that every state has more beds in nursing homes than in hospitals. Yet, conditions in many nursing homes are such that one would not wish himself or herself or a loved one cared for there. Nursing is the one health profession in a unique position to help persons use advances in scientific health care and reasonable self-care practices to increase their control over health-care decisions. The use of tax dollars to finance tertiary care is just one illustration that broader ethical issues related to health care are difficult to resolve. Resolution would require a profound social commitment and national priority for equality of human rights and valuing of individual persons.

| ACCOUNTABILITY

As the previous discussion suggests, accountability to the profession to uphold its standards is an ethical issue. Accountability is also a major introductory legal concept. From your life experiences, you have internalized an everyday definition of accountability. Being answerable for professional conduct extends the concept to another dimension.

Standards

Accountability means responsibility or the obligation to account for one's behavior or acts. Persons are generally held accountable in relation to a peer group: a group of like educational preparation, experience, licensure, specialization, certification, etc. Standards are both professionally and legally defined. Novices or learners are held to different standards than licensed experts.

In the introductory clinical nursing course of one baccalaureate nursing program, faculty members have identified the following general behavioral objectives related to accountability and reliability.

The student will

- assume responsibility for his or her own actions.
- demonstrate self-discipline in meeting commitments and obligations, for example, keeping appointments, submitting written assignments on time.
- prepare in advance for clinical experience.
- report unsafe client-patient practices.

- demonstrate awareness of client-patient rights.
- demonstrate commitment in meeting client-patient needs.
- follow standard regulations and rules.
- apply safety measures to nursing interventions.

The first objective, to assume responsibility, takes on new meaning for the professional nursing student. Although being a student gives a licensure to learn, certain prudent behavior is expected nevertheless, as indicated by the other objectives. the principle of reasonable care is considered in determining whether one has exercised such prudent behavior.

Hemelt and Mackert, in their book *Dynamics of Law in Nursing and Health Care,* defined **reasonable care** as "that degree of skill and knowledge customarily used by a competent health practitioner of similar education and experience in treating and caring for the sick and injured in the community in which the individual is practicing or learning his profession" (1982, p 11). Thus, just as a faculty member is expected to exercise appropriate judgment in making clinical assignments and supervising a student, so too is the student expected not to proceed without appropriate supervision if uninformed or unable to perform a certain skill. Clients have a right to expect a student to perform at a safe level, even if not as skillfully as a licensed practitioner. Licensed practitioners themselves demonstrate accountability through consultation with informed peers as well as in a number of other ways.

Professional **nursing standards** are an element of the professional regulation of nursing practice by which nurses regulate nursing. Poyss described a nursing standard as "an agreed upon level of excellence promulgated [published] by the professional association" (1988, p 16). Licensed registered nurses are understandably held to high professional standards. The ANA first published general standards of nursing practice in 1973. Since then, a variety of standards of specialty practice have also been published.

The state provides another form of regulation, that is, legal regulation through practice acts and licensure. The relationship of professional and legal regulation of nursing practice is shown in Figure 11–2.

Simms and Lindberg, in *The Nurse Person: Developing Perspectives for Contemporary Nursing,* presented yet another perspective on accountability. They wrote:

> To be accountable means to be responsible for something within one's power, control, or management. Power is often given by others but control and management of self is certainly within the grasp of every professional nurse. Legal responsibilities are well-documented and made understandable by such nursing and legal experts as Creighton in *Law Every Nurse Should Know.* We are considering an accountability made more ambiguous by the very uniqueness of individuals. This is also an accountability concerned with practical consequences. It urges us to contribute to our own and each other's growth, nurse-to-nurse, person-to-person. It holds us responsible as individuals to prepare for our futures, both personally and professionally, to be our unique selves within nursing and the general community beyond. This means to be accountable to move in the direction of improving situations for both self and clients, not in martyr fashion but in risk-taker style, moving in the direction of least resistance to effect the smallest or largest possible change consistent with decreasing problems/constraints which impinge upon the nurse role. Accountability invites us to develop our own individualities in ways that are meaningful to ourselves as well as to others. (1978, p 230)

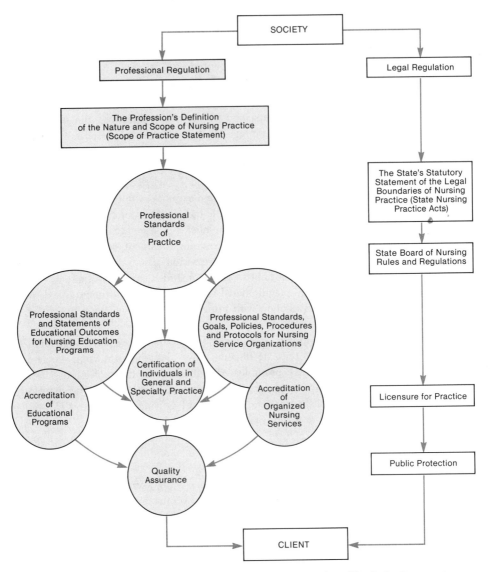

Figure 11–2 Professional and legal regulation of nursing practice. (Hirsch IL: Statement on nursing's scope describes how two levels of nurses practice. The American Nurse, April 1988, p 13)

Accountability is a demanding professional and legal responsibility to assume. However, as the previous discussion suggests, accountability has many dimensions. The expectations about its demonstration change over the course of both professional education and career development. Potential nurses who wonder about whether they can meet these ethical and legal obligations are not alone in their concerns. Probably most nurses, as well as other professionals, have had such questions early in their careers. Most practicing professionals as well as educators can provide reassurance. There are many safeguards built into both educational and professional systems to make ethical and legal practice less troublesome. Legal security for the nurse is enhanced by such diverse strategies as record keeping and documentation, contracts in education and practice, effective interpersonal communication as discussed in Chapter 9, Good Samaritan Laws, and professional liability insurance.

Documentation

Documentation is literally the collecting or supplying of written information for future reference. A diploma signifying educational achievement and a state license to practice as a registered nurse fit this definition. These credentials document an initial competency attested to by experts or their representatives. Nurses document their actual clinical practice in written narratives about patients' conditions and the administration of medications and treatments. They also document accountability with signatures or initials indicating access to controlled substances. Students, practicing under both direct and indirect supervision, could be thought of as practicing under the professional license of the supervising educator. It should come as no surprise then that even introductory clinical courses hold students to course objectives of beginning accountability.

Health-care records, which vary greatly among agencies, are legal records and provide documentation about health care given. They are admissible in legal court proceedings to document care given. Care and observations not documented are assumed not to have occurred. Responsible health-care providers demonstrate their professional accountability with such documentation. Therefore, such documentation needs clear entries that include the nurse's name, date, time of entry, any significant change in the person's progress, and the nurse's observations and actual interventions.

Documentation in the past has often, if not usually, taken the form of handwritten notes. Increasingly, computerization enable documentation to occur electronically at the client's bedside. In this day and age of continuous commercial surveillance, one can image video documentation of provider care as a realistic possibility.

| PRACTICE ACTS AND LICENSURE

The laws that govern nursing practice are state laws. The first nursing practice act was made state law in North Carolina in 1903. It was a permissive or voluntary law. Such permissive licensure laws permitted nurses to practice without a license if they did not claim licensure or use the RN initials. Currently, mandatory licensure for nurses requires all persons who nurse for compensation to be licensed. Many state practice laws underwent major revision in the 1970s. In 1972, New York's nursing practice act boldly defined nursing's professional practice as "diagnosing and treating human responses." This or similar wording has been a model for many other state law revisions. This definition was also central to the social policy statement by nursing's professional organization (ANA, 1980).

Nursing practice acts define nursing practice and requirements for licensure in the particular state. They also create a board of examiners and specify their responsibilities. One of the requirements of licensure is passage of the National Council Licensing Examination (NCLEX). All the state Boards of Nursing contract with an independent agency, the National Council of State Boards of Nursing (NCSBN), for the provision and scoring of the test. The national passage rate for first-time takers is approximately 86%.

Having the same examination for all states now facilitates state-to-state movement of RNs. The rationale of having one examination taken by graduates of associate degree, diploma, and baccalaureate programs was debated for many years. Perhaps there was one redeeming argument for a single examination: the purpose of licensure is to protect society by making sure that professionals demonstrate a *minimal* level of competence. Remember, according to the state, *RN* is intended to designate the professional nurse in a legal sense only. *RN* is not intended to mean professional according to the definition and criteria for a profession as previously discussed. Movement to have different examinations for different levels of preparation is in progress. Some states have been more receptive than others.

Many states are considering ways to test competency for RN relicensure. It is, however, proving particularly difficult to find a definition of professional nurse competency about which there is agreement. It is even more difficult and threatening to decide how competency should be measured. Nurses have a moral obligation, if not a legal one, to update their knowledge of nursing science and practice through some form of continuing education or learning.

| NEGLIGENCE AND MALPRACTICE

Before beginning this discussion, it is necessary to consider some basic legal terminology. *Laws* are the civilized principles and processes by which people in society seek to resolve disputes and problems. *Criminal law* is concerned with behavior detrimental to society as a whole. *Civil law* deals with legal rights and duties of private persons. A *legal right* is a claim that is recognized and is enforceable by law. Nurses and clients have legal *constitutional rights*. For example, persons who are hospitalized retain their constitutional rights, including those granted by amendments related to freedom of thought and speech, due process of law, and protection of minorities and the handicapped. An illustration of the contrast between criminal law and civil law is as follows: criminal law is basically the State versus John Doe; whereas if Nurse Naylor were sued by Client Smith, the civil case would be Smith versus Naylor.

Generally, health professionals are concerned with the category of law called torts. This concern is added to the legal rights and responsibilities the professionals retain as private citizens. *Torts* are civil wrongs that may be intentional or unintentional. The underlying concept of torts is the violation of reasonable behavior.

Two commonly confused terms relating to torts and reasonable behavior are negligence and malpractice. *Negligence* is the more general concept. Although we often think of being negligent as being careless, the two are not necessarily synonymous. For example, Student Baker, who injured Client Jones by attempting a new procedure for which he had not received instruction, would be negligent even if he did it carefully. Negligence applies to laypersons as well as professionals. **Malpractice** involves negligence in carrying out professional services by persons who are licensed to perform such services. Technically, malpractice applies only to the professional already actually licensed to practice.

The term **liability** means responsibility because of position or particular circumstances. Thus, health professionals are liable or legally responsible for their professional behavior. Even though they proceed carefully, they could be found negligent as students or licensed professionals. Their performance must be prudent in comparison with what similarly prepared health professionals would have done in the same circumstances. Again, the standard for judgment is that of the reasonable and prudent person. However, the reasonable and prudent standard for malpractice makes a comparison with other similarly

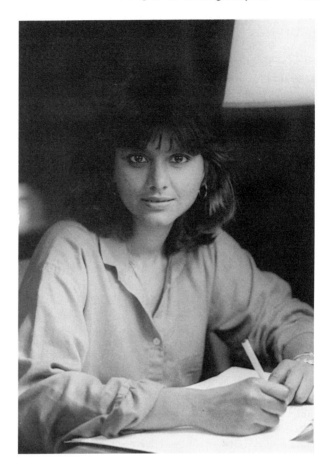

Nursing ethics and legal requirements demand careful documentation.

licensed practitioners. Malpractice is the specific type of negligent behavior for which professionals are uniquely liable because of their education and licensure.

Common Problems

Negligence related to nursing commonly includes such acts as failure to take appropriate precautions, failure to recognize dangers, or failure to report hazardous conditions. The nurse is responsible both for error in dependent nursing functions, such as administering medications, and in professional judgment regarding more independent functions, such as assessing client responses. The duty to take affirmative action when presented with a deteriorating situation (e.g., unusual bleeding) refers to taking positive steps to bring such a situation under control. Common problems related to legal issues can be the result of such seemingly simple errors as the failure to properly identify persons who are the recipients of care. These identification errors could result in wrong medications and diagnostic tests or untherapeutic interventions by a variety of health-care workers.

Avoiding Litigation

Although opportunities for negligence abound, a formal charge is likely to be brought and a trial to occur only if harm results. Such a trial in court to settle issues is called **litigation**. Increasingly, clients pursue litigation if they believe they have suffered mental or physical harm. Therefore, even careful students and registered nurses need the protection of liability insurance. Both the professional organization, the ANA, and the student organization, the National Student Nurses' Association, provide such insurance service to their members at a reasonable cost.

While liability insurance is strongly advised, some of the strategies for avoiding litigation are surprisingly simple and often overlooked. A most basic strategy is not to undertake, without supervision, any procedure or intervention for which you have not received appropriate instruction or assurance that you are able to practice on your own. This advice is equally true for students and licensed practitioners. An extension of this strategy is not to practice or proclaim practice for which you are not licensed. For example, nurses cannot practice as licensed midwives or pediatric nurse practitioners unless they are legally licensed for that expanded practice. Neither can nurse practice medicine in ways restricted by law or practice nursing in states in which they are not licensed.

Nurses, as well as other health professionals and ordinary citizens, are afforded protection to act in emergencies by what are called *Good Samaritan Laws*. Under these laws, which vary from state to state, persons who give emergency care — such as at the site of an automobile accident — are regarded as a protected class.

Another often neglected strategy for avoiding litigation is effective interpersonal communication as indicated earlier. The importance of this strategy cannot be overestimated. Faulty communication can create both ethical and legal problems. For example, informed consent is required for clients' participation in both varied therapies and also research investigations. Informed consent has both ethical and legal dimensions. Even when informed consent has been appropriately obtained, something occasionally goes wrong. Nevertheless, certain clients are less likely to take their disappointment and frustration to a court of law for minor problems. Often, these are the clients who believe they have been treated humanely and thoughtfully and communicated with appropriately. Some actions in the care of clients might be considered assault (threat to do bodily harm) or battery (committing bodily harm). These are actions taken when the client's consent has not been obtained or his or her communication to resist the nurse's action has gone unheeded.

| LEGISLATIVE PROCESS

Affecting Nurses

Perhaps the preceding discussion has suggested that all manner and detail of nursing practice is indeed legislated or comes into being by making laws. In reality, "custom and usage" may be equally important. As Hemelt and Mackert acknowledge, "the law itself generally follows actual practice. That is, the 'custom and usage' community standards may permit a certain act, such as nurses starting intravenous fluids or removing surgical sutures, before legislation has been passed regulating the act" (1982, p 21).

With such notable exceptions as midwifery and nurses administering anesthesia, the law generally does not prohibit nurses from functioning in more independent ways consistent with their education.

Nurse Training Acts in 1943 and 1971 authorized the creation of the U.S. Nurse Cadet Corps in the Public Health Service which supported and expanded the training of nurses. With the nursing shortage of the 1980s, Kalisch (1988) suggested: Why not launch a new cadet nurse corps? Clearly, such action would affect nurses and would make a statement about the kind of health-care policy needed for transition to the 21st century.

Shaping Policy

Political participation can benefit both nursing and society. Policy changes that appear to be primarily self-serving for any professional group are understandably suspect. However, the detailed discussion of this chapter has identified a number of bioethical issues that may be, by their very nature, of more concern to nursing than to other health professions. These relate primarily to preserving the essence of persons amidst ever-increasing technology and economic pressures.

Although the decades of the 1970s and 1980s have been characterized by their attention to personal welfare over social welfare, nursing offers an outlet for social expression. Nursing also offers a community of professionals who value social welfare, especially as it relates to health concerns. Nurses are prepared by education and privileged by social mandate to promote social welfare. To do so fully, nurses will need to become partners in the legislative process. Nurses shape policy when they vote, inform themselves and legislators about health-care matters, and offer resources to political candidates evidencing ethical and humanistic support of pressing health-care issues.

Nursing students can make a difference in the professional and legal systems that apply to nursing. Professionalism is important both for the future well-being of the profession and its practitioners, and for society. As students adhere to professional standards, including an ethical code, they renew the professional commitment of nursing to society. As they practice ethically and legally, they encourage society's reaffirmation to the nursing profession of its valued place in society. Baccalaureate-prepared nurses and students who practice to the full extent of their educational background make an important professional statement. They demonstrate the value of this level of education, that is, society's investment in them. They also demonstrate that society will be enriched by making this level of educational investment in all nurses who aspire to serve society as professionals.

Baccalaureate nurses (and students) who practice to the full extent of their education also serve society in other ways. They innovate practice in ways that change the legal boundaries of practice. This expansion furthers the profession but, more importantly, benefits society by giving it the full range of nursing's potential service (e.g., nurses in independent practice who collaborate with physicians).

Students can also make a difference in the legal system by influencing and shaping legislative process. Aspiring nurses can work for candidates who are nurses or who support nursing's position in health-care issues; equally important, they can inform the voting public about nursing's potential as a profession and its political health-care agenda.

I CONCLUSION

This chapter introduced nursing ethics by presenting a person focus for bioethics and indicating a number of bioethical issues that are of concern to nurses. The topic of values was revisited from an ethical perspective. Various ethical conflicts arising from personal and professional values, client and professional values, and value differences among health professionals were suggested. Several theoretical models were briefly mentioned before presenting a practical strategy for analyzing ethical problems. A number of major health-care issues needing ethical resolution were identified as relating to burgeoning technology, access to and quality of care, and control of health-care decisions.

Accountability was introduced in both an ethical and legal context. Other legal aspects related to practice acts and licensure. Negligence and malpractice and legislative process were mentioned briefly.

| STUDY QUESTIONS

1 How do you feel about clients making ethical decisions with which you do not agree?

2 What ethical responsibilities does nursing have as a profession for collective action of its members?

3 What responsibilities does the nursing profession have to influence health-care legislation?

| REFERENCES

American Hospital Association: Patient's Bill of Rights. Chicago, American Hospital Association, 1970

American Nurses' Association: A Social Policy Statement. Kansas City, MO, American Nurses' Association, 1980

American Nurses' Association: General Standards of Nursing Practice, 1973. Kansas City, MO, American Nurses' Association, 1973

ANA comments on withholding food and fluid. Am Nurse 26, 1988

Barbus AJ: The dying person's bill of rights. Am J Nurs 75:99, 1975

Davis AJ, Aroskar MA: Ethical Dilemmas and Nursing. New York, Appleton-Century-Crofts, 1978, 1983

Harvard Medical School: Report of the Ad Hoc Committee of the Harvard Medical School to Examine the Definition of Brain Death: A definition of irreversible coma. JAMA 205:8588, 1968

Hemelt MD, Mackert ME: Dynamics of Law in Nursing and Health Care. Reston, VA, Reston Publishing, 1982

Hirsch IL: Statement on nursing's scope describes how two levels of nurses practice. Am Nurse 13, 1988

Kalisch BJ, Kalisch PA: Politics of Nursing. Philadelphia, JB Lippincott, 1982

Kalisch PA: Speaking out: Why not launch a new cadet nurse corps? Am J Nurs 88:316–317, 1988

Kétéfian S: Moral behavior in nursing. Adv Nurs Sci 9:10–19, 1987

Kittrie NN: The Right to Be Different, pp 400–408. Baltimore, Johns Hopkins University Press, 1971

Kohlberg L: Child Psychology and Childhood Education: A Cognitive-Developmental View. New York, Longman, 1987

Kubler-Ross E: On Death and Dying. New York, Macmillan, 1969

Mappes TA, Zembaty JS: Biomedical Ethics. New York, McGraw-Hill, 1981

Maraldo P, Solomon SB: Nursing's window of opportunity. Image: J Nurs Scholarship 19(2):83–86, 1987

Poyss A: Cited in McCarty P: National standards are a guide to excellence. Am Nurse 16, 1988

Rogers CR: On Becoming a Person. Boston, Houghton Mifflin, 1961

Simms LM, Lindberg JB: The Nurse Person: Developing Perspectives for Contemporary Nursing. New York, Harper & Row, 1978

Steele SM, Harmon VM: Values Clarification in Nursing. New York, Appleton-Century-Crofts, 1983

Thompson JB, Thompson HO: Ethics in Nursing. New York, Macmillan, 1981

Thompson JE, Thompson HO: Bioethical Decision Making for Nurses. Norwalk, CT, Appleton-Century-Crofts, 1985

United Nations: Declaration on Rights of Mentally Retarded Persons. New York, The Association, 1971

United Nations: Declaration on Rights of Disabled Persons. New York, The Association, 1975

United Nations: Declaration on the Rights of the Child. New York, The Association, 1979

Wasserstrom R: The legal and philosophical foundations of the right to privacy. In Mappes TA, Zembaty JS (eds): Biomedical Ethics, pp 109–116. New York, McGraw-Hill, 1981

PART FOUR

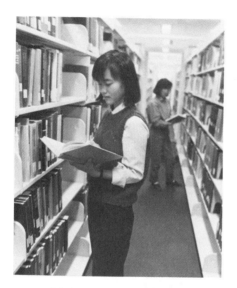

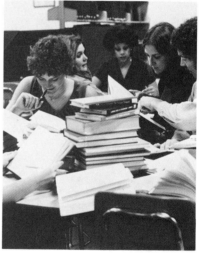

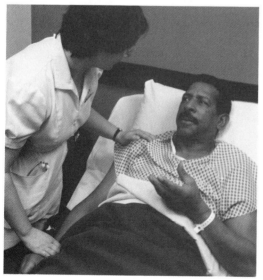

12 | OPPORTUNITIES AND CHALLENGES

KEY WORDS	After completing this chapter, students will be able to:
Clinical trial Dual career Entrepreneur Experiments Innovation Intervention research Intrapreneur Understanding	Identify several career and personal opportunities available to professional nurses. Identify several challenges facing the nursing profession. Explain how the challenge to humanize health care also offers an important opportunity for the nursing profession. Identify personal characteristics and attitudes that are compatible with professional nursing.

Nurses have served a social need during all of recorded history. Nurses have sometimes been men although more often they have been women. Throughout history, nurses have been educated in a variety of ways: history has recorded nurses who were self-taught as well as nurses who pursued all avenues of formal education. Regardless of gender or education, interpersonal care has been the hallmark of nursing service. What nursing will become in the future is a function of social need and also influenced, to a great extent, by nurses themselves.

This chapter provides a summary of some of the opportunities and challenges facing nurses and the nursing profession currently and in the future. A hypothetical advertisement for professional nursing aspirants follows.

WANTED—diverse, quality persons to make a difference in the health care of the future. Unlimited opportunities and challenges in all health-care settings. Applicants must like people and analytical thinking. No experience necessary but maturity and adaptability helpful.

Nurses fulfill a myriad of career aspirations in general practice and by specializing within nursing. Or they may blend nursing with other fields or unique personal abilities for "dual careers."

The challenges presented in this chapter can also be viewed as opportunities of a different nature. Under the challenge to humanize health care, two explicit health problems (AIDS and care of older persons) receive brief but special emphasis. These health problems create particular windows of opportunity for organized nursing.

The self-assessment tool at the end of the chapter is an inventory to assist you in determining how your interests and abilities compare with the authors' perceptions of nurses and nursing.

| OPPORTUNITIES

The selected opportunities are briefly described and only illustrative of the many available. To review the traditional practice options available in clinical specialties and functional areas, the reader is directed to Chapter 3.

Develop a Secure Career

Nursing offers wide-ranging opportunities to develop a secure career. *Secure* means dependable and long-lasting. Persons need nursing care from birth to death, so nurses have clients of all ages; also, the geographic need for nursing is universal and timeless. Presently and for the foreseeable future, the demand for nurses will exceed the supply at all levels of educational preparation.

Nursing is nursing wherever it happens. Many health-care settings need nurses around the clock, increasing both the number of jobs available and the compensation offered. Interstate relocation for nurses is facilitated by a national licensing examination. Licensure in a new state is usually expedited by endorsement of previous licensure.

Nursing, in contrast to most careers, offers professional status after baccalaureate education. Smaller initial investments of both money and education provide beginning entry to the occupational field, and this entry enables early gainful employment and relevant experience. Recent widespread shortages of RNs have brought sharp economic gains for nurses in entry-level positions. The similarity of nursing across settings and specialties also enhances career security and the number of opportunities for movement and variety within nursing practice. Additionally, persons entering nursing can become advanced specialty practitioners, scientists, administrators, teachers, and business entrepreneurs.

Practice Creative Nursing in Unlimited Settings

Guilford wrote that, "Creativity is not any one thing. It is many things and takes many forms" (1970, p 157). To *create* is to evolve from one's own thoughts. Few answers exist about the specifics of creativity as a thought process. People have creative ideas, perceptions, and experiences. Creativity is both a process and a product of creative behavior. Because creativity is a uniquely human quality, creativity or creative potential undoubtedly exists to some degree within each of us. Nurses can be as creative as other professionals; they can be creative in the ways that they both practice nursing and expand nursing practice.

Nursing urgently needs creative leadership and creative practice: in a cost-conscious health-care world, both nursing leaders and practitioners must create ways to demonstrate efficient and effective nursing care. That is, nursing care must produce the desired effect with a minimum of effort, expense, or waste. This demonstration will require creative problem solving and innovation. **Innovation** is the introduction of new methods; thus, the

National Center for Nursing Research gave a top priority to funding research about both AIDS (HIV) and innovative nursing care delivery patterns.

Innovative professionals shape their practice arenas within the limits of law and policy, but creatively extend their control and influence. Creative ideas and behavior start with one person. No one can tell someone else how to be creative. Each individual's most immediate sphere of influence is over oneself, but sharing creative approaches may stimulate creativity in others, so influence can be far-reaching. Innovation in nursing will come from nurses.

Innovation is also uniqueness in the way of doing things. As Peters noted the "value of uniqueness as a source of empowerment is the basis for market value" (1987, p 142). This distinction suggests that creative nurses will convince the public about what creative nursing is worth. Nurses as professionals must assume responsibility for demonstrating their value to society and must say, "This is what we have to offer!" Even beginning nursing students must learn about nursing's unique service. Innovation in nursing care will come especially from new persons entering the field with new perspectives. How would you be creative in nursing? The opportunities are twofold: for you to strive to increase your creativity and to bring innovation to nursing.

Extend Nursing Science Through Research and Theory Development

Few aspiring nurses are aware of the opportunities in nursing to be a research scientist or theories. Given that not many nurses may choose this role, perhaps this point seems minor. However, such a lack of awareness suggests that many practicing nurses do not recognize and publicize the scientific potential of nursing. Therefore, young persons who aspire to health science careers generally may not realize the particular opportunities in nursing for exciting scientific investigation. Furthermore, the loss to nursing of such scientific personpower is unfortunate at this stage in nursing's scientific development.

Nursing needs to increase its ability to predict what the outcomes of specific nursing interventions will be in actual practice. The research to support such prediction is known as **clinical trials, intervention research**, or **experiments** conducted in the real world of practice. Theory development is needed, as indicated earlier, to both guide research and increase nursing's scientific credibility.

Nursing is now evolving a scientific community with national visibility and political influence. In a strange twist of fate, the nursing shortage has indeed created a window of opportunity for nursing as a science, that is, to help solve many current and future health-care dilemmas. National research funding is increasing rapidly for nursing science. Scholarly societies, research forums, and journals unite nurse scientists. Nursing, as Meleis said, "is one of very few disciplines that isolates the components of research design and methodology and helps students develop necessary skills to undertake a research career" (1985, p 304). Yet, because not all nurses consider themselves scientists, nurse-scientists have unique opportunities within the professional nursing community. Also, because nursing is a new science, there is much uncharted territory. Opportunities to extend nursing science through research and theory development are particularly rich for interested professional nurses.

Manage or Administer Health-Care Organizations

Health care encompasses medical and nursing care as well as a number of other clinical disciplines. Nurses represent the largest number of health-care providers and nurses have always been excellent and practical problem solvers. Increasingly, nurses are recognizing that complex health-care organizations require contemporary nurses to have additional skills related to management, leadership, and fiscal responsibility. Long gone are the days when the "head nurse" on a hospital unit was concerned only with nursing care. With recent consolidation of middle-management positions, even traditional titles like "head nurse" are being changed. However, the need to "manage" and "administer" nursing and health care is more crucial than ever before.

Some corporate directors of health might argue that nursing is best done by nurses and managing is best done by professional managers. However, management and administration are not foreign concepts for nurses. Baccalaureate nursing programs offer courses that focus on nursing management; social, political, and professional issues that affect nursing practice; and leadership. Students learn how to assess a health-care setting, analyze nursing within the setting, and design planned change. Students learn individual and collective strategies to influence professional nursing practice and health-care delivery. They also learn management theory and organizational principles. Increasingly, opportunities for beginning-level management positions in nursing are being filled by baccalaureate-prepared nurses. In settings where nurses with advanced nursing preparation are available, they fill these positions.

Management and administrative positions at the corporate level require more sophisticated skills and knowledge related to budgeting and general business matters. This preparation is available in master's and doctoral programs in nursing, although many nurses have sought advanced degrees in business administration. Such preparation, from either source, opens the door to the corporate board room. Here nursing has the potential to participate in senior management decisions. The unique perspective that nurses bring to the board room is the understanding of nursing care requirements.

In many health-care settings, for example, nursing homes, home-care agencies, and community health agencies, nurses may be the only health professional consistently on site or available in the agency. Clearly, it is in nursing's best interest to assume leadership in many of these situations, and it may also be in society's best interest for nursing to do so. As Meleis commented, "Nursing goals are generally congruent with those of the recipients of its care; nursing operates from a health and holistic approach and purports to enhance coping and harmony with one's environment" (1985, p 305).

Teach Consumers or Professionals

In addition to practicing, researching, and administering, nurses teach. In the past, the particulars of this teaching role were more often derived from physician prescription or doctor's orders than is currently the case. With the ANA's publication of its Social Policy Statement in 1980, nursing was defined as "the diagnosis and treatment of human responses to actual or potential health problems."

As Mundinger wrote:

> Unhealthful responses, or the absence of some healthful responses, often can be the primary reason for nursing care. . . . Teaching and counseling for resolution and

self-care of disease or pathology are unique elements of professional nursing. Pathology resolution is the scope of medicine; resolution of responses to pathology is nursing. . . . Nursing is one of the only professions using primary physical and emotional data and intellectual and hands-on skill to identify and resolve unhealthful responses. . . . Only nurses have the full scope for identification and care to resolve health problems. (1980, p 58)

The functional abilities that define health are in part those abilities needed to perform the activities of daily living. The necessary knowledge and skill learning may be related to such basic activities as eating, sleeping, and exercising. Additionally, persons may need to learn basic information about body structure and function to promote and maintain health or to fully rehabilitate after medical intervention for disease.

In the future, many more opportunities will exist for nurses to teach clients outside the hospital setting. With hospital stays decreasing in length and increasing in acuity, much health teaching by nurses will be done preadmission and postdischarge and in alternative health-care settings. Increasingly, nurses will be teaching family members about how they can play a more active role in home health care for clients of all ages, but especially for the elderly. They will teach basic physical care as well as how to do treatments and dressings and manage pain, diets, and medications.

Many nurses find themselves drawn to the role of teacher as a way to greatly increase their influence on the improvement of nursing care. A heavy demand will remain for teachers of nurses in all levels of basic and continuing educational programs. In baccalaureate and higher degree programs, the role of teacher will be combined with that of researcher-scientist.

Be a Health-Care Entrepreneur

Throughout this book, "health" has been consistently claimed as the domain of nursing. An **entrepreneur** is a contractor and also someone who undertakes projects requiring unconventional activity and some risk. Nurses are logical persons to be health-care entrepreneurs. Private duty nurses who provided nursing care at home during the early 20th century may have been some of the first health-care entrepreneurs. Seventy years later, Lewis might have been describing nurse entrepreneurs when she wrote about "New Breed" nurses:

> They have no patience with bureaucratic routines, accepted ways of doing things or playing the game to accomplish what they believe needs to be done. . . . They know their own worth and skills and if they don't have an opportunity to use the latter to their fullest, then they're off to another position with more potential. (1974, p 685)

Perhaps a difference between turn-of-the-century nurses and the nurses described by Lewis is that early entrepreneurs usually worked independently of institutions. Today's nurse-entrepreneurs work both independently of and within institutions and formal organizations. A new word has been coined: *intrapreneur*. **Intrapreneurs**, in the health-care industry as in other businesses, offer nontraditional services within traditional organizations. These services not only provide opportunities for creative nurses but also enable large health-care agencies to market health care competitively. Traditional acute care centers are diversifying their "product lines" to offer services that meet nursing needs beyond the period of hospitalization. Such services may include screening, counseling, and instruction prior to same-day surgery, home health care planning and coordination, extended skilled nursing care, and individualized home care. Additionally, the alternative birthing arrangements originally offered by enterprising nurse-midwives are now being sponsored by hospitals eager to meet consumer demand and claim a market share.

The rent-a-nurse agencies of the 1980s supplied temporary nurses to meet hospitals' permanent staffing needs. These agencies were a distortion of the early nurses registries (listing of RNs available for service). Commercial non-nurse agency pools were also a forerunner of legitimate nurse-entrepreneurs working collectively. Such nurse-entrepreneurs now contract more permanently with institutions for nursing services.

Lucille Kinlein was a prominent independent nurse-practitioner whose entrepreneurial practice activities made headlines in the 1970s (Kinlein, 1977). Since then, many other less-publicized nurses have set up entrepreneurial services to help clients manage chemical dependency and severe pain, for example. Nurses are also consultants to retirement communities and businesses such as organizational management and accounting firms, insurance companies, architects, and manufacturers of health-care equipment. Orem (1971), described earlier as a theorist, set up a consulting firm based on her unique perspective. One nurse incorporated cruise travel for dialysis patients into her services for persons with kidney disease (Clark and Quinn, 1988).

By their very nature, entrepreneurial opportunities arise over time through the originality of professionals entering the field. Who knows what opportunities your generation of practitioners will conceive?

Apply Computer Skills to Nursing

Although computers are not new to health care, their importance has escalated rapidly in recent years. It is now apparent that computerization throughout the health-care industry affects nursing profoundly. To ignore this reality is to enter the next century walking backward. Just as the industrial revolution affected manufacturing, computerization has affected information processing. Computerized information processing is the key that enabled a costing of health care related to medical DRGs. Now, much client-related information is collected and processed via computers as the basis for important health-care decisions.

Nursing was late to recognize the need to integrate nursing information with other client-related information, and the complexity and nature of nursing information contributed to the lag in translating it to computer format. The recent attempts to standardize nursing diagnoses have been important advances toward nursing computerization. Identification of the nursing Minimum Data Set (Werley and Lang, 1988) was an important effort to compile comparable uniform data across clinical settings. Nursing needs such integrated information to determine nursing costs per client, per medical diagnosis, per nursing diagnosis, per care delivery unit, etc.

Nurses with computer skills will find varied opportunities to use these in the health-care world of today and tomorrow. The full array of skills will be needed. Thiele suggested such a range in the 1988 article, "There's a Computer in the Curriculum!" These skills range from word processing to file management to accessing information. More advanced skills enable the computer to be a management tool using data base and spread sheet strategies.

The most important computer skill is openness to learning the basics of a technology that will have applications in both professional and personal life. Computers can make many personal and professional tasks easier. The same word processing skills used to write

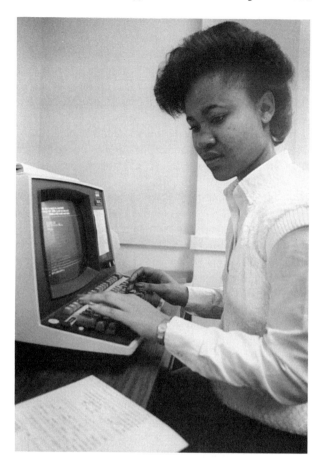

Nurses use computers as an integral part of client care.

personal letters and term papers help nurses create computerized care plans; while accessing information can be accessing a college academic record, on-line personalized student evaluations from an instructor, professional literature, or client data bases. In 1980, the first personal computer-based information system, NurseSearch, allowed searching literature in 60 journals via author, title, topic, etc. In a basic educational program, such technological capacity enables students to orient rapidly to the field. Practicing nurses can apply computer skills to access the continuing education information that will keep practice current through lifelong learning.

In spite of nursing's rather late interest in computing, there are many software programs that fit nursing's many clinical specialties and functional areas. These include general education in basic areas, for example, physiology, safety, medications, and case simulations. The latter help nurses practice problem-solving skills in preparation for clinical activity or State Board licensure exams: applying basic computer skills with user-friendly programs, students can review for state boards in either a tutorial or practice test mode. Basic computer literacy also includes being able to read basic computer-generated reports.

Other applications of computer skills include data management for staffing and scheduling, accessing expert practice consultants, writing resumes, constructing tests, authoring papers and presentations, and finding appropriate educational materials for client-patient use. Interactive computer instruction, which combines computer program basics with videotape examples, holds much promise for learning both manual skills (psychomotor) and feeling (affective) responses. Nurses can apply computer skills as both consumers and creators of such media.

Working collectively, nurses could plunge nursing into profession-wide computer literacy that would do wonders for nurses' intelligence gathering in the world of health care. User groups, message systems, and public domain software sponsored *by* nurses and *for* nurses would be very helpful.

Use of computers is less a technical skill problem and more a mental attitude opportunity. It is not the equipment per se but what it allows you to do that offers the great potential. In the past, nurses used mechanical lifts to augment their muscles in lifting and moving clients; now robots do such lifting and also hospital delivery tasks that nurses once did. Now data management requires that nursing expand its collective brain power to work smarter by applying computer technology. Commitment to doing this will assure that nursing as a profession is not left behind in this mind-boggling age of health-care technology. Such technology will always require that nurses supplement the technology with human perception and analysis. And as Naisbitt (1984) claimed, increased technology (hi-tech) will only increase the importance of human caring (hi-touch).

Promote Sports Health and Physical Fitness

Given the increasing interest in health and physical fitness, nursing has also been late to recognize the professional service opportunities in this area. Sports medicine and sports injuries have dominated the scene. There is even a well-established journal, *The Physician and Sports Medicine*. Interest in prevention usually follows rather than precedes interest in cure. Perhaps a journal titled *The Nurse and Sports Health* will be forthcoming.

Much interest in this area is focused on amateur and professional competitive sports. However, health and fitness related to lifetime individual sports offer potential involvement of an entire society. Consultancy to retirement communities suggests exploration in this area may be underway and nurses will develop this window of opportunity.

Two nurses did seize an entrepreneurial opportunity related to fitness of pregnant women. A childbirth educator and a nurse studying exercise physiology pooled their experience to create a maternity fitness package. The total program package was then marketed to hospitals and grew from a single maternity class in one hospital in 1980 to over 50 hospitals within 7 years (Clark and Quinn, 1988).

The physical fitness of children as well as mothers has come under increasing scrutiny and criticism in recent years. When funds for public school education diminish, societal interest in nonacademic aspects of public education wanes. Art, music, and physical education programs are often at risk of cuts or closures. However, given the overall increased interest in sports, other segments of society may assume responsibility for children's health and physical fitness. As they do, nurses have much valuable information and many insights to share. It could be argued that the needs for physical fitness and sports health is important for all youth even before formal public education begins. To accommodate this concern, nurses may increase their consulting about physical fitness and health to the growing preschool child-care industry.

Fitness facilities in the workplace are also gaining increasing prominence. The traditional occupation health nurse's role is changing from focusing only on injury prevention and treatment in factory settings to health consultation in all kinds of business enterprises.

Pioneer In Space Health

In a 1985 article entitled, "Space" nursing: A Professional Challenge," Perrin noted

> It is essential for man to understand his limited tolerance of the space environment and the create strategies for the promotion of safety, well-being, comfort and productivity during the extended space missions. . . . An active health care/maintenance program with clinical studies will become essential to promote physiologic and psychologic well-being for space crews. (p 497)

The nurse is a uniquely appropriate health-care specialist to staff either a traveling spacecraft or a permanently based space station. For the space nurse, the traditional nursing skills of expert care and sensitive communication will be basic to prolonged confinement. Nurses have the ability to assess and improvise solutions for novel problems of health maintenance and altered health. Carefully selected space travelers will need basic instruction about health maintenance and activities of daily living that a nurse is well-suited to provide. Of course, modifications will need to be made for the confined quarters and zero gravity of space flight.

The manned space activities have produced an enormous amount of new information, especially regarding physiology and communication. Humans' physiologic responses in space include parallels to the known changes after bed rest, for example, loss of skeletal calcium. New problems that accompany weightlessness include the pooling of blood in upper body parts rather than lower extremities. Sleep, nutrition, exercise and mobility, common concerns for nurses, will become everyday concerns for space travelers. Human psychosocial responses in space will increase the need for purposeful interventions to decrease stress, counteract boredom and isolation from loved ones, and facilitate constructive interpersonal activity.

Space travel is a high-tech enterprise whose health-care equipment will include that to sample and analyze various body products and processes. Data from laboratory samples, imaging, and psychological testing will be beamed to earth for interactive computer analysis; while computerized instruction and electronic stimulation can be beamed back to maximize the person's adaptive capabilities for biopsychosocial processes. Computer smart cards will contain complete individual health histories to assist space and earth personnel. Computer literacy for health specialists will be a given and as important as for early pilot-astronauts. Because computer literacy will be increasingly required in earth health-care settings, it will seem commonplace to space travel. Just as computer science is now making its way into nursing curricula, space science with attention to physics and bioengineering will not be far behind. Although very little of nursing's present scientific literature speaks directly to space nursing today, that too will change. If aspiring nurses want to be health-care providers in space, they will need to agitate for the necessary education and preparation. Other life scientists are already partners in planning for the activities and equipment that will support space travel and work stations, now nursing needs to assert its interest and expertise to be included. How exciting it will be to test Martha Rogers' theoretical principles about energy fields that transcend time and space in actual space travel!

The applications of early space travel, for example, Velcro, dehydrated food, etc., are now so overshadowed by new marvels of bionics, robotics, and artificial intelligence that it is difficult to imagine what new space-age marvels will soon dominate health care. These will literally bring space nursing to earth in your professional lifetime.

Arthur C. Clarke's *July 20, 2019: Life in the 21st Century* (1986) opens a window on astounding technological predictions for space and earth based on present science and futuristic speculation. If you're looking for a yet to be publicized career option that blends concern for people with space-age technology, read his fantasy and dream, and then remember that some of these space-age technologies — for example, computer-assisted self-medication, odorless human waste disposal, and muscle stimulators — already exist.

Gain Personal Understanding

Long before women generally made commitments to professional careers and work outside the home, nursing was considered a good preparation for living and family life. Although times have changed, nursing remains a scientific discipline and a clinical practice experience which contributes much to personal understanding. Through interactions with clients and their families, nurses expand their life experiences greatly. Many persons entering nursing have not experienced birth and death, poverty or wealth, fatal diagnosis or chronic disability, and pain or suffering. They probably have not observed a rescue from the brink of despair by nurses, the wonder of surgical reconstruction by surgeons, or the togetherness of families in crisis. Although the potential of such experiences may seem frightening, fear of the unknown is perhaps the greatest fear of all. By thoughtful observation and guidance from others, nurses learn ways to help professionally without having lived through experiences personally. In doing so, they gain personal understanding

Understanding is a thinking function that combines knowledge with comprehension and application. It implies analysis and evaluation. Personal understanding brings awareness of personal self, interpersonal interactions, and the relationship between these. Nurses are privileged to witness life's most tender and intense moments. Doing so enables one to work through thoughts and feelings about how you would respond if it were your life being so affected, thus, in this way it is possible to confront dilemmas you might otherwise not have anticipated. It is possible to gain personal understanding as a participant-observer in the lives of other persons; doing so enriches your own life.

Create Dual Careers

There is an often-unrecognized opportunity in nursing to blend nursing with unique personal abilities for a **dual career**. "The holistic concept of man all too often is applied more to the other' person or client than to the person who is becoming a nurse. . . . If individuals are seen as unique, each student's individuality can be a most valuable asset for personal fulfillment and contribution to society" (Simms and Lindberg, 1978, p ix).

Many unique abilities will combine with nursing knowledge and skill to find expression in nursing. Some of us are more artistic while others are more analytic. For example, some practitioners use music, art, or drama regularly in their nursing (e.g., pediatric and psychiatric mental health nurses), while, other practitioners' verbal skills may predominate over their mathematical abilities. And, some of us write better than we speak and relate more comfortable one-on-one than in groups. Some nurses are fascinated with high-tech equipment and critical care, while others are primarily people-persons and prefer interpersonal interaction in ambulatory care settings to high-tech drama in the operating room. Nursing needs all kinds of practitioners. All can find their special niche in direct care, management, teaching, research, and administration.

Nursing is also, as indicated above, solid preparation for living and self-understanding. Nurses learn stress and time management, broad problem-solving techniques, communication techniques, strategies for dealing with ethical dilemmas, and teaching skills. With this educational foundation and self-understanding, nurses are qualified candidates for additional education in other fields. Two of the more common fields entered by nurses are law and business. The combination of nursing and law lends itself to careers ranging from health-care policy to plaintiff.'s (complainant's) attorney. The combination of nursing and business lends itself to careers ranging from entrepreneurial endeavors, as described above, to corporate health-care management. The transition to professional person involves maximizing personal potential. Nursing education in combination with personal abilities or other education offers many opportunities to satisfy the individual and enrich nursing, health care, and society.

| CHALLENGES

Some of the selected challenges have been stated explicitly or alluded to in previous discussion. All professions present challenges to their practitioners and certainly nursing is no exception.

Humanize Health Care

Perhaps one of the greatest fears of both health-care professionals and their clients is that modern technology will dehumanize health care. Health-care professionals fear that some of their professional skills (e.g., diagnosing) may be replaced by automation. Clients fear the loss of human compassion. They worry that they will lie alone amidst whirring and ticking machines to be tended by robots and monitored via computers and television.

Two currently prominent health-care problems may fuel these concerns. These problems are AIDS (HIV) and the increasing demand for health-care services by the elderly.

AIDS is frightening because of its fatality, transmission to unsuspecting persons, and the continuing misunderstanding about how persons become infected. AIDS turns independent adults into physically wasted and dependent beings.

Aging is frightening to some because it is a situation from which no one escapes and is often accompanied by chronic disease and diminishing functional abilities. There is continuing misunderstanding about the usual abilities and deficits of healthy older persons. Additionally, the increasing priority given to youth, physical attractiveness, and stamina causes some older persons to question their worth and to fear that they have outlived their usefulness to society.

Both AIDS clients and the elderly dread being unable to exercise their will and also becoming a burden on society and loved ones. They also worry that their diminishing physical beings will cause them to be devalued as persons.

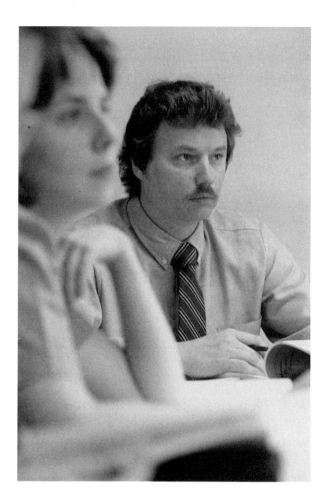

Individual nurses hold the key to nursing's future.

Care of AIDS clients and elderly persons presents challenges for health professionals in general. However, because nursing's domain is both health and caring, nursing is the one health profession which has the most to contribute to "care" of persons in both these circumstances.

Interestingly, "Proud to Care" was the theme of the 1988 Biennial Convention of the ANA. With this theme, nurses publicly reaffirmed their commitment to care. Aspiring nurses seem to respond to this theme also: a beginning nursing student wrote in an anonymous course evaluation, "Clinicals were always exciting and fun. I never realized how many people need care."

Before further highlighting some aspects of both AIDS and elder care for their challenges and opportunities, let us consider each briefly.

AIDS

In the mid-1980s, aspiring nurses and their loved ones voiced explicit concerns about nurses contracting AIDS from clients. Following are some significant developments in the emergence of AIDS as a health-care issue.

1983 — The first major article about AIDS for the general public appeared in Science Magazine (Marx, 1983).

1985 — The first international professional conference occurred in Atlanta.

1986 — The Surgeon General's Report to the people of the United States on AIDS was issued in October.

1987 — The Centers for Disease Control (CDC) issued what were called "universal precautions" to be followed by health-care providers caring for infected clients.

1988 — The Surgeon General and the CDC prepared a brochure titled *Understanding AIDS*. It was sent to all known households. Perhaps this event signaled a turning point for AIDS (HIV) information available to all citizens.

AIDS challenges all care-givers, including aspiring nurse, to understand several facts.

- AIDS is a difficult disease to catch.
- The CDC universal precautions are easy-to-understand guidelines that will protect health-care workers — including nurses — if followed. The highlights of these are: handwashing, preventing needle sticks, and using gloves for all invasive procedures and handling all body substances. Interestingly, similar precautions have been used for years for other infections.
- A government agency, the Occupational Safety and Health Administration, is enforcing the CDC guidelines in health-care workplaces.
- The care required by AIDS clients is not unique.

"People with AIDS require the kind of care and skills that all nurses learned" (Bennett 1987, p 1152). In caring for AIDS clients, one of the identified challenges is avoiding burnout from the psychological stress. This challenge is not unique for AIDS clients but applies elsewhere in nursing and in many other professions and occupations. As one nurse remarked, "I didn't know what I was getting into, but it certainly has been the most challenging, rewarding, and fulfilling nursing job I've ever had" (Bennett, 1987, p 1153).

Health Care of the Elderly

The elderly segment of our population is not well understood by society in general or health-care professionals in particular. "The number of Americans over age 85 is expected to total 5 million by the end of this century. At present, 80 percent of such people live outside nursing homes. The 'oldest old' are four times more likely to require daily care than persons between 75 and 85 years old" (*Ann Arbor News,* June 1, 1988).

Although the proportion of elderly persons is increasing in society, these persons are often isolated by early retirement, the trend away from extended families, and the trend toward segregated retirement communities.

Myths about aging and elderly persons arise partly from the fears of growing older and partly from generations of tales and jokes, but mostly from inexperience in dealing with elderly people (Table 12–1). Gerontological research has produced a variety of perspectives about how persons age. Older persons are variously described as the vulnerable or fragile elderly, or more optimistically as the hale elderly. Diverse descriptors are undoubtedly appropriate in different circumstances. One is reminded of a psychological screening tool that asks subjects to describe a drinking glass containing water: Is it half full or half

TABLE 12-1
MYTHS AND REALITIES

Myth	Realities
Old age equals sickness.	Although the probability of having chronic disease is higher in older people, most older people are adapting successfully in their homes and communities with the help of their families and health-care professionals as needed.
After 65, people age dramatically.	Many body functions vary enormously throughout old age, depending on heredity, diet, occupation, environmental factors, life style, and mental attitude.
Older people form a homogeneous group.	There is no such single entity as "the elderly."
Older years are tranquil, golden years of pleasure.	Old age is a challenge of adaptation and some persons may be lonely, poor, and frustrated.
Older persons are rigid, fixed, and unable to change.	Many social, environmental, and personal factors affect adaptability.

empty? Perhaps whether one chooses to focus on persons' strengths or problems will determine what labels are used.

There are both developmental tasks of aging (e.g., retirement) and adaptation tasks to biophysical changes of aging. A few of the biophysical changes are as follows:

- Respiratory and cardiovascular systems produce less efficient ventilation and circulation.
- Skin changes increase its fragility.
- Nutrition and elimination needs vary greatly according to activity levels.
- Vision and hearing changes may increase environmental hazards and decrease sensory pleasures.

The most pervasive security need among the elderly derives from a common fear of neglect, especially in crisis. Love and belonging needs are also important for older persons.

The longer a person survives in this world, the greater the number of losses he or she will encounter in terms of family, friends, meaningful roles, and possessions. As meaningful roles are lost, so may self-esteem be lost. When an older person loses decision-making control over his or her life, he or she is also at risk for suffering lowered self-esteem and feelings of helplessness, hopelessness, and worthlessness. Self-actualization, the highest of Maslow's needs, is perhaps the most elusive for the elderly. One prerequisite of self-actualization, however, is the satisfaction of basic and preceding needs. For this satisfaction, many elderly persons depend on nursing services to keep them healthy and to help them adjust to change.

Elders worry about not staying healthy, and especially about the devastation of catastrophic illness. In 1988, both houses of Congress were finally able to agree on the largest expansion of Medicare in the program's 23-year history. This expansion was hailed as a landmark piece of legislation that would bring peace of mind to millions. Hospital coverage increased sixfold in length-of-stay provisions. Also included were doctors' bills, drug costs, hospice care, and skilled nursing care. Another major step forward was a change in Medicaid to prevent impoverishment of a spouse caused by nursing home care of a mate. These expansions also brought a variety of unanticipated problems.

Perhaps with fear of devastating illness diminished, more attention can be focused on staying healthy. And perhaps elder abuse, an increasingly serious societal problem, may subside if some frustrations related to management of health-care problems of the elderly are decreased.

In summary, many similarities exist between the health-care needs of AIDS clients and the elderly. Both populations have been misunderstood and in many ways ostracized by society. Both will experience decreasing functional abilities and increasing dependency on others for assistance. To maintain independence will require maximizing remaining functional abilities. Susceptibility to infection is increased for both groups because of compromised immune systems (AIDS) or decreased adaptability (elderly). Loneliness from isolation is a potential threat to both populations. The living of both groups are survivors and need care to continue to survive.

For both groups, nurses can be care-givers, respecters of personhood, advocates, and teachers to the affected as well as to their informal caregivers. AIDS clients and elderly persons represent a challenge to society, health care, and nursing. As has been indicated, nurses have the knowledge, caring skills, and compassion to make a difference in the care of these persons. Nursing as a health profession can use this opportunity: Nurses can demonstrate both the essence of nursing and also the value of the care nurses provide. If nursing chooses to do so, it can make a powerful professional statement: Nurses meet the challenge to humanize health care in a most significant way.

Continue Professionalization of Nursing

Although professions arise from the needs of society, they flourish under the nurturance of the professionals themselves. On the one hand, such nurturance can obviously be viewed as self-serving to the profession. On the other hand, it should be obvious that the profession itself is best able to develop its services and make them known. In spite of nursing's name and the nurturance of its clients, nurses have been remarkably slow to nurture their profession. To do so will require the concerted and collective efforts of both new and established professionals who are convinced of nursing's value, while these nurses must also be comfortable with their own self-worth so they can be assertive with a purpose.

Society's need for nursing is not going to go away, but whether this need can be fully met by organized nursing is a real question and challenge. When the shortage of nurses in hospitals reached alarming proportions in the late 1980s, physicians became concerned. An element of physicians' concern was obviously a genuine interest in their clients' welfare because nurses, as 24-hour care-givers, are often the first professionals to recognize a deteriorating client condition which may require medical intervention. Physicians also know that the availability of quality nursing care may influence the choice of a hospital for elective medical procedures.

Interestingly, but perhaps not surprisingly, the medical profession's solution to problems caused by the nursing shortage was to propose a new category of health-care worker, called a Registered Care Technologist, who could be a physician extender after only a few months of training. An alternative solution would have been to support nursing in its recruitment efforts. A clear message in the action chosen is that the challenge to continue professionalization of nursing belongs to nursing, not to another profession like medicine.

It could be argued that medicine proposed to intervene in a way that was logical for medicine. Clearly, medicine addressed the problem in a way that would protect medicine's professional interest. However, that such a solution will not really meet the increased public demand for "nursing care" is clear. Nonetheless, nursing need not face the nursing shortage challenge alone. The public is ready to be a partner and must be asked to help. Prospective nurses and the public might also be concerned that with the medical proposal, potential nurses would be siphoned from nursing and exploited while the underlying nurse shortage problem remains unsolved.

Extend Practice Through Research

The National Center for Nursing Research has featured a phrase, "Nursing Science: Serving Health Through Research." The research programs of the National Center for Nursing Research focus on both actual and potential health problems: these include health promotion and disease prevention — decreasing the vulnerability of persons to illness and disability throughout life; acute and chronic illness; and approaches to nursing care delivery that include quality, cost, and ethical issues. Buerhaus (1986) argued that nurses will also need to research the meaning and value of care by directly querying their clients. Even beginning nursing students recognize the importance of care as noted in the anonymous comment cited earlier: "I never realized how many people need care." But predicting and controlling the outcomes of care are another matter. Being able to do this will require a sophisticated level of nursing research as well as a greatly increased quantity of research. In effect, this major challenge will require large numbers of well-qualified nurse-scientists. The challenge will await nurses entering the profession and established practitioners for decades to come.

The challenge to extend practice through research will be met in part by individual nurses believing in their own problem-solving skills and identifying problems from actual clinical practice. Some of the needed studies will be very sophisticated, while others will be quite straightforward. In the latter category, McCorkle (1988) found that home care nursing (in contrast to visits to doctors' offices) benefited persons with cancer. Home care nursing enables clients to minimize their distress and maintain their independence longer. The home health nurses relieved symptoms of fatigue, nausea, and shortness of breath, and also helped clients with activities of daily living like eating and bathing.

Increase Public Awareness of Nursing's Contributions to Health Care

Nurses need to make the public aware of nursing's contribution to health care. This awareness is particularly important in an era when nurse demand exceeds nurse supply and various remedies are proposed to alleviate the shortage. Nurses could make more of a public impact in this regard if they would publish in newspapers for laypersons and in popular magazines. Such topics as women's health, sexuality, coping with life's stressors in healthy ways, dangers of substance abuse, sexually transmitted disease, care of the elderly and chronically ill in the home are all within nursing's expertise. For the public to see such topics widely and expertly discussed by nurses would increase nurse credibility and greatly expand the public's knowledge of nursing.

Sometimes others, outside nursing, speak for nurses. George F. Will, a political commentator, made such a statement in Newsweek regarding "the dignity of nursing." He further commented, "The nursing profession must be nurtured with financial and emotional support. Otherwise, someday when you are in a hospital and are in pain or other need you will ring for a nurse and she will not come as soon, or be as attentive as you and she would wish" (1988, p 80). In their verbal presentations and everyday conversations, nurses can also increase public awareness of nursing's contribution to health care. In addition to dispensing information in community forums as indicated above, they can make clear that well-educated nurses are prepared to offer care that is scientific and up-to-date, and they can differentiate between medical care and nursing care. Because the public often fails to do this, it may attribute to medicine that for which nursing deserves credit, for example, close, around-the-clock observation for untoward responses to surgery or recognition of early deviations from health.

The public needs to know that nurses care for persons of all ages and in all levels of sickness and wellness, and that nurses do this in ways that maximize their clients' strengths so that they can maintain optimal independence in activities of daily living. The public also needs to know nursing's commitment to give comforting care in those situations where "cure" is not currently possible, as illustrated previously with AIDS and the elderly. And in all settings, nurses advocate on the client's behalf for the fullest possible client control of health-care decision making.

Increase Nursing Influence on Health-Care Policy and Delivery

Several strategies for nurses to increase nursing influence were enumerated in some detail in Chapter 3. In summary, it is appropriate to recall the individual strategies as: using information to advantage, planning ahead, participating, and personally demonstrating professional competence. Nurses need to empower themselves and their nurse colleagues so that collective nurse strategies can have the greatest possible impact on health-care policy and delivery. Nurses can do this through informal peer groups, formal organizations, and through political participation. These strategies, coupled with increasing the public's awareness of nursing's contribution to health care, can be very powerful.

A high order of response to political pressure is action by organized government at the national level. In 1987, U.S. Health and Human Services Secretary Oits Bowen appointed a national commission on nursing to address strategies related to recruitment and retention of nurses. Recognition of the nurse shortage as a national issue shows the influence of nurses on health-care delivery; part of this influence is related to economics. Aydelotte, testifying before the Bowen Commission in 1988, stated, "Hospital administrators must recognize that nurses are not only a cost; they earn income for the institution. If nurses were not income producing, concern about the nursing shortage would not be identified as urgent." In other testimony, the representative of Sigma Theta Tau International, Honor Society of Nursing, suggested that national policy decisions about both the cost and the scope of services to be included in the country's health agenda need to be examined (Norby, 1988). Furthermore, the nursing shortage was identified not as a nursing issue but as a health-care issue. Felton likened nursing to a public utility that was a national necessity (Felton G: Personal communication, April 7, 1988).

The old adage that "money talks" may well be true, and, regardless of the reason for the recognition, it is important to have others outside nursing (e.g., *Newsweek's* George

Will) aware of nursing's contribution to health care. The real challenge, however, is for organized nursing as a single powerful voice, speaking for nursing and in the public interest, to lead the way in increasing nursing's influence on both health-care policy and delivery.

Increase the Number of Nurses in Health-Care Leadership and Administrative Roles

Nurses have the appropriate problem-solving and interpersonal skills to represent the public interest in health-care leadership and administrative roles. However, to date nurses have been underrepresented in these roles. Two major reasons for this situation have been nurses' failure to assert themselves and others' failure to acknowledge nurses' abilities. Nurses themselves are largely responsible for both of these situations. As the most numerous of health-care professionals, nurses should exert more influence just by sheer numbers alone.

The rationale for taking up this challenge is not merely to bring prestige to nursing. Rather, the public interest would be served by humanizing health care and bringing economies of cost. Although it is quite clear nursing could provide leadership for the former, it is less clear to those outside nursing that nurses could do the latter. Clearly, the gauntlet has been thrown, especially by the public; it remains to be seen whether nurses of the future will rise to the challenge.

Some might interpret this challenge as confrontational to medicine, which is not the intent. Rather, perhaps nurses have not assumed their fair share of responsibility for collaborative action on the wide range of challenges facing health care. It is partly because *cure* has been so successful in prolonging life that many of the *care* problems now loom large. Care to stay healthy and care to comfort humanely are now assuming ever larger roles in health services delivery. As this happens, the potential for leadership by nurses will grow dramatically.

Increase the Number of Ethnic Minority Persons and Men in Nursing

In recent years, the nursing profession has become acutely aware of cultural variations and their impact on providing person-centered care. Official statements have been published, recognizing nursing's contribution toward meeting the "health needs of a diverse and multicultural society" (National League for Nursing, 1977, p 13) and toward considering "individual value systems and lifestyles" (American Nurses' Association, 1976, p 4).

As discussed in Chapter 5, ethnic origin and racial background have a great influence on how a person reacts and is reacted to by others in the health-care environment. Ethnicity is "affiliation due to shared linguistic, racial, (religious), and/or cultural background" (Werner, 1979, p 343). Other cultural variables important in the health-care setting include value orientation, family system, healing beliefs and practices, and nutritional behavior. In addition, nurses should have knowledge of how biophysical variations among ethnic minority groups influence their own ability to carry out appropriate and accurate physical assessments as well as other aspects of the nursing process for clients different than themselves.

Nurses should also be aware of both differences and similarities cross-culturally as a way of developing sensitivity to persons with varied cultural backgrounds and avoiding stereotypic approaches in relieving psychological and physical stress. Especially in the last decade, there has been an influx of culturally sensitive nursing education literature to enable the nurse to learn about cultural and ethnic differences. Yet nursing exhibits relatively little cultural diversity within its ranks: in the late 1980s, blacks — the largest minority group in nursing — represented roughly 5% of students graduating from basic RN programs. Other groups were also underrepresented: men, less than 5%; Hispanics, about 2%; Native Americans, less than 1% (Rosenfeld, 1987, p 64). Real-life diversity of professionals contributes a rich multicultural sensitivity to practice issues that cannot be duplicated in any other way.

A large number of ethnic minorities (i.e., blacks, Hispanics, Native Americans, and other poor ethnic minorities) are part of a low socioeconomic – poverty group characterized by high unemployment, low income, poor housing and living conditions, and low educational standards. These socioeconomic conditions have a profound effect on the level of health among ethnic minorities. Blacks and other minorities suffer proportionately greater rates of death and illness than the population as a whole. The 1985 Report of the U.S. Department of Health and Human Service's Task Force on Black and Minority Health cited excess deaths from heart disease and stroke, homicide and accident, cancer, infant mortality, chemical dependency, and diabetes. In addition, AIDS is disproportionately found among black populations (Bakeman and colleagues, 1986).

Clearly, the current health-care system is woefully inadequate for the health care of blacks and other ethnic minorities. To enrich its multicultural sensitivity and better serve the country's health-care needs, nursing requires both ethnic and gender diversity.

Undoubtedly, some of the same socioeconomic conditions that are decreasing access to the health-care system also decrease access to educational preparation for health-care professions like nursing. For example, blacks comprise less than 4% of the total RN population. Some very capable minority scholars are unaware of career options in nursing or are being recruited to other professions. Other minorities may not recognize their potential for nursing or realize the access available through community college programs.

The benefits of recruiting more minority persons to nursing are multiple: providing more sensitive nursing care to minorities, increasing health-care access for minorities in the population, providing secure employment in an area of demand, and increasing sensitivity of all health-care professionals to diverse population groups. Furthermore, because all minorities are underrepresented in nursing, minorities are an untapped pool for recruitment to fill critical nursing vacancies in all health-care settings.

The number of men in nursing has changed relatively little in spite of social change and the entrance of women into traditionally male-dominated fields. The rationale for needing men in nursing is both different from and similar to that for needing ethnic minority persons. Obviously, unlike ethnic minorities, men are not generally disadvantaged as a group; however, like ethnic minorities, men are grossly underrepresented in nursing proportionate to their health-care needs.

In the past, men have been heavily concentrated in care populations that have been primarily male, that is, the military. Growing prison and substance abuse populations suggest such populations will continue to be available and will need increasing health-care services; however, caring men would be an asset to all areas of nursing.

Balancing the gender distribution of nurses would be likely to increase the sensitivity across the sexes to nursing's goals and challenges, and such balance might also decrease the likelihood that the profession's problems would be viewed as women's problems. Also, it would seem that expanding scientific and technological opportunities available in nursing would be intriguing to men as well as to women.

| SELF-ASSESSMENT

The final section of this chapter presents an informal self-assessment tool for the reader. You are asked to agree or disagree with each statement presented. There are no right or wrong answers here: The statements simply ask you to reflect on certain personal characteristics and attitudes that the authors believe are compatible with professional nursing. After the list of statements, the statements are repeated with a brief rationale for each. The more the rationales make sense to you and seem comfortable, the more likely you are to find satisfaction, opportunity, and challenge in the wide-open profession of nursing. These statements may suggest others that you might wish to discuss with an academic advisor, career counselor, or nursing faculty member.

| DO YOU AGREE OR DISAGREE WITH | EACH OF THE FOLLOWING?

1   I like people.
2   I have a curiosity about human life.
3   I am a sensitive and caring person.
4   I want to learn to express my caring for another person.
5   I can accept and value persons who are unlike me.
6   I can be accepting of individual persons even when I disagree with or do not understand their behavior.
7   I want to interact comfortably with persons who are unlike myself.
8   I am self-directed.
9   I adapt well to change.
10 I can pay attention to details.
11 I can keep confidential those communications told to me in trust.
12 I expect to work collaboratively with others.
13 I am interested in developing my interpersonal communication skills.
14 I am interested in helping others to learn.
15 I am interested in helping persons to care for themselves.
16 I find satisfaction in helping others.
17 I understand that nursing is a health profession different and separate from medicine.
18 I am more interested in health than disease.
19 I recognize AIDS and care of the elderly as health problems of growing concern to nurses.
20 I am looking for a challenging occupation.
21 I expect my chosen life work to sometimes be demanding of my personal resources.
22 I accept responsibility for my individual actions and judgments.
23 I expect to confront ethical issues in nursing that do not have easy answers.

24 I am willing to adhere to a professional code of ethics.
25 I expect to be a lifelong learner.
26 I expect to participate in the continuing development of nursing as a profession.
27 I am a healthy person.

STATEMENTS WITH RATIONALES

1 I like people.
In addition to being an art and a science, nursing is a profession that focuses its concern on people. Although it is not necessary to "like" all clients, persons who do not have a genuine interest in other people will probably not enjoy nursing as a life work.

2 I have a curiosity about human life.
Nursing care of the holistic person offers unlimited opportunities to satisfy curiosity about all aspects of human life.

3 I am a sensitive and caring person.
Nursing needs persons who can demonstrate sensitivity and caring as well as scientific abilities.

4 I want to learn to express my caring for another person.
Nursing is an interpersonal process that requires the demonstration of caring.

5 I can accept and value persons who are unlike me.
Each person needing nursing care has inherent worth as a human being, regardless of his or her personal values and behaviors.

6 I can be accepting of individual persons even when I disagree with or do not understand their behavior.
Nurses give care based on the awareness that persons can be accepted even when their behavior is not fully understood or socially acceptable.

7 I want to interact comfortably with persons who are unlike myself.
Nurses provide care to all clients, with special regard for clients' beliefs, feelings, and personal needs.

8 I am self-directed.
As a profession, nursing needs independently functioning practitioners who are self-directed in decision making and in professional development.

9 I adapt well to change.
Nursing is a rapidly changing science and health care is one of the most rapidly changing industries.

10 I can pay attention to details.
Nursing requires practitioners who are careful in their observation, diagnosis, planning, care activities, and documentation of their work.

11 I can keep confidential those communications told to me in trust.
The communication between nurses and their clients is confidential as is that of other professionals and their clients.

12 I expect to work collaboratively with others.
Nurses work collaboratively with their clients to determine and meet nursing needs. Nurses also work collaboratively with other members of the health-care team.

13   I am interested in developing my interpersonal communication skills.
      Communication is a major component of nursing practice in all settings
      and specialties.

14   I am interested in helping others to learn.
      A major professional responsibility of nurses is to facilitate learning about
      health for their clients.

15   I am interested in helping persons to care for themselves.
      Nurses recognize and foster their clients' inherent strengths and self-care
      abilities rather than encouraging their dependency.

16   I find satisfaction in helping others.
      True caring is based on an attitude of helping another or others to grow
      and be healthy.

17   I understand that nursing is a health profession different and separate from
      medicine.
      Identification with one's profession is important both to the development of
      the professional nurse and the nursing profession.

18   I am more interested in health than disease.
      Because nurses believe in the strengths of even sick persons, health — not
      disease — is the primary concern of nurses.

19   I recognize AIDS and care of the elderly as health problems of growing
      concern to nurses.
      Nurses will increasingly be expected to provide the health care that AIDS
      patients and older persons need.

20   I am looking for a challenging occupation.
      Nursing will be most satisfying for those who accept the challenges facing
      nurses in their everyday practice and those facing the profession as an
      occupation.

21   I expect my chosen life work to sometimes be demanding of my personal
      resources.
      Over the span of a nursing career, various demands will be placed on your
      mental, psychological, and physical resources. However, most nurses believe
      that the personal rewards from a nursing career far exceed the personal
      demands.

22   I accept responsibility for my individual actions and judgments.
      Nurses are legally accountable for the professional practice based on their
      education and licensure.

23   I expect to confront ethical issues in nursing that do not have easy answers.
      Many bioethical issues relate to "What is health?" and "When is a person
      a person?" Because both health and person are concerns of nursing, such
      issues are inescapable in professional practice although nurses have many
      sources of support to help them cope with ethical dilemmas.

24   I am willing to adhere to a professional code of ethics.
      Practice according to a Code of Ethics is an expectation for professionals.

25   I expect to be a lifelong learner.
      Nursing, like other sciences and professions, requires continuous updating
      of scientific information for competent practice.

26   I expect to participate in the continuing development of nursing as a profession.

As a developing profession, nursing needs new members who are willing to make this commitment.

27   I am a healthy person.

Persons who consider themselves healthy in meeting their own basic human needs may find it easier to focus their energy and concern on the needs of other persons.

| CONCLUSION

This chapter has addressed a number of opportunities and challenges that await today's professional nurses. Opportunities to gain security and display individuality are included. The professional challenges that were detailed were portrayed as opportunities of a different nature, and the challenge to humanize health care was given special priority. Care of the elderly and AIDS clients were singled out as ways to demonstrate nursing's unique contribution to meeting this challenge. An informal self-assessment tool provided the reader with a way to assess personal characteristics and attitudes for their compatibility to professional nursing.

| STUDY QUESTIONS

1   How might your unique personal abilities find expression in nursing?
2   Which of the challenges presented do you think has the highest priority, and why? (Give a rationale for your answer.)
3   Compare responses to the self-assessment questions with a classmate or friend.

| REFERENCES

American Nurses' Association: Code for Nurses with Interpretive Statements. Kansas City, MO, American Nurses' Association, 1976

American Nurses' Association: A Social Policy Statement. Kansas City, MO, American Nurses' Association, 1980

Aydelotte MK: Testimony before the Department of Health and Human Services Secretary's Commission on Nursing. Chicago, March 7, 1988

Bakeman R, McCray E, Lumb JR, Jackson R: AIDS among Blacks and Hispanics, MMWR 35(42):655–666, 1986

Bennett JA: Nurses talk about the challenge of AIDS. Am J Nurs 87:1150–1155, 1987

Buerhaus PI: The economics of caring: Challenges and new opportunities for nursing. Top Clin Nurs 8(2):13–21, 1986

Clark L, Quinn J: The new enterpreneurs. Nurs Health Care 9(1):7–15, 1988

Clarke AC: July 20, 2019: Life in the 21st Century. New York, Macmillan, 1986

Guilford JP: Creativity: Retrospect and prospect. J Creative Behav 4(3):149–168, 1970

Kinlein ML: Independent Nursing Care with Clients. Philadelphia, JB Lippincott, 1977

Lewis EP: The new breed. Editorial. Nurs Outlook, 22(11):685, 1974

Marx JL: Spread of AIDS sparks new health concern. Science 219(4580):42–43, 1983

McCorikle R: Key aspects of comfort. National Sigma Theta Tau Conference held in Chapel Hill, NC, March, 1988

Meleis AI: Theoretical Nursing: Development and Progress. Philadelphia, JB Lippincott, 1985

Mundinger M: Autonomy in Nursing. Germantown, MD, Aspen Systems, 1980

Naisbitt J: Megatrends: Ten New Directions Transforming Our Lives. New York, Warner Books, 1984

National League for Nursing, Department of Baccalaureate and Higher Degree Programs: Criteria for the Appraisal of Baccalaureate and Higher Degree Programs in Nursing. Pub. No. 15-1251, 4th ed. New York, National League for Nursing, 1977

Norby R: Testimony before the Department of Health and Human Sevices Secretary's Commission on Nursing. San Francisco, May 24, 1988 pp E2

Number of Americans over age 85. Ann Arbor News, June 1, 1988 pp E2

Orem DE: Nursing: Concepts of Practice, New York, McGraw-Hill, 1971

Perrin MM: Space nursing: A professional challenge. Nurs Clin North Am 20(3):497–503, 1985

Peters T: Thriving on Chaos: Handbook for a Management Revolution. New York, Alfred A Knopf, 1987

Rogers ME: An Introduction to the Theoretical Basis of Nursing. Philadelphia, FA Davis, 1970

Rosenfeld P: Nursing Student Census with Policy Implications, 1986. National League for Nursing, Division of Public Policy and Research, Pub. No. 19-2175. New York, National League for Nursing, 1987

Simms LM, Lindberg JB: The Nurse Person. New York, Harper & Row, 1978

Thiele JE: There's a computer in the curriculum! Computer Nurs 6(1):37–40, 1988

U.S. Department of Health and Human Services: Report of the Secretary's Task Force on Black and Minority Health, Vol 1.—Executive Summary. Washington, DC, Pub. No. 0-487-637 (QL-3), August, 1985

U.S. Department of Health and Human Services: Surgeon General's Report on Acquired Immune Deficiency Syndrome. Supt. Docs. No. HE 20.2:Ac 7/3. Washington, DC, 1986

U.S. Department of Health and Human Services: Understanding AIDS. HHS Pub No. (CDC) HHS-88-8404. Rockville, MD, Public Health Service Centers for Disease Control, 1988

Werley H, Lang N: Identification of the Nursing Minimum Data Set. New York, Springer, 1988

Werner EE: Cross-Cultural Child Development: A View from the Planet Earth. Monterey, CA, Brooks/Cole, 1979

Will GF: The dignity of nursing. Editorial. Newsweek, May 23, 1988, p 80

GLOSSARY

Accomodation. The alteration of internal schemes to fit reality; reconciling new experiences or objects by revising the old plan to fit the new input (Piaget).

Active listening. The cultivated skill of deriving meaning from the words and nonverbal vocalization of another.

Actual problem. A problem that can be identified clearly from the data at hand.

Adaptation. (1) The dual process of assimilation-accommodation (which leads to adaptation) is a continuing process of learning from the environment and learning to adjust to alterations in the environment (Piaget). (2) The process of changing throughout life by persons when faced with new, different, or threatening experiences without loss of health, sense of wholeness, or integrity of self.

Affirmative action. Positive steps to bring a deteriorating situation under control, for example, intervening to control unusual bleeding.

Aggregating. The process of collecting and summarizing many nursing interventions and their outcomes and determining relationships among the outcomes such that predictions can be made about the most effective interventions for a given age, sex, culture, health concern, life style, and so forth.

Asepsis. Freedom from infectious agents.

Assertiveness. A verbal communication skill that states one's own rights positively without infringing on the rights of others.

Assessing. The collection of information, data or facts about the person so that the nurse may better understand his or her feelings, ideas, values, and biophysical responses.

Assimilation. Reality data or input from the real world are treated or modified in such a way as to become incorporated into the structure of the person (Piaget).

Authority. An assumed right to control someone or something.

Autonomous. Independent; self-governing.

Bioethics. A subspecialty of the discipline of ethics; issues of an ethical nature that concern health professionals.

Body image. How one views or thinks of the physical part of the self.

Civil law. Law concerned with legal rights and duties of private persons.

Client.   A person who engages the professional advice or services of another; a person served by or using the services of an agency; a person who has contracted for services from another who is qualified to provide those services.

Climate.   Average weather conditions at a place over a period of years, including factors such as average temperature, humidity, precipitation, and wind velocity.

Closed system.   A system that cannot exchange matter, energy, or information with its environment.

Communication.   A complex process in which two (or more) persons exchange messages and derive meanings. It is both verbal and nonverbal.

Community.   A group of persons living in the same locality and under the same government; having common norms and cultures, health interests, and needs.

Consent.   Voluntary granting of permission, for example, for treatment procedures or research.

Consumer.   An individual, a group, or a community that uses a commodity or a service.

Coordinator of care.   One of the roles of the nurse; the act of helping the client use appropriately all resources available to him or her.

Coping behavior.   Adaptive or maladaptive responses consisting of cognitive function, motor activity, affect, and psychological defenses. Consists of actions or reactions in response to stress.

Criminal law.   Law concerned with behavior detrimental to society as a whole.

Crisis.   A turning point, a crucial period of increased vulnerability and heightened potential; may be biological, psychological, or social; individual experiences disequilibrium when usual coping behaviors are not operating.

Cultural healing belief.   Belief that reflects a specific cultural orientation toward health and illness.

Cultural variables.   Characteristics that a person exhibits or identifies with from a particular cultural group.

Culture.   A system of symbols shared by groups of humans and transmitted to upcoming generations; a group's design for living.

Culture shock.   Profound disorientation suffered by the person who has plunged without adequate preparation into an alien culture.

Defining characteristic.   Sign or symptom that can be observed in the client.

Deontological.   A classification of ethical theory; belief that the moral right or wrong of an act is considered separately from the goodness or badness of consequences.

Dependent nursing behavior.   Those activities performed under delegated medical authority or supervision or according to a priori routines.

Development.   The patterned, orderly, lifelong changes in structure, thought, or behavior that evolve as a result of the maturation of physical and mental capacity, experiences, and learning and that result in a new level of maturity and integration.

Developmental task.   A growth responsibility that arises at a certain time in the course of development (Erikson).

Diagnosing. Investigator analysis of the cause or nature of a condition, situation, or problem. The act of reaching a conclusion about the nature or cause of some phenomenon. The phase of nursing process that involves analyzing assessment data and making a nursing diagnosis.

Diagnosis. A statement or conclusion concerning the nature or cause of some phenomenon.

Diagnostic-related groupings. A system of classifying health-care needs according to an accepted list of diagnosed illnesses and conditions of health deficits; used to determine Medicare payments for health-care services, and thus affect the extent of services provided by many institutions.

Distress. A state induced by unpleasant stimuli.

Ecology. The study of the relationship between humans and the external environment.

Empathy. Ability to participate in the life of another individual and to perceive his or her thoughts and feelings.

Environment. An open system composed of the social, natural, and human-made subsystems and their variables; the external system.

Ethics. A discipline concerned with social, political, and legal philosophy and principles of good and bad, moral duty, obligation, and values; rules of conduct.

Ethnicity. A group's affiliation due to shared linguistic, racial, religious, or cultural background.

Eustress. A state induced by pleasant stimuli.

Evaluating. The act of determining the client's progress toward the outcomes established in the planning step of the nursing process.

External environment. Anything external to a system's (person's) boundaries, including all stimuli, objects, and other persons impinging on a person.

Family. A group of persons who are emotionally joined, who live in close geographical proximity.

Function. The kind of action or activity proper to a person in a certain role, for example, functions of a professional nurse.

Geography. The physical features of an area; the physical components of land, sea, air, and the plant and animal life that are supported by these physical features.

Good samaritan law. A state law intended to encourage health professionals to offer assistance in emergency situations.

Group. An assembly of persons who share specific functions or goals and who interact over a period of time.

Growth. An actual biological or quantitative increase in physical size, that is, the enlargement of any body component by an increase in the number of cells.

Health. A state of complete physical, mental, and social well-being, not merely the absence of disease or infirmity (World Health Organization definition).

Health behavior. Actions by persons who believe they are well to avoid an encounter with illness.

Health maintenance organization (HMO). A group health-care practice whose major distinguishing feature is prepayment.

Health-care delivery. The methods of and approaches to health care, sometimes described as a system or as an industry.

High-level wellness. "An integrated method of functioning which is oriented toward maximizing the potential of which the individual is capable within the environment in which he is functioning" (Dunn, 1959, p 447).

Holism. A theory that the universe, and especially living nature, is correctly seen as interacting wholes that are more than the mere sum of elementary particles; a theory that describes the parts of a person as dependent upon each other and coordinated in a systematic fashion (Smuts, 1926).

Homeodynamics. A reciprocal interaction of living systems that maintains a balance within each system and a balance among them.

Illness. A dynamic process, a disturbance in equilibrium between humans and their environments. Illness is a reaction of the whole organism, a consequence of factors in a reaction—internal and external stimuli as well as predisposition of the individual.

Illness behavior. The initial response of the person to psychological and somatic cues that are perceived as incapacitating, therefore, signs of illness.

Implementing. The activation of the plan of care.

Independent nursing behavior. Those activities initiated as a result of the nurse's own knowledge and skill rather than as a result of delegated authority from another, for example, a physician.

Influence. The power of producing effects by invisible or insensible means.

Intercultural communication. A process that occurs whenever a message producer is a member of one culture and a message receiver is a member of another.

Interdependent nursing behavior. Those activities that overlap functions or activities of other health professionals; this type of nursing behavior recognizes the desirability of collegial relationships in which each profession contributes according to knowledge, skills, or focus.

Internal environment. Anything internal to a system's boundaries.

Interview. An interaction with a purpose.

Intuition. The ability to obtain knowledge without the apparent use of rational processes; involves direct cognition and rapid insight.

Legal right. A claim recognized and enforceable by law.

Liability. Responsibility or obligation because of position or particular circumstances; a legal responsibility for professional behavior.

Litigation. A trial in court to settle legal issues; a lawsuit.

Maladaptation. The process of using inadequate ways of dealing with stress in an attempt to maintain equilibrium.

Malpractice. Negligence in carrying out professional services; improper professional action.

Mandatory licensure. A kind of state law controlling nursing practice; requires all persons who nurse for compensation to be licensed.

Maturation. Development of cells until they can be completely utilized by the organism.

Maturational (normative, developmental) crisis. Expected life changes such as birth, puberty, marriage, pregnancy, etc.

Medicaid. Title XIX of the Social Security Act, which provides health-care insurance for certain needy and low-income persons.

Medicare. Title XVIII of the Social Security Act, which provides health-care insurance for persons over 65 years of age and for certain other persons.

NANDA. The North American Nursing Diagnoses Association, formerly known as the National Group for the Classification of Nursing Diagnoses.

National health insurance. A proposed insurance program that would provide guaranteed coverage so that health care could be obtained by everyone.

Negligence. Failure to exercise that degree of care required by law for the protection of others.

Noise. Unwanted sound.

Norm. Expected behavior that provides rules about standards of appropriate behavior in particular situations.

Nosocomial infection. Infection that originates in a hospital or medical facility.

Nursing diagnosis. The conclusion drawn by the nurse or the nurse and the person from the data collected in the various functional areas; may represent a strength, a need, or a problem.

Nursing process. A series of five scientific steps that assist the nurse in using theoretical knowledge to diagnose the strengths and the nursing needs of persons and to implement therapeutic actions to attain, maintain, and promote optimal biopsychosocial functioning and to evaluate the client's progress.

Nursing research. Scientific study or investigation about nursing practice.

Nursing theory. The systematic abstraction or formation of mental ideas about nursing practice reality.

Object permanence. Realization by the child that objects can exist apart from himself or herself; understanding that even though he or she may not see the object, it still exists.

Open system. A system that can exchange matter, energy, and information with its environment.

Operation. An interiorized action or an action performed in the mind (Piaget).

Paternalism. Fatherly interference with a person's autonomy or independence.

Pathogens. Microorganisms that are capable of causing disease.

Patient (adjective). To bear pains or trials calmly and without complaint; to be steadfast despite opposition or adversity; to be able or willing to bear.

Patient (noun). An individual awaiting or under medical care and treatment; the recipient of any of various person services.

Permissive licensure.   A kind of state law controlling nursing practice; it permitted nurses to practice without a license if they did not claim licensure or use the RN initials.

Person.   A unique human being who has some characteristics in common with others as well as his or her own individual thoughts, feelings, and ways of responding.

Planning.   Decisions by the nurse and client about the outcomes to be achieved and the actions both need to take.

Politics.   Power and control; promotion of an interest using whatever resources are available to protect and advance it.

Position.   Synthesis of related roles that represents the location of persons in a social system.

Possible problem.   A problem for which some data have been obtained but not enough to identify it as an actual problem.

Potential problem.   A problem the person is at high risk of developing, given his or her particular situation.

Power.   The ability to secure a particular outcome.

Preventive health care.   Activities that promote health by reducing factors that contribute to illness and by reinforcing a person's strengths.

Primary preventive health care.   Intervention with persons who have no symptoms but who are at risk for developing behaviors that could diminish their health.

Problem.   A situation that requires specific action to be taken.

Professionalism.   Professional character, spirit, or methods; also, activities found in various occupational groups whose members aspire to be professional.

Professionalization.   The process of acquiring or changing characteristics in the direction of a profession.

Professions.   Traditionally, the occupations of medicine, law, and the ministry.

Reasonable care.   That degree of skill and knowledge customarily used by a competent health practitioner of similar education and experience in treating and caring for the sick and injured in the community in which the individual is practicing or learning his or her profession.

Responsible consumerism.   The act of controlling and providing input into those things that affect one as an individual; it is an obligation as well as a right.

Role.   Set of expected behaviors, normatively defined, that serves to make behavior predictable.

Schema.   A more complex mental image, an action organization that a person uses to explain what he or she sees and hears (Piaget).

Science.   Knowledge gained by systematic study.

Secondary preventive health care.   Education, counseling, and treatment that assist persons to minimize factors that are a part of their life styles and that could affect their health.

Self-care.   Activities that individuals personally initiate on their own behalf in maintaining or enhancing life, health, and well-being (Orem).

Self-concept. A collection of notions, feelings, and beliefs about the self with which one identifies and through which one relates and communicates with others and interacts with the environment.

Self-esteem. One's personal judgment of one's own worth.

Self-ideal. How one believes he or she ought to function and behave given his or her personal value system and set of personal standards.

Sensory overload and sensory deprivation. Syndromes caused by too much or too little sensory stimulation, characterized by altered perception and disorientation.

Situational (accidental) crisis. Unexpected or hazardous events such as illness, catastrophic circumstance, natural disasters.

Standard. Something set up and established by authority as a rule for the measure of quantity, weight, extent, value, or quality.

Strength. An internal resource; a biological, psychological, social, or spiritual quality that contributes to a person's character, integrity, and uniqueness and that can be mobilized to cope with a problem or to attain a goal.

Stress. The nonspecific response of the body to any demand made on it. Everyday wear and tear of living.

Stressor. Anything that induces stress; the stimulus that places demands on persons to prepare for change, for example, pain, cold, a test.

Structure. The way in which information is organized within the person to make a simple mental image or pattern of action (Piaget).

System. "An organized unit with a set of components that mutually react" (Abbey, 1978, pp 20–21).

Teleological. A classification of ethical theory; belief that ends justify the means.

Tertiary care. Health care that takes place in highly specialized institutions that provide sophisticated diagnosis and treatment.

Tertiary preventive health care. Care that focuses on persons who have encountered a specific stressor that has already compromised their health.

Torts. Civil wrongs that may be intentional or unintentional; violations of reasonable behavior.

Value. A belief or a custom that frequently arises from cultural or ethnic backgrounds, from family tradition, from peer group ideas and practices, from political philosophies in one's country, and from educational and religious philosophies with which one identifies.

Value. Intrinsic belief about the worth of an entity or concept.

Value judgment. A personal decision about whether something is right or wrong.

Variable. "A characteristic or attribute of a person or object that varies (i.e., takes on different values) within the population under study (e.g., body temperature, age, heart rate)" (Polit and Hungler, 1987, p 538).

Utilitarianism. An approach to ethics that advocates the greatest good for the greatest number.

Wellness. A dynamic process, a condition of change in which the person moves toward a higher potential of functioning.

INDEX

Page numbers in *italics* indicate illustrations; those followed by t indicate tables.

A

Abdellah, Faye, 219, 221t
Abortion, and bioethical issues, 302
Accidents. *See also* Health problems
  prevention of, 114–117, 120, 121t–122t
Accommodation, 99
Accountability, 34, 316–319, *318*
Acquired immunodeficiency syndrome, 339–341
Activities of daily living, and data collection, 219–
    220, 220t
Adaptation, 150–161
  case example of, 163–164
  definition of, 17, 150
  vs. maladaptation, 157
  nursing implications of, 163–165
  process of, 155–161
  theories of, 150–155
Adaptation model, Roy's, 9t, 49, 52
Adaptive model, of health, 147, 149
Aesthetic needs, 86
Affective learning objectives, 286, 288t
Aggregation, in nursing process, 208–210
Aging, health care for, 339–340, 341–343, 342t
AIDS, 339–341
Air quality, 111–112, 115t
Alcohol, Drug Abuse and Mental Health
    Administration, 182t
American Association of Occupational Health
    Nurses, 113
American Indians. *See* Ethnic minorities
American Nurses' Association, 71
  Code for Nurses of, 34, 35t
  standards of practice of, 33–34, 212, *213*
Anxiety, 156
  and communication, 262
Appearance, professional, 266
Applied Nursing Research, 52
Asceticism, 24, *24*
Asepsis, 117
Asians. *See* Ethnic minorities
Assertive behavior, 272–273

Assertive communication, 272–273
Assessment, in nursing process, 208, *209*, 211,
    212–225. *See also* Data collection
Assimilation, 99
Associate degree programs, 32–33, 66
Auscultation, *217*, 217t
Authority, definition of, 71
Automobile accidents, safety precautions for, 122t
Autonomy, client, 295–296

B

Baccalaureate programs, 32–33, 60, 66
Beard, Richard, 32
Behavior
  assertive, 272–273
  coping, 156–157
  definition of, 149
  health, 149–150
    variables influencing, 194–196
  illness, 150
  nonverbal, and communication, 265–268
  testing, 257–258, *259*
Behavioral objectives, clarification of, 285–286
Behaviorism, 278–279, 282t
Behavior modification, 279
Beliefs, definition of, 134
Benemortasia, 306
Bernard, Claude, 150, 151t
Bioengineering, 303–304, 308t
Bioethical issues, 299–308, 308t, 309t. *See also*
    Ethical issues
  and bioengineering, 303–304, 308t
  and death and dying, 306–308, 308t, 309t
  and neonatology, 303, 308t
  and pregnancy, 301–303, 308t
  and psychological competence, 304–305, 308t
Bioethics
  definition of, 295
  person focus for, 299–308, 308t
Blacks. *See* Ethnic minorities
Body image, and self-esteem, 87–88